The Dreams of Mabel Dodge

"History comes alive, as we are drawn into the dream life of Mabel Dodge, an articulate woman who played a significant role in the history of psychoanalysis in America. It is 1916 and we listen as she recounts dreams and associations to her analyst, Smith Ely Jelliffe, and he responds. Through impeccable scholarship and priceless historical documentation, Patricia Everett contextualizes a psychoanalytic adventure. Unconscious meets conscious, patient meets analyst, and reader meets author, as this fascinating story unfolds. Patricia Everett gives us privileged access to their exciting, spirited, even thrilling interplay as they explore a realm of dreams."

—**Sandra Buechler**, PhD, Training and Supervising Analyst at
the William Alanson White Institute,
author of *Psychoanalytic Approaches to Problems
in Living* (Routledge, 2019)

"If I hadn't seen it with my own eyes, I'd find it hard to believe that such a book actually exists. Everett presents us with the dreams of Mabel Dodge, recorded during her analysis with Smith Ely Jelliffe, one of the most influential and creative of the first American psychoanalysts. We are whisked, as if by a time machine, deep into a lost world of a century ago. And what is revealed is the inner life of an extraordinary woman, the contours of the American avant-garde, of which she was a central figure, and the workings of psychoanalysis in an early, crucial period of its history."

—**James William Anderson**, PhD, Professor of
Clinical Psychiatry and Behavioral Sciences,
Northwestern University

In 1916, salon host Mabel Dodge entered psychoanalysis with Smith Ely Jelliffe in New York, recording 142 dreams during her six-month treatment. Her dreams, as well as Jelliffe's handwritten notes from her analytic sessions, provide an unusual and virtually unprecedented access to one woman's dream life and to the private process of psychoanalysis and its exploration of the unconscious.

Through Dodge's dreams—considered together with Jelliffe's notes, annotations drawn from her memoirs and unpublished writings, and correspondence between Dodge and Jelliffe during the course of her treatment—the reader becomes immersed in the workings of Dodge's heart and mind, as well as the larger cultural embrace of psychoanalysis and its world-shattering views. Jelliffe's notes provide a rare glimpse into the process of dream analysis in an early psychoanalytic treatment, illuminating how he and Dodge often embarked upon an examination of each element of the dream as they explored associations to such details as color and personalities from her childhood.

The dreams, with their extensive annotations, provide compelling and original material that deepens knowledge about the early practice of psychoanalysis in the United States, this period in cultural history, and Dodge's own intricately examined life. This book will be of great interest to psychoanalysts in clinical practice, as well as scholars of the history of psychoanalysis and students of dreams.

Patricia R. Everett is a psychologist in private practice in Amherst, Massachusetts and the author of *Corresponding Lives: Mabel Dodge Luhan, A.A. Brill, and the Psychoanalytic Adventure in America* (Karnac, 2016) and *A History of Having a Great Many Times Not Continued to be Friends: The Correspondence Between Mabel Dodge and Gertrude Stein, 1911–1934* (University of New Mexico Press, 1996). Since 1983, she has researched the Mabel Dodge Luhan archives at the Beinecke Rare Book and Manuscript Library, Yale University.

The History of Psychoanalysis Series
Series Editors
Professor Brett Kahr and Professor Peter L. Rudnytsky

This series seeks to present outstanding new books that illuminate any aspect of the history of psychoanalysis from its earliest days to the present, and to reintroduce classic texts to contemporary readers.

Other titles in the series:

What is this Professor Freud Like?
A Diary of an Analysis with Historical Comments
Edited by Anna Koellreuter

Corresponding Lives
Mabel Dodge Luhan, A.A. Brill, and the Psychoanalytic Adventure in America
Patricia R. Everett

A Forgotten Freudian
The Passion of Karl Stern
Daniel Burston

The Skin-Ego
A New Translation by Naomi Segal
Didier Anzieu

Karl Abraham
Life and Work, a Biography
Anna Bentinck van Schoonheten

The Freudian Orient
Early Psychoanalysis, Anti-Semitic Challenge, and the Vicissitudes of Orientalist Discourse
Frank F. Scherer

For further information about this series please visit https://www.routledge.com/The-History-of-Psychoanalysis-Series/book-series/KARNHIPSY

The Dreams of Mabel Dodge

Diary of an Analysis with Smith Ely Jelliffe

Patricia R. Everett

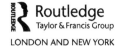
Routledge
Taylor & Francis Group

LONDON AND NEW YORK

First published 2021
by Routledge
2 Park Square, Milton Park, Abingdon, Oxon OX14 4RN

and by Routledge
605 Third Avenue, New York, NY 10158

Routledge is an imprint of the Taylor & Francis Group, an informa business

British Library Cataloguing-in-Publication Data
A catalogue record for this book is available from the British Library

Library of Congress Cataloging-in-Publication Data
A catalog record has been requested for this book

ISBN: 978-0-367-74933-0 (hbk)
ISBN: 978-0-367-74932-3 (pbk)
ISBN: 978-1-003-16041-0 (ebk)

Typeset in Times New Roman
by codeMantra

To Zael and Django,
for giving me more than I ever could have dreamed of

To Gary,
for answering an undreamt dream

And to Paul,
for teaching me about play, and the deep pleasures of dreams

Contents

Acknowledgments		xi
Series editor's foreword		xiii
Prelude		xxii
PAUL LIPPMANN		
Author's preface		xxv
List of abbreviations		xxix

1	**Mabel Dodge**	**1**
	Childhood, marriages, and salons 1	
	Mabel Dodge's first contact with Smith Ely Jelliffe 3	

2	**Smith Ely Jelliffe**	**5**
	Childhood 5	
	Education and first love 8	
	Beginning medical practice and turn to neurology	
	and psychiatry 11	
	Conversion to psychoanalysis 13	
	Jelliffe's patients 14	
	Psychoanalytic Review 20	
	"Technique of Psychoanalysis" papers 22	
	Diseases of the Nervous System 23	

3	**Mabel Dodge in psychoanalysis with Smith Ely Jelliffe**	**27**
	Jelliffe's "Technique" papers and Dodge's analysis 27	
	Jelliffe's approach to psychoanalysis and dream interpretation,	
	as presented in Diseases of the Nervous System 30	
	Mabel Dodge in analysis with Jelliffe 31	
	Mabel Dodge on dream interpretation 45	
	The Dreams of Mabel Dodge 46	

4   **Cast of characters**   50

5   **The Dreams of Mabel Dodge**   67
    A note on how to approach the dreams 67

Appendices   243

**Appendix A: Mabel Dodge, "Mabel Dodge Writes About the
Unconscious":** *The New York Journal,* **1917 (Excerpted)**   244

Appendix B: Mabel Dodge, "A Game of Cards—Hearts"
***Psychoanalytic Review,* 1918 (vol. 5, pp. 442–444): Reprinted
with the permission of Guilford Press**   246

References   249
Index   253

Acknowledgments

I first read Mabel Dodge's dreams in 1989, an impossibly rich and intimate encounter with her archives at the Beinecke Rare Book and Manuscript Library at Yale University, a discovery made even more startling by her psychoanalyst Smith Ely Jelliffe's notes from her sessions describing her dream associations. I am forever grateful to Patricia Willis, then curator of American literature at the library, for granting me early access to these extraordinary documents.

This book would never have appeared in print if Peter Rudnytsky had not shown exquisite appreciation for the rareness of such historical material, and his subsequent careful reading and wise guidance. I am enormously grateful to him for ushering me through. In addition to introducing me to Peter, James Anderson's contribution to this project is immeasurable, as his immense curiosity and enthusiasm about Mabel Dodge's early contributions to psychoanalytic history through her dreams and letters propelled me further. As editor, he was the first to publish some of Dodge's dreams in *The Annual of Psychoanalysis* in 2015. The late John Burnham expressed a faith in me that surprised and emboldened me. The late Bruce Kellner was the earliest supporter of my research on Mabel Dodge, teaching me the grace and beauty of mentorship, how doors can open if you ask.

At the Beinecke Library, Nancy Kuhl has always been a brilliant resource with her unfailing energy and beyond generous support. She remains a reason to continually return to the library for more research. I greatly appreciate the staff at the Beinecke who played such a significant role in making the archives available, as well as the staff at the Manuscript Division of the Library of Congress who facilitated access to the Jelliffe papers.

Paul Lippmann took the manuscript of this book with him to Truro over a decade of summers ago and devoted precious time to reading it and then writing an associative and poetic response. As a teacher about dreams, Paul is a master of play and passion. If he loves something you've done, you forever have his gaze. I cherish the places we have gone together and still have much to learn from his curiosity and irreverence.

Julie Westcott was the first to read an early version of this book in 2008 and leave me an expansive phone message (that I luckily had the forethought to write down) confirming that the dreams were a treasure, and created a captivating world when read with their annotations. I'm forever grateful for her initial excitement that helped me keep going.

For permission to publish Dodge's dreams, Jelliffe's notes, and correspondence between Dodge and Jelliffe, and to reproduce photographs, I am grateful to the Yale Collection of American Literature, Beinecke Rare Book and Manuscript Library, Yale University.

At Routledge, I am thankful for the responsiveness of Russell George and Alec Selwyn who were always available to answer questions, and for Jeanine Furino and Rebecca Dunn who graciously guided my manuscript through copy editing to publication.

With a writing project that has mostly been in the background for three decades, my friends and family have nonetheless kept me company with their questions and interest, and that has meant the world to me. During editing and proofreading this manuscript, I greatly missed my late mother, Jean Halverson, as her impeccable eye for detail and her companionship in getting things just right were essential for completing my last book. Mark Elin heard my dreams and provided all the space I needed to inhabit and explore them. My sons, Zael and Django Ellenhorn, writers themselves, are each living out their dreams in ways I deeply admire and respect. Finally, I could never be grateful enough for the way dear Gary Bivona protects (and even feeds me during) my solitude, so that my writing time can be a true refuge. I am indebted to him in all good ways, forever.

Series editor's foreword

The present volume forms a "prequel" to Patricia R. Everett's *Corresponding Lives: Mabel Dodge Luhan, A.A. Brill, and the Psychoanalytic Adventure in America* (2016), also published in the History of Psychoanalysis series. In that book, Everett told the story of the relationship between her heroine and the preeminent first-generation American psychoanalyst, which began in 1915 when Dodge (as she was known at the time of the second of her four marriages) invited Brill to conduct a "Psychoanalysis Evening" at her salon at 23 Fifth Avenue in New York City. The relationship was transformed in the summer of 1916 when Dodge became Brill's patient, and it continued Möbius-like on an interwoven personal and professional plane until their last epistolary exchange in March 1944, four years before Brill's death and eighteen years before Mabel Luhan's.

While making its appearance after *Corresponding Lives*, *The Dreams of Mabel Dodge: Diary of an Analysis with Smith Ely Jelliffe* rewinds the clock because Dodge first sought out Jelliffe on a night in 1914 when she and a group of Greenwich Village friends took peyote together and one of them underwent a psychotic episode. On December 27, 1914, Jelliffe, who in 1913 had left his clinical appointment at Fordham Medical School and would have had an eye to increasing his private practice, sent Dodge the first extant letter of their correspondence along with two offprints, a friendly missive in which he thanked her for "having turned to me at a time when it seemed I might have been able to serve." And so it came to pass that, probably on January 1, 1916, Dodge, then thirty-seven with a fourteen-year-old son from her first marriage, having survived five suicide attempts and in the throes of a torturous love affair with the painter and sculptor Maurice Sterne, who became her third husband in August 1917, wrote to Jelliffe, "I want very much to see you to discuss the possibility of your analysing me," which led to their first session two days later.

Dodge remained in analysis with Jelliffe between two and four times a week for a little over five months, until June 7, 1916. Then, when Jelliffe, whose wife, Helena Leeming Jelliffe, had died unexpectedly of a brain hemorrhage on March 3, was on vacation, Dodge—who can in hindsight be seen

to have emitted rumblings of discontent about her experience with Jelliffe—
appealed to Brill, who despite some misgivings yielded to her entreaties and
took her on as a patient on the condition that she stop seeing Jelliffe. This,
not surprisingly, caused hard feelings in the latter, who told Dodge in a valedictory session on October 23, "It was duress. I had no quarrel c. [with]
M.D. but I did not take it right in part of A.A.B. & would have nothing to
do c. him. He had done the same thing for several patients & I was through
c. him."

Notwithstanding his irritation at having been poached, Jelliffe remained
on friendly terms with Dodge, with whom he continued to correspond and
sporadically to see until 1939, six years before his death. With Brill, too,
things righted themselves over time, to the point where in an address to
the New York Psychoanalytic Society, "Glimpses of a Freudian Odyssey"
(1933), Jelliffe expressed his "unstinted praise and admiration for the essential spirit of this Society" (p. 327), the founding of which in 1911 its members
had gathered to celebrate.

In her two books in this series, Patricia Everett has provided a portal
through which to enter into the multidimensional encounters between a
distinguished American woman of letters and the two most important
American psychoanalysts of the first half of the twentieth century. Although
Brill is more often referred to than read nowadays, the cognoscenti will
at least be able to recall that he was Freud's first disciple and translator
in the United States, but opposed Freud on the question of lay analysis.
Jelliffe, conversely, although he and Brill share the honor of being the only
two founding fathers of American analysis accorded biographical entries in
Psychoanalytic Pioneers (Alexander, Grotjahn, and Eisenstein, 1966), has
by now receded almost entirely from collective psychoanalytic memory. To
the degree that Jelliffe is still remembered, it is, in the title of Nolan D.C.
Lewis's chapter (1966) in *Psychoanalytic Pioneers*, for his groundbreaking
contributions to "Psychosomatic Medicine in America," and through the
superlative study of his life and work by John Burnham, *Jelliffe: American
Psychoanalyst and Physician* (1983), a volume which includes Jelliffe's complete correspondence with both Jung and Freud, spanning the years 1912 to
1939, edited by William McGuire. (Burnham, however, errs in stating that
Dodge was Jelliffe's patient "shortly before World War I" [p. 144].)

Everett's first signal contribution in the present book, therefore, is to give
Jelliffe a much-deserved new lease on life. Burnham's volume is now closer
to forty than thirty years old, while that of Alexander & Co. is truly from
a bygone era. I venture to predict that I will not be the only reader of *The
Dreams of Mabel Dodge* to have been motivated to pluck these classic works
from the shelf, and to dip my toes in Jelliffe's own vast waters, and thereby
to bring to the surface of my consciousness one of the most prodigious and
fascinating lost continents in the history of psychoanalysis.

Burnham (1983) allows us to see that the waning of Jelliffe's influence is due to two converging factors. On the one hand, Jelliffe staked a claim to fame "in four different major roles: neurologist and psychiatrist, pioneer psychoanalyst, a founder of psychosomatic medicine, and editor" (p. 41). On the other, he for the most part lacked the institutional base or other channels through which creative thinkers commonly perpetuate their legacies, such as "students who spread both the teacher's viewpoints and his reputation" or being known for having "originated some specific idea or ideas that are more or less easy to trace" (p. 155). In psychosomatics, Jelliffe has been almost completely overshadowed by Groddeck. As Burnham adds, "the only institution with which he could be identified was the *Journal of Nervous and Mental Disease*," of which he served as the editor from 1902 to 1944, "and the publications associated with it: the [Nervous and Mental Disease] monograph series and the *Psychoanalytic Review*" (p. 157).

These last two ventures were undertaken jointly with William Alanson White, who became Jelliffe's closest friend and collaborator after they met in 1896 at the Binghamton State Hospital: the monograph series was launched in 1907, and the *Review*, the first psychoanalytic journal in English, followed in 1913, with White at the helm. Despite having been superintendent at St. Elizabeths Hospital in Washington, D.C., from 1903 until his death in 1937, White looms largest in the contemporary imagination as the namesake of the interpersonal institute in New York City cofounded in 1943 by Harry Stack Sullivan, while the library of the New York Psychoanalytic Institute is named after Brill, whom Jelliffe met in 1910 at the New York Neurological Institute and later credited, in Burnham's paraphrase, with having "converted him to psychoanalysis" when they "walked home from their clinic there across Central Park" (p. 45). Of these three legends, only Jelliffe does not have a monument to his memory, not even at what is now known as the Institute for Living in Hartford, to which he sold his professional library of more than 10,000 volumes in 1941.

Although, as Burnham notes, the cosmopolitan and erudite Jelliffe, who knew all the major figures in European psychiatry—including Kraepelin, Bernheim, Janet, Dubois. Déjérine, Oppenheim, Ziehen, and Babinski—"discussed Freud's views in two book reviews in a manner that suggested that everyone ought to have known about Freud's teachings" (p. 70) as early as 1905, the key point is that Jelliffe first came into direct contact with psychoanalysis through Jung, whom he met in September 1907 at the First International Congress for Psychiatry, Neurology, Psychology, and the Nursing of the Insane, where Jung stepped forth as Freud's champion and clashed with Gustav Aschaffenburg. After the Congress, Jelliffe's travels across Europe took him to Zurich, where, with White and M.S. Gregory, he had lunch with Jung and his associates Alphonse Maeder and Franz Riklin. It was thus natural that when Jelliffe, then affiliated with

Fordham University, helped to organize an international speaker series in September 1912 he should have invited Jung, and indeed hosted him at his house. By a twist of fate, however, Jung's lectures, although they bore the title *The Theory of Psychoanalysis*, actually threw down the gauntlet to Freud by criticizing his sexual theory of the libido, and thereby became a catalyst for the rupture between the two men. To make matters worse, not only were Jung's Fordham lectures immediately serialized in *The Psychoanalytic Review*, but the inaugural issue also featured a congratulatory letter from Jung, while Jelliffe (1913–1914) hailed his handiwork with White as "the only journal in English ... which aims to be catholic in its tendencies, a faithful mirror of the psychoanalytic movement, and to represent no schisms or schools but a free forum for all" (p. 444).

As a consequence of these perceived displays of support for Jung at precisely the juncture when the formerly anointed crown prince metamorphosed into the pariah of the psychoanalytic movement, Jelliffe was viewed by Freud's adherents as a renegade. A peek behind the curtain is afforded by Brill's letter to Freud on December 12, 1913: "Jelliffe is a very ardent worker for psychoanalysis, but of course he is thoroughly Jung. He is one of those persons who can make believe that he knows it all when as a matter of fact he knows very little. I have occasion to see one of his cases and I am satisfied that he had no idea what he was doing" (qtd. in Everett, 2016, p. 38). (Might this case have been among those Jelliffe had in mind when he complained to Dodge about Brill's purloining of his patients?) While Brill expressed himself thus unreservedly to Freud, Ernest Jones wrote diplomatically to Jelliffe on November 24, 1913, "It seems quite impossible for Vienna and Zurich to come to any kind of terms, so it will be better if they separate altogether, when each can develop without personal emotions on the lines that suit him best—and the best man win!" (qtd. in Burnham, 1983, p. 193). William McGuire is doubtless correct in surmising that "Jones's uncharacteristic evenhandedness may reflect his growing belief that Jelliffe was becoming a Jungian" (p. 193), though this "evenhandedness" was no more than a ploy that concealed his true feelings toward Jelliffe, who was not only "becoming a Jungian" as far as the loyalists were concerned, but had made it clear that he belonged to the enemy camp.

From Jelliffe's perspective, however, he was not taking sides in a conflict, but simply promoting and practicing psychoanalysis as he understood it in an ecumenical spirit. In the first of a series of papers titled "The Technique of Psychoanalysis" (1913–1914), which appeared in the maiden issue of *The Psychoanalytic Review* together with Jung's letter and the first installment of *The Theory of Psychoanalysis*, Jelliffe observed that the need had been evident since the "days of Charcot" to "unite into a genetic or dynamic concept these data of psychopathology," and that "it remained for Freud to forge the tools of psychoanalysis, and make them of value for every student of psychical phenomena" (p. 70). By 1914, moreover, when Rank's *The Myth of the Birth of the Hero*, co-translated by Jelliffe, appeared as the eighteenth work in the Nervous and Mental Disease Monograph Series, it had been preceded by Freud's *Selected Papers on Hysteria and Other Psychoneuroses* and *Three Contributions to Sexual Theory*, both translated by Brill, as well as by Karl Abraham's *Dreams and Myths* and Eduard Hitschmann's *Freud's Theory of the Neuroses*. Indeed, Freud's polemic against the unholy trinity of Jung, Adler, and Stekel, *The History of the Psychoanalytic Movement*, as it was called in Brill's translation, was itself published in 1916 in *The Psychoanalytic Review* and the following year as the twenty-fifth monograph in the Nervous and Mental Disease series.

Notwithstanding Jelliffe's services to the cause, a journal aligned with Jung and that sought "to represent no schisms or schools" but instead to be "a free forum for all" was the last thing that Freud would have wanted to countenance while he was in the throes of expelling the heretics from the fold. Inevitably, therefore, when White wrote to Freud in September 1913 to solicit a contribution to *The Psychoanalytic Review*, his reply, as Jelliffe (1933) recalled two decades later, was "not very cordial" (p. 326), although the rebuff came as a disappointment to the petitioners.

The turning point occurred in August 1921 when Jelliffe, on his first trip to Europe after World War I, met Freud for the first time in the Austrian spa town of Bad Gastein. In a letter to White, Jelliffe reported that Freud had been "very nice" to him and they "spent the afternoon talking about everything" (Burnham, 1983, p. 205). Synchronously, Freud had met Groddeck for the first time the previous year at the congress of the International Psychoanalytical Association in the Hague, and Jelliffe went on to inform White that Freud "was very much interested in our organic work and told me of one of his pupils in Baden-Baden who was carrying on quite a similar type of analyses and with the same ideas we have been working on." Indeed, Freud in subsequent publications twice coupled Jelliffe's name with Groddeck's, and once also with that of Felix Deutsch, as therapists who have attested that "the psycho-analytic treatment of serious organic complaints shows promising results" (1924, p. 209; see also 1923, p. 250).

Freud's signs of favor were simultaneously efforts to peel Jelliffe away from Jung and to cement the ties of personal loyalty to himself. Whereas Jung fulminated to Jelliffe on December 18, 1920 that "the Pope in Vienna is most revengeful and tries his best to extinguish any trace of myself" (Burnham, 1983, p. 204), Freud dropped a hint almost exactly a year later that he was available should Jelliffe wish to come to Vienna for analysis: "American physicians who wish to take up self-analysis with me are advised to sign up for 1 October of the coming year and to allow sufficient time, at least four to six months, for the course" (p. 207). Jelliffe never took Freud up on this offer—writing on November 26, 1929 that "what analysis I have had has been from [White] chiefly" (p. 230)—just as Freud never accepted Jelliffe's renewed invitations to contribute a paper to *The Psychoanalytic Review*.

But through the years the relations between the two grew increasingly cordial. Most uncharacteristically, Freud repeatedly apologized to Jelliffe for his previous coolness. On April 11, 1926, he explained that he "was at first very suspicious" of Jelliffe and White, and that his "distrust carried over to the *Psychoanalytic Review*," because he had initially heard Jelliffe's name "from Jung, who spoke emphatically of you as his friend at a time when I was already convinced of his hostile attitude toward me" (p. 224). Freud added that he had met Jelliffe at Bad Gastein "in the company of Dr. Stekel ... and that again was no recommendation in my eyes," although he now recognized that Jelliffe, "as an outsider, could have had no exact knowledge of these personal relations." In a later letter, on February 10, 1933, Freud reiterated that he "was suspicious, because I had seen you in the company of Stekel," and underscored how he had subsequently "learned to esteem you for the breadth of your interests and knowledge, the freedom of your thinking, and your worth as one of the strongest pillars of analysis in America" (p. 253). Finally, on February 9, 1939, in his last letter to Jelliffe, Freud made a joke of the matter: "I now often laugh in remembrance of the bad reception I gave you at Gastein because I had first seen you in company of Stekel" (p. 279). In agreement with a comment made by Jelliffe, he appended the now-classic remark, "I am by no means happy to see that Analysis has become the handmaid of Psychiatry in America and nothing else."

Jelliffe reciprocated wholeheartedly. Replying to Freud's April 1926 letter, he recalled that during a visit to Jung two years earlier he "was amazed to learn how narrow his vision was ... and how one-sided he had developed in his interests," to the point where Jelliffe "felt that he had ceased to be a physician" (p. 225). For good measure, he castigated a recent publication by Stekel for being "'stupid.'" In response to Freud's February 1933 letter, Jelliffe took the responsibility for their having gotten off on the wrong foot:

> I have long since felt that I was perhaps more to blame in re. our first meeting than you. In true American simplicity—perhaps stupidity—I was not alert to the contrary winds of doctrine that were blowing in the psychoanalytic movement, and it has only been after my contacts with X [Stekel] that I realized and have increasingly come to feel that he was not very trustworthy as a scientist. A clever, inspirational, intuitive personality maybe, but hardly the one who had much to offer save a bright gathering of material made possible by another's ideas.
>
> (p. 254)

Freud's valedictory letter elicited from Jelliffe a lingering backward glance over his own life, which concluded by defending Freud against the reproach to which he was most vulnerable: "I never have been sympathetic to a very widespread accusation of your intolerance" (p. 282).

One could scarcely imagine a marriage of truer minds. Freud found in Jelliffe the ideal disciple, one who recognized the errors of his former ways and pledged his fealty where it properly belonged. On September 2, 1938, Freud told his devoted analysand Smiley Blanton (1971), "Brill apparently is the only friend I have in the New York group—or perhaps I should include Dr. Jelliffe" (p. 108). Jelliffe, for his part, found in Freud an intellectual hero whose chastisement concerning *The Psychoanalytic Review*, he said in his final letter, he and White learned to accept in "the spirit of the wrongly accused little boy—'We'll show papa we were not as bad as he thought'" (Burnham, 1983, p. 281). Not for nothing did Jelliffe title his address to the New York Psychoanalytic Society—Brill's bastion of orthodoxy to which, after being dropped from the rolls for more than a decade and unsuccessfully applying for reinstatement in 1920, he was finally readmitted to membership in 1925—"Glimpses of a *Freudian* Odyssey." Nor is it happenstance that this paper was published not in *The Psychoanalytic Review*, or even in Jones's *International Journal of Psycho-Analysis*, founded in 1920, but rather in the *Psychoanalytic Quarterly*, a rival to both journals established in 1932 by a cadre of conformists in New York "to fill the need for a strictly psychoanalytic organ in America" (qtd. in Smith, 2002, p. 1).

* * *

In contrast to the epic sweep heralded by the title of *Corresponding Lives*, which tracks the "psychoanalytic adventure in America" across swaths of time and space, *The Dreams of Mabel Dodge* takes the reader on a journey into the interior delimited by the first six months of 1916 when Dodge was in analysis with Jelliffe. In addition to restoring Jelliffe to his rightful place on the psychoanalytic map, Everett's second signal achievement in this book is to have compiled the record of one particular psychoanalytic adventure, documents of immense historical interest that illuminate what is at once an intersubjective and an intrapsychic experience.

The fruition of extensive archival research, the "diary" as Everett has presented it, is a veritable palimpsest that makes Dodge's analysis with Jelliffe into something mutual, or at least co-constructed, a window into his psyche as well as hers. Reading this symbiotic text can be compared to the effect produced by juxtaposing Elizabeth Severn's account of her mutual analysis with Ferenczi in *The Discovery of the Self* (1933) with Ferenczi's rendering of their entanglement in the *Clinical Diary* (Dupont, 1985). Uncannily, Severn had previously been in treatment with Jelliffe contemporaneously with

Dodge, and, as Everett shows, her testimony on what it was like to be his patient echoes that of Dodge but in a harsher key.

Augmenting her unabridged transcription of all 142 of Dodge's dreams recorded by either one of them during this brief period, Everett furnishes salient extracts from Jelliffe's voluminous notes on their sessions, Dodge's associations to the dreams, and (in sections she calls Interludes) all the letters they exchanged while she was his patient, along with valuable ancillary materials. That Jelliffe at this stage of his psychoanalytic journey did not conceive it as a "Freudian odyssey," for instance, comes through beautifully in Dodge's memoir *Movers and Shakers* (1936), where she recalls how he began their first session:

> "Jung has taught us," he said, "that when one reaches an impasse, it is because he is unable to function in the way his own particular nature wishes. When we try to force ourselves to go in directions contrary to the psyche, she rebels. You do not like your present life. Why?"
>
> (p. 439)

Everett annotates the primary sources with two tiers of notes: factual identifications of people, events, allusions, and so forth—buttressed by the "Cast of Characters" in her Introduction—and interpretative. The latter, of course, although extremely insightful, are by no means definitive, but are rather invitations to the reader to ponder and come up with his or her own formulations. I find it impossible not to be impressed by the frankness with which Dodge and Jelliffe discussed her sexual life and functioning, as well by the degree to which Dodge's dreams and associations lend credence to what Freud (1908) called the "sexual theories of children" in which breast—penis—feces—baby—semen—milk—urine—blood—rice—snake, and so on *ad infinitum* are part of a vast symbolic network in which anything can, and often does, turn into anything else.

Shortly before she abandoned Jelliffe for Brill, Dodge became pregnant by Maurice Sterne, but wrote to Jelliffe on May 26, 1916, "If ever was a psychoanalytic baby—this is one.... It has brought about the submission of the female organs." In thus ascribing symbolic paternity to Jelliffe, Dodge repeated a pattern established when she became pregnant with her son John by (as she believed) having an involuntary orgasm during intercourse with her first husband Karl Evans while fantasizing about her gynecologist Dr. John Parmenter, with whom (to top it off) she and her mother were both having affairs. Fittingly, she gave the name of her lover rather than her husband to this pre-psychoanalytic baby. Whether Dodge would have named her second child Ely—or, indeed, whether it would have been a boy or a girl—we shall never know, because the story ends with her decision to abort her baby and her analysis with Jelliffe simultaneously. But what we are left with is a true psychoanalytic baby in the form of an imperishable record of how Freud's mad invention was lived and dreamed by one incomparable dyad in America more than one hundred years ago.

Peter L. Rudnytsky
Series Co-Editor
Gainesville, Florida

References

Alexander, F., Eisenstein, S., & M. Grotjahn, eds. (1966). *Psychoanalytic Pioneers.* New York: Basic Books.

Blanton, S. (1971). *Diary of My Analysis with Sigmund Freud.* New York: Hawthorn Books.

Burnham, J.C. (1983). *Jelliffe: American Psychoanalyst and Physician & His Correspondence with Sigmund Freud and C.G. Jung.* W. McGuire (Ed.). Chicago, IL: University of Chicago Press.

Dupont, J., ed. (1985). *The Clinical Diary of Sándor Ferenczi.* M. Balint & N. Zarday Jackson (Trans.). Cambridge, MA: Harvard University Press.

Everett, P.R. (2016). *Corresponding Lives: Mabel Dodge Luhan, A.A. Brill and the Psychoanalytic Adventure in America.* London: Karnac.

Freud, S. (1908). On the Sexual Theories of Children. In James Strachey et al. (Eds. and trans.). *The Standard Edition of the Complete Psychological Works* (hereafter *S.E.*). 24 vols. London: Hogarth Press, 1953–1974. 9: 205–226.

Freud, S. (1923). Two Encyclopaedia Articles. *S.E., 18*: 233–260.

Freud, S. (1924). A Short Account of Psycho-Analysis. *S.E., 19*: 189–210.

Jelliffe, S.E. (1913–1914). The Technique of Psychoanalysis. *The Psychoanalytic Review, 1*: 63–75, 439–444.

Jelliffe, S.E. (1933). Glimpses of a Freudian Odyssey. *Psychoanalytic Quarterly, 2*: 318–329.

Lewis, N.D.C. (1966). Smith Ely Jelliffe, 1866–1945: Psychosomatic Medicine in America. In Alexander, Eisenstein, and Grotjahn 1966, pp. 224–234.

Severn, E. ([1933] 2017). *The Discovery of the Self: A Study in Psychological Cure.* P.L. Rudnytsky (Ed.). New York: Routledge.

Smith, H.F. (2002). Editor's Introduction. *Psychoanalytic Quarterly, 71*: 1–3.

Prelude

by Paul Lippmann

You hold in your hands a psychoanalytic treasure: a book of dreams dreamt in 1916 by Mabel Dodge during her psychoanalysis with Smith Ely Jelliffe, and richly accompanied by his session notes containing her associations to her dreams. Dodge was an extraordinary woman in her engagement with the extraordinary intellectual-social movement and treatment method of psychoanalysis in its early days on the American continent. For Freud and the psychoanalytic pioneers, dreams were the royal road to an understanding of the unconscious mind. This book of dreams immerses us in that world and carries us to the deepest experiences of Mabel Dodge and of psychoanalysis.

First, a word about this book's design. Frequently, the text—filled with a dream, the analyst's comments, and amplifying footnotes—reminds me of pages from the Talmud, in which Jewish scholars, separated by centuries, wrote to each other in intimate exchange and commentary on the central Torah text. The Talmudic design characteristically consists of a central core surrounded in circular fashion by a discussion across centuries of thought. Patricia Everett has constructed pages in a similar pattern—the dream as core surrounded by the analyst's notes, and both enriched with clarifying context provided by the editor. The design allows the reader access to dreams and analytic response from almost a century ago. The reader then supplies the final layer as the dreams are permitted into his or her consciousness and unconsciousness. They may even become part of one's own dream world.

It is conceivable that one's own dreams can respond to Mabel Dodge and her nighttime imagination. Some weeks after reading this book for the first time, I found myself, in a dream, *in my own analytic office arranged strangely and in the company of a very old woman who was both highly nervous and hugely pregnant. I felt somehow responsible for this pregnancy* and awoke in puzzlement. Who did this woman remind me of? Was she like my mother? Was she Abraham's old Sarah, the biblical matriarch? Was she Mabel Dodge? In my mind, my own mother, Sarah, and Dodge combined with my own old, childhood pregnancy wishes, leading me to think further about Dodge as tragic mother both in terms of her relationship with her son and her own later lost pregnancy, a pregnancy suggested in her dreams and then revealed in letters to Jelliffe, and a pregnancy that Dodge attributed to the success of her analysis in making her receptive, thereby holding Jelliffe responsible for the conception. In such ways, my own dream may have been engaged in a further circling Talmud-like discussion with Mabel Dodge and her life. I like to think that, under the surface, it is possible to engage with the emotional life of the subject of this book. In sleep, without conscious design, we meet each other across the generations. In ancient times, the idea was common that we traveled in our dreams and passed through the lives of others, and they through our lives—an entire social world of intimate interaction during sleep time. Our modern ideas, however, have it that our dreams are more insular (like much of our actual contemporary lives).

As you read these dreams, along with their associations and related material, let the dreams enter your being and see what happens as Mabel Dodge's inner life comes out to meet you. Bit by bit, dream by dream, something begins to happen. There is a shape to her soul that slowly enters your experience. Through the prism of dreams, we look at the life and times of Mabel Dodge.

What an extraordinary idea, to view life through the prism of dreams! In our highly materialistic times, this restoration of the place of dreams in coming to know someone merits our appreciation and gratitude. Our modern culture with its emphasis on the technological has turned away from dreams. Once upon a time, long before we lit up the night with our own designs, dreams were a more significant part of individual and communal experience. Long before we became addicted to the external screen, life on the inner screen was our passion. Long before 500 TV channels, we looked at the stars and the dome of heaven at night. We watched babies as we sat around the kitchen table. And we talked about our dreams. But that was long ago, in ancient times, long before the industrial and electronic revolutions changed our lives, inside and out, long before the cell phone touched our ear. At the beginning of the twentieth century, psychoanalysis was born on the wings of dreams and dreams entered that century on the wings of psychoanalysis. To its lasting credit, psychoanalysis turned once again to dreams, to the ancient mind, to the sleeping mind for inspiration and knowledge about unconscious life. Freud's *Interpretation of Dreams* (1900) was and remains the central text of psychoanalysis. Mostly through the study of Freud's own dreams, psychoanalysis found its beginnings. More than one hundred years later, this book on Mabel Dodge's dreams is firmly in that tradition.

In this book, we meet up with the beginnings of the psychoanalytic movement in the United States prior to the beginning of World War I. On one side of Europe, the Bolshevik Revolution fired the imagination. On the other side of Europe and in America, the internal revolution fired the imagination. The power of the unconscious mind and the power of the proletariat matched each other. In the intellectual, bohemian, upper-class circles that served as background for Mabel Dodge, both revolutions were the topic, and Dodge plunged into the interior revolution. We can glimpse some of the power, single-mindedness, and hubris of the early analysts. In the realm of the mind, they were no less heroic or convinced of their rightness than were Lenin and Trotsky. Dodge is alternately dominated by and independent of Jelliffe's certainty about his convictions. At times, when her sense of herself is strong, she educates him about the best way to approach her, and she can be stubborn in her instructions. Since these early days, analytic therapists have learned much about letting patients teach us about how best to treat them.

Bit by bit, dream by dream, we come to feel Mabel Dodge's heart—the lonely little girl left alone, even hated, by her father and mother, the child who finds comfort in her own thoughts and imagination, the jealous and anxious young woman unable to find happiness in love, the adventurous and independent mind that pursues stimulation and connection, the lover seeking security—and her bittersweet struggle and search for self-understanding. Her rich social and intellectual life is intermingled with dreams of despair and deepest loneliness. We find in her dreams the shadows of death and the rays of life intermingled and bleeding into each other. Welcome to the dream world of Mabel Dodge.

Author's preface

This collection of Mabel Dodge's dreams represents the complete and unedited extant record of the 142 dreams written down during her psycho-analysis with Dr. Smith Ely Jelliffe in New York during the first six months of 1916. These dreams date from January 2 to June 2, 1916 and appear in three different forms: handwritten by Dodge; typewritten by Dodge; or handwrit-ten in red by Jelliffe in his case notes of her treatment. Because the major-ity of the dreams are written in Dodge's hand, I have only indicated those that appear in the two other forms. For typewritten dreams, I have included "[typed]" beneath the date of the dream. For dreams that appear in Jelliffe's notes, I have noted "[written in red in Jelliffe's notes from _____, 1916]," with the date of the analytic session filled in, beneath the date of the dream. If more than one dream is recorded for a specific date, I have indicated the number of dreams for that night preceded by the numerical order of each dream, such as "(1 of 3)." At times, Dodge wrote down her own comments about and associations to her dreams, notes that appear in the margins, between lines, or at the end of the recorded dream.

All of Dodge's dreams, as well as Jelliffe's case notes, are located in the Mabel Dodge Luhan (her name from her fourth marriage) Collection at the Beinecke Rare Book and Manuscript Library, Yale University. In ad-dition, the archives contain a significant correspondence between Dodge and Jelliffe, beginning in 1914 and continuing until 1939 (six years before his death in 1945). There are 47 letters from Dodge to Jelliffe, circa 1915 to 1939, with 14 from the period of her treatment with him, three appearing as fragments of letters in Jelliffe's case file. Jelliffe wrote 35 extant letters to Dodge, 1914 to 1939, two written during her analysis. One of these two letters from Jelliffe to Dodge from 1916 is reprinted in her memoirs but not found in the archives. I transcribed Dodge's dreams, Jelliffe's notes, and their correspondence from the original documents. I have not individually cited the location of these dreams, notes, or letters, as all are from the Mabel Dodge Luhan Collection. These papers also include an August 5, 1947 letter from Luhan to Dr. Eric Hausner, her physician in Santa Fe, that explains how she acquired this material: "Dr. Jelliffe's wife Belinda sent me these

2 vols. of case history he made while I worked with him. I had them here but have never gone through them! Too <u>boring</u>! But I feel people see them when they come here....Do you want them? If not get them burned up. Still they might have something of interest in them—very old stuff maybe dating back 30 years! His letters & mine—his notes on the case, my dreams! Heavens!" Dr. Hausner clearly did not heed her wish to burn the records, as they remained among his files when Dr. Richard Streeper assumed his medical practice in 1959. Dr. Streeper donated the material to the Beinecke Library in 1979, where Luhan herself had bequeathed her papers.

In my transcriptions of Dodge's dreams, I have tried to remain loyal to the original written word. I have presented the dreams exactly as they are recorded, with all their misspellings, non-standard number of ellipsis points (such as ".." or ".....”), occasional lack of capitalization and punctuation, grammatical errors, and repeated words. I have included "[*sic*]" when appropriate, have added punctuation in brackets, such as "it[']s," and have added letters in brackets for sense, such as "clim[b]." Where Dodge's handwriting has continually baffled me and made the recognition of a word difficult, I have substituted "[illegible]" for the elusive word or passage.

To accompany the dreams, I have included relevant selections from Jelliffe's extensive handwritten notes from Dodge's analytic sessions, drawn from 50 separate entries from January 3 to June 7, 1916. Given their form and the way they read, these notes appear to have been taken verbatim during the sessions, as Dodge associated to her dreams. Jelliffe writes with much shorthand, many abbreviations (some of them quite idiosyncratic), a number of recurring symbols, a lack of standard punctuation, an affection for colons, hashtag marks, and forward slashes to mark the end of a thought, and inconsistent capitalization. Jelliffe's notes recording Dodge's associations to her dreams appear most consistently in his case notes, although occasionally his writing appears in the margins, between lines, or at the end of the pages containing Dodge's handwritten dreams, most frequently in his characteristic red ink. I have indicated when Jelliffe's notes are written at the end of a dream.

My transcribing of Jelliffe's notes seeks to represent accurately the original document. However, given the number of abbreviations, confusing punctuation and capitalization, and often indecipherable handwriting, it is challenging to present a fluent record of his notes. In order to make them flow more consistently, I have occasionally deleted words or passages, indicated by ellipses, and added punctuation or the end of a word, such as "apolog[ize]."

For dating the dreams, I have relied primarily upon Dodge's own inclusion of dates. At times when a dream is simply identified by the day of the week, such as "Wednesday," I have used the dates of surrounding dreams as well as Jelliffe's dated notes in order to arrive at a date. When I have been unable to determine the date, I have presented the dream as "undated, circa _____." When the text of a dream comes directly from Jelliffe's case notes, I have written "circa" preceding the date of the case note to identify the dream.

Dodge's dreams are presented in the following format to distinguish the various sources of information: The dreams themselves appear in standard black text; Dodge's comments on or associations to her dreams *appear in black italics* and Jelliffe's notes about her dreams (both from his writing on the pages containing the dreams and from his records of her analytic sessions) *appear in grey italics.*

In a chapter before the dreams, "Cast of Characters," I provide brief biographical sketches of the most significant of Dodge's friends and family who frequently appear in her dreams. In sections between the dreams, entitled Interludes, I present the complete and essentially unedited correspondence between Jelliffe and Dodge from January to May 1916 (only three letters have minimal deletions of text, for the sake of flow and clarity, as indicated by [...] to distinguish them from Dodge's frequent use of ellipses; her first letter appears in full in the introduction), as well as relevant letters from others, such as Leo Stein to Dodge, William Alanson White to Jelliffe after his wife's death, and excerpts from letters to Dodge from Alfred Stieglitz and Hutchins Hapgood. In Dodge's letters, ellipses are part of her writing style and thus not an indication of missing text. In reading letters from this period, keep in mind that there was mail delivery several times a day in New York in 1916. Also included in these Interludes are three of Maurice Sterne's dreams, my commentary on confidentiality between analyst and patient in 1916, and excerpts from a letter Dodge wrote in 1914 to Morton Prince trying to understand her father's severe moods.

The dreams are primarily annotated with notes that draw their material from Mabel Dodge's voluminous autobiographical writings and her extensive correspondence with others. I have also consulted contemporary newspapers, memoirs by friends such as Hutchins Hapgood and Max Eastman, and historians of the period. If not already included in the "Cast of Characters" chapter, I have identified all other individuals the first time they are mentioned in one of Dodge's dreams or in Jelliffe's case notes. I have tried to determine the identity of all persons named and have provided biographical information for all with whom I have succeeded. However, a number of individuals have eluded all efforts at identification and are referred to in the footnotes as "unidentified." The annotations present *in bold italics* ideas about dream interpretation that would have been popular at the time that Dodge was dreaming her dreams, and also at the forefront of Jelliffe's approach to working with dreams, with his enthusiasm for Freud's *Interpretation of Dreams* (1900) and its analysis of typical dreams and dream symbols.

An excerpt from this book appeared as "The Dreams of Mabel Dodge" in *The Annual of Psychoanalysis: Psychoanalysis and Dreams* (2015). Several of Dodge's 1916 letters to Jelliffe and one from Jelliffe to her in 1916 were excerpted in my article "Letters in Psychoanalysis and Posttermination

Contact: Mabel Dodge's Correspondence with Smith Ely Jelliffe and A.A. Brill," *The Annual of Psychoanalysis* (1999). As mentioned earlier, one of Jelliffe's 1916 letters to Dodge was reproduced in her memoir *Movers and Shakers* (1936). In *The Suppressed Memoirs of Mabel Dodge Luhan* (2012), Lois Rudnick devotes a ten-page section to Jelliffe's notes, including edited excerpts of two of Dodge's 1916 letters to Jelliffe. None of the rest of the material has been previously published.

With two exceptions, Mabel Dodge's autobiographical and psychoanalytic writings were produced after she married Antonio Luhan in 1923, so all references to her published and unpublished works are cited as Luhan, not Dodge. These exceptions are her 1917 article, "Mabel Dodge Writes About the Unconscious" (Appendix A), and a 1918 piece in *Psychoanalytic Review*, "A Game of Cards—Hearts" (Appendix B), authored by "M. Dodge."

Abbreviations

For manuscript collections

GLSC: Gertrude and Leo Stein Collection, Beinecke Rare Book and
Manuscript Library, Yale University
LOC: Library of Congress
MDLC: Mabel Dodge Luhan Collection, Beinecke Rare Book and
Manuscript Library, Yale University
SFA: Sigmund Freud Papers, Library of Congress
SJA: Smith Ely Jelliffe Papers, Library of Congress

With no exception, all of Mabel Dodge's dreams, all correspondence to Mabel Dodge/Luhan, and all of Smith Ely Jelliffe's case notes, as well as his letters to and from Dodge are in the Mabel Dodge Luhan Collection, so no citation is indicated in the text.

Chapter 1

Mabel Dodge

In her dream world, where anything is possible, Mabel Dodge, an only child, can have a brother. She can be pregnant (and then become so in real life), and she can attempt to convince her father to try psychoanalysis. Her son, John Evans, can bite her hand and then transform into a dog. She can rescue a pony hanging from its reins. Dodge herself can be bundled in upholstery and fall down the stairs. Her nosebleed can soak the bed with blood, and her father can actually be cheerful. A piece of excrement can be yards long and a woman can have three light green eyes. Dodge can light dynamite and explode it in a confined place. And sheep covered in manure can jump into the sea and become white again.

Childhood, marriages, and salons

Born on February 26, 1879 to a wealthy family in Victorian Buffalo, Mabel Ganson was an only child whose parents were drastically unhappy and deeply estranged, their vast economic privilege derived solely from inheritance. Her father's despair and violent moods permeated her childhood years, and the atmosphere in her home was barren of any closeness or warmth. Her mother was characteristically absent, both when she was actually home and when she was away, leaving her daughter to fend for herself in her dreaded state of inactivity. In a passage from the first published volume of her memoirs, *Intimate Memories: Background* (1933a), which covers her upbringing in Buffalo, after describing her discovery of her mother's unhappiness, Dodge explains: "My mother, a speechless woman herself, had set an example of mute endurance and I had modeled myself upon her. So it was, in our house, as though we believed that by ignoring and never speaking of the misery we caused each other we would thereby blot it out from our hearts" (p. 37). Mabel searched for excitement outside her house, determined to flee its emptiness and secrets, as well as "escape the *fear* of the pain of idleness" (p. 42). She admitted: "To be alone in a room or, worse, alone on a whole floor of a house, to be only one, has a feeling of doom in it….doom of separateness and immobility….All my life has been, then, an attempt to escape

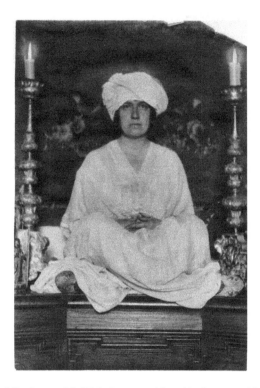

Figure 1.1 Mabel Dodge at 23 Fifth Avenue, New York, circa 1915. Courtesy of the Beinecke Rare Book and Manuscript Library.

from this" (p. 34). These three early themes—flight from boredom, silence about anguish and melancholy, and fear of being alone—were central to Mabel's life struggles and her eventual turn to psychoanalysis—a process that likely felt familiar from her crucial childhood experience of playing the game of Truth with friends in Buffalo: "We grilled each other, probing into the most hidden corners, laying bare preferences, analyzing each other and ourselves until we were in a tingling excitement. But it helped us by letting off steam and it helped us, too, to call by name the vaguer thoughts and feelings that we carried about inside us, as well as by airing those secrets that were all too defined for comfort. The unloading of secrets—what a pleasure that always was!" (p. 10).

Mabel Dodge (Figure 1.1) eventually married four times. (Had she retained all her names, she would have been Mabel Ganson Evans Dodge Sterne Luhan.) Her first husband, Karl Evans, the presumptive father of her son, was killed in a hunting accident in 1903. She then married Edwin Dodge the following year and became a patron of the arts, establishing active salons at their Villa Curonia outside of Florence and at their home in

New York. An early supporter of modernist art and a pioneer in her fascination with psychoanalysis, she began hosting evenings at her 23 Fifth Avenue apartment in January 1913, where artists, intellectuals, and activists met to exchange ideas with revolutionary fervor until 1917. She held a Psychoanalytic Evening around 1915 at which the psychoanalyst A.A. Brill spoke about Freudian theory, thereby providing many of her guests with their first glimpse of psychoanalysis. As a columnist for the Hearst newspaper chain from 1917 to 1918, Dodge added to the popularization of psychoanalysis with articles such as "Mabel Dodge Writes About the Unconscious" (Appendix A).

At this searching and dynamic time in New York, Smith Ely Jelliffe and A.A. Brill were two of the most prominent psychoanalysts. Dodge was in analysis twice, with Jelliffe for the first six months of 1916, and then with Brill beginning that summer (when Jelliffe was away for vacation) and continuing somewhat regularly until she moved to New Mexico in December 1917 (where she soon met Antonio Luhan, a Pueblo Indian, marrying him in 1923, after divorcing her two previous husbands, and remaining with him until her death in 1962).

Mabel Dodge's first contact with Smith Ely Jelliffe

Dodge had urgently consulted Jelliffe in 1914, following a disastrous experimentation with peyote at her 23 Fifth Avenue apartment. In her autobiographical account of her New York years, *Movers and Shakers* (1936), Dodge devotes a chapter to describing this evening during which she and a number of friends, including the artist Andrew Dasburg, the scenic designer Robert Edmond Jones, and the writers Max Eastman, Hutchins Hapgood, and his wife Neith Boyce, along with an actress named Genevieve Onslow, all participated in chewing peyote buttons provided by Boyce's cousin, who had recently arrived in New York from Oklahoma where he had been living and working with Native Americans. In the spirit of curiosity and with interest in expanding their experiences of reality, the group of friends engaged in a peyote ceremony, resulting in a night filled with intense perceptions and feelings, and ending with Genevieve's impulsive flight and disappearance into the streets of New York. She eventually arrived at Eastman's apartment, full of panic, speaking gibberish, and making odd movements. Worried about Genevieve's disorganized state, Hapgood arranged for her to consult with Dr. Harry Lorber, who had not heard of peyote but wondered if the drug they took could have been mescal. Although Dodge does not mention Jelliffe in this section of her memoir, she does introduce her chapter entitled "Dr. Jelliffe" with the following: "I decided I must have help from outside and I thought of Dr. Jelliffe, whom I had been to see when Genevieve Onslow frightened us so that night we experimented with *peyote*" (p. 439). Jelliffe's first extant letter to Dodge, dated December 27,

1914, concerns this consultation: "I am taking the liberty of adding to the paper which I promised you on Mescal, one of my own in an entirely different field.[1] That both are dealing with 'mankind' is my chief justification, but added thereto is my desire to thank you for having turned to me at a time when it seemed I might have been able to serve. In adding the little folder I am presuming on furthering an interest, the [sic] which has been brought to my attention by some that know and admire you." No other letters between them exist to suggest any more contact until Dodge started her analysis with him in January 1916.

Note

1   It is quite possible that Jelliffe sent Dodge a paper he wrote with "Zenia X—," "Compulsion Neurosis and Primitive Culture: An Analysis, a Book Review and an Autobiography," published in *Psychoanalytic Review* in October 1914 (*1:* 361–387).

Chapter 2

Smith Ely Jelliffe

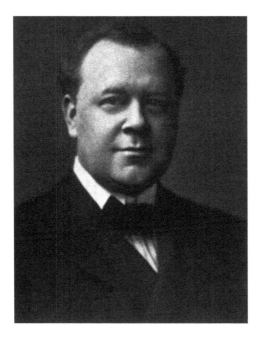

Figure 2.1 Smith Ely Jelliffe, circa 1910. Courtesy of the U.S. National Library of Medicine.

Childhood

Smith Ely Jelliffe (Figure 2.1) was born October 27, 1866 on West 38th Street in New York, and spent his childhood years in Brooklyn. He was the son of Susan Emma Kitchell, a school teacher, and William Munson Jelliffe, an influential public school principal in Brooklyn who received a doctorate in pedagogy from the City University of New York in 1891, and was well known for establishing the first organized kindergarten in Brooklyn in

1886, as well as for his elocution and entertaining public readings ("Public School No. 45," *The Brooklyn Teacher*, February 1898, pp. 1–2). In an unfinished, undated, and unpublished "autobiographical sketch" located among Jelliffe's papers at the Library of Congress—and quoted from at length in John Burnham's biography of Jelliffe (1983, pp. 8–12)—he reports that his birth "must have been a very anxious time in my parents['] life. My next older brother Samuel had died the April of the year previous and the next older brother William Rushby died when I was but 7–8 months old" (p. 27). Jelliffe offers a different angle on these events in an autobiographical article, "The Editor Himself and His Adopted Child" (1939), a reference to his "journal baby," *Journal of Nervous and Mental Disease*. He reflected that, in the midst of their losses, "I must have been very much loved by my parents" and considers "I was probably saved from being absolutely spoiled by the birth of a brother a year and a half later and thus I became the special ward of a sister nine years older" (pp. 546–547). Jelliffe came into a world already defined by a significant loss that would soon be magnified by his older brother's death.

Before recounting memories of his childhood in this "autobiographical sketch," Jelliffe offers a context for them informed by psychoanalysis: "It is a fairly well understood principle of psychology that no early experiences are totally lost and the psychoanalytic technique is one whereby much of this early imagery may be recalled. It is often glimpsed in the dream life and in many illnesses bits of one's infantile experiences come into activity" (pp. 26–27). Although Jelliffe himself was never in psychoanalysis, he did analyze his dreams and himself with his friend and fellow analyst William Alanson White for more than a decade (Jelliffe, 1933, pp. 327–328). In his autobiographical sketch, Jelliffe records a few passages from his own dreams. He reports that his "occasional night mare [*sic*] of 'horses hoof's [*sic*] and sparks of fire'" is a "clear cut illustration of an eidetic memory occurring in a dream" since his sister told him that he "was nearly run over by a fire engine while she was leading me across the street when I was 2–4 years of age" (pp. 27–28). He also names two images from his dreams—a "wistana vine" that he identifies from his childhood home, and a second-story porch that "I have never been able to locate. It is a cover memory of some sort" (p. 28)—to illustrate the work of finding meaning through dream interpretation.

In this sketch, Jelliffe characterizes himself as a "quickly learning" child who played running and chasing games in their Brooklyn neighborhoods and was "very agile and fleet of foot" (pp. 28, 31). "As for sickness, I knew little of it," he claims, and from a young age, remembers being "a stoic" who tended then, and throughout his life, "rarely to complain" (pp. 32, 33). He reports "an idiosyncrasy concerning my lessons": "For the most part I preferred to get them all done Friday. This left me all day Saturday and Sunday with no tasks ahead. It was, if I do not mislead myself[,] a general tendency to get the disagreeable or necessary task out of the way first. This trend has persisted all my life to some degree" (p. 39). Jelliffe valued a balance of work and play, as he was serious about his studies but also passionate about both his active life outside and his free time.

If Jelliffe's dreams were the subject of this book instead of Dodge's, evocative images in his autobiographical sketch would provide memories to inform interpretations. He enters a pigpen dressed in his best clothes, naturally soiling them, and his mother finds him there (p. 29). He remembers his uncle's factory where high heels were manufactured from wood: "The mill wheel and the belts were a constant source of pleasure" (p. 29). He pictures a chestnut tree, a cherry tree, and an outhouse at his family's house in Darien, Connecticut (p. 30). The sound of rain on the roof "came to me for years as a soothing memory as I would fall asleep" (p. 30). He recalls "a peculiar excitement when for the first time, when I was about 7–8[,] I saw a bull mount a cow. I did not know what it was all about, but something within me must have known. I was, so far as I recall, singularly inattentive to such matters" (p. 32). He stole cherries and pears from the trees of neighbors and reports having "no recollection of sadness" about his actions (p. 36). And, even though Jelliffe declares "I think I was a happy child. I have no recollection of unhappy experiences" (p. 29), he writes at length about one crucial upsetting event:

> One sad memory of childhood is important, since it carried with it, for years, a mood of sorrow with a specific nuance of suffering. I cannot bring anything but the feeling to memory but the probable reconstruction is not difficult. Christmas stocking[s]...were hung up. I could not have been more than four years of age. On one Christmas, mine was empty. A sadness, unaccompanied by anything but a dull heaviness of loneliness[,] was my response.
>
> I seem to remember I have been told[,] although this may be a phantasy reconstruction[,] it was because I had hit my little brother on the head with a hammer. On several occasions in my later life when I have done some mean or unworthy action, or have had a severe rebuff,...this same mood of deep sadness has come over me, but I have rarely felt it save associated with some wave of self[-]reproach for some antisocial act. At all events I feel it is no rationalization to say that this punishment has served as a censorship throughout my life.
>
> (pp. 33–34)

He is candid about his distress when he behaves badly or is rejected, showing his capacity for self-reflection and his use of this unhappy memory to set his actions right. And the loneliness that Jelliffe describes here is a theme that he will come back to, over and over, in his love letters to his fiancée.

Education and first love

Jelliffe entered the Brooklyn Collegiate and Polytechnic Institute misguided by his father to study civil engineering—"the only criticism I had of my father" (1939, p. 547)—since his passion lay instead with geology and zoology, and graduated in 1886 with a degree in engineering. During this time, he met Helena Dewey Leeming (Figure 2.2) whom he would marry in 1894: "Already at the age of sixteen I had found my first object choice. It was an enduring one and a long grueling time of conquering the anxiety of tension followed. Twelve years we waited and worked together" (p. 553). In high school, he admitted that her "definite literary gifts" rescued him from an assignment, as "she wrote that French oration, for I was helpless" (p. 553). As part of their romance, they shared a rich intellectual life, reading Emerson, Thoreau, Darwin, and George Eliot, among others, and pursued their mutual passion in botany, "collecting winter buds and arranging our herbarium sheets" (p. 548).

Smith Ely Jelliffe's path to practicing psychoanalysis was a convoluted one. After high school, he went directly to Columbia University's College of Physicians and Surgeons, completing his medical degree in 1889. He then did a year internship at St. Mary's General Hospital in Brooklyn, where he attributed his beginning interest in the field of psychology to the experience

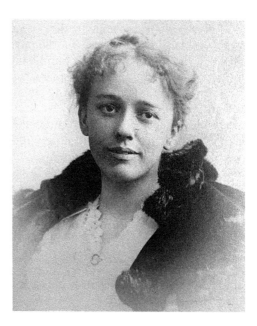

Figure 2.2 Helena Leeming Jelliffe, circa 1894. Courtesy of the Library of Congress.

of being immersed in a Catholic environment, as he relates in his autobiographical essay, "Glimpses of a Freudian Odyssey" (1933): "At first a bit bewildering, it ultimately became of signal service in getting a better orientation to emotional values and was distinctly serviceable in wearing down narrow prejudices and scotomata of all kinds" (p. 319). He recalled an event from this time that served as his "early introduction to 'dream' psychology which has kept me amused at myself for many years." In the hospital there was a "charming hysterical patient, a somnambulist....a Spanish type, beautifully classic, vivacious and alluring." Jelliffe apparently dreamed of this patient and then reports: "I well remember my going to the Mother Superior and virtuously telling of my being visited in my room by this charming creature after midnight. The calm, easy and serious way in which this very superior woman assured me I should not be disturbed again has always made me smile at my early ignorance of the wish fulfilling function of the dream" (1933, p. 320). Early in his training, he was also compelled to consider psychological factors when evaluating and diagnosing diseases of the body: "I felt I wanted to know a little more about brain than blood; more about the things of the spirit as I had been too long immersed in the things of the body.... I was firmly convinced they were the same. There was no antithesis of body and mind. They were one and inseparable but, above all, function determined structure and then structure directed function" (1930, p. 153). This conviction about the interconnection between mind and body led Jelliffe to develop theories and practices that became the basis for psychosomatic medicine, ideas advanced in 1915 when he published his first textbook with psychiatrist William Alanson White.

After St. Mary's, Jelliffe traveled in Europe for a year, a *Wanderjahr* devoted to cultural education and postgraduate classes in medicine and botany. At medical centers in cities such as Berlin and Vienna, he studied ear and eye diseases, internal medicine, and pathology, but not neurology or psychiatry. While he was away, he also immersed himself in learning German and French and made sketches of the art and architecture he encountered. Many of his letters to Helena Dewey Leeming from this time are illustrated with these drawings.

When he left for Europe in 1890, he was 25 years old: "Neither my fiancée nor I relished this year's separation made more bearable however by an almost daily mutual correspondence. Six volumes of this on thin paper await the autobiographer or biographer's efforts" (1939, p. 549). In Jelliffe's papers at the Library of Congress, two volumes of correspondence from Jelliffe to Leeming contain 548 numbered letters, from 1890 to 1893, with 298 letters from this first trip in 1890–1891. (There are also four volumes of letters from Leeming to Jelliffe from 1890 to 1891.)

In this extensive correspondence, Jelliffe reveals to his fiancée his devotion to her, and his vulnerabilities and passions. In his first letter, on the day of his departure, October 25, 1890, he addresses "My precious darling Lelie":

> From the bottom of my heart I feel & know that love's omnipotence has done more for me & my growth than any other thing could have done & now comes my testing time to prove my lessons & see if I am strong & steadfast, for the right & wisest thing. To see if I can be what I want to be & what you want me to be. Heart has been developing at the expense of head—now it's head's turn to develop, but not at the expense of heart: for heart[']s growth has been true & steadfast & now it is ready to wait for full fruition.... I love you with a love that is stronger than myself.

He expands on this idea a month later, this time prioritizing the lessons of heart over head: "I am becoming more and more of the opinion that love in a life, carried throughout, is worth far more than intellect or distraction or any other element, it is becoming more and more impressed upon my mind that my last year spent with you—in love—little spent in much else—has been a greater growing year in almost all respects than any growth I have had before." He then admits his struggle with loneliness away from her: "You have never known & may be [sic] never will know just how much of my life is entirely bound up in you; for I have always been a lonely boy and a lonely man; and through you my all comes; dearest truly I should not care to live if I had not the promise & hope of a life to be spent with you as a helper & lover. To love me supremely—passionately & with your whole life. Is it asking more than you care to give?" (November 30, 1890). Jelliffe's loneliness persisted, as he wrote her on January 31, 1891: "Dearest I have been so homesick for you....I am very, very lonely." His letters are filled with longing and romance: "I was kissing you in wish & thought" (November 4, 1890); "tell me how much you love me as often as you want to: tell me that you long to put your arms around my neck & draw me close to you & long to kiss me—dearest tell me all this. I am so lonely all the livelong day with no one to tell my love to except to these white pages" (November 26, 1890); he "kissed the pages [of her letters] over and over, silly boy that I was" (March 12, 1891). Jelliffe's tender letters to Leeming lay bare the primacy he placed on his love for her and its central place in his life, revealing the longing and vulnerable side of a wildly curious and impressionable physician; reading this correspondence adds layers to understanding his humanity. (In addition, the themes of loneliness and immersion of one's life in another's are also central emotional preoccupations for Mabel Dodge. To connect Jelliffe's internal life with that of Dodge's along these lines enriches the possibility of imagining what may have been going on in each of their psyches as they sat in a room together years later and analyzed Dodge's dreams.)

Beginning medical practice and turn to neurology and psychiatry

Jelliffe returned to New York from Europe, struggled to start a medical practice (admitting "my first year profits...were just $75" [Jelliffe, 1933, p. 321]), supplemented his income with teaching pharmacognosy and materia medica at Columbia University, returned to his interest in botany (eventually getting a doctorate in 1899), wrote numerous articles on topics as diverse as "Some Dangers Resulting from the Use of Cows' Milk" (1894a) and "A Report of Two Cases of Perforating Ulcer of the Foot" (1894b), and was frustrated by his inability to find a consistent direction, as he struggled to combine his training in medicine and botany to forge a career.

Then, crucially, in the summer of 1896, he met William Alanson White when they were both working at the Binghamton State Hospital in New York, where he had direct experience with psychiatric patients, and, as he reports, "began the downward path to the subterranean depths of psychiatry" (Jelliffe, 1933, p. 321). He then expanded his knowledge of neurology and psychiatry by working at the Vanderbilt Clinic at Columbia and in the Neurological Wards at the City Hospital. In 1897, the beginning of his lifelong involvement in medical journalism, Jelliffe became responsible for editing abstracts for the *Journal of Nervous and Mental Disease*, a publication that featured articles emphasizing the growing interest that neurologists were taking in mental diseases. In 1899, he became the associate editor of the journal and then, in 1902, managing editor.

Jelliffe's encounter with White resulted in an enduring friendship and professional collaboration, an association that Brill asserted "was destined to exert the greatest influence on his life" (1939, p. 529). Years later, when Jelliffe was fervently practicing and writing about psychoanalysis, he and White (who, in 1903, became the superintendent of St. Elizabeths Hospital in Washington, D.C., where he remained for his entire career) informally analyzed each other, as Jelliffe recalls:

> I had had no didactic analysis but my patients were analyzing me from hour to hour and I had had the rare association, especially during the summer months[,] with Dr. White. For some ten or more years almost uninterruptedly he had spent a month or so at my summer home [in Lake George, New York] with me and my family. We were continuously at each other, our dreams, our daily acts and aberrations, not for an hour but sometimes all day. I owe much more than I can tell at this time to these contacts not alone psychoanalytically but in many other relations.
>
> (1933, pp. 327–328)

In 1907, Jelliffe and White founded the Nervous and Mental Disease Monograph Series, publishing works such as A.A. Brill's translation of Jung's *Psychology of Dementia Praecox* (vol. 3, 1909) and his translations of Freud's *Selected Papers on Hysteria and Other Psychoneuroses* (vol. 4, 1909) and *The Three Contributions to the Theory of Sex* (vol. 7, 1925).

Jelliffe reports that 1907 was his "first personal contact with psychoanalysis" when he met Carl Jung at the First International Congress for Psychiatry, Neurology, Psychology, and the Nursing of the Insane in Amsterdam in September. Jelliffe was already familiar with Jung's application of Freud's ideas to the treatment of the psychoses in his 1907 book, *The Psychology of Dementia Praecox*, which Jelliffe had positively referenced in a paper he delivered at the American Medical Association meeting in June 1907, "Some General Reflections on the Psychology of Dementia Praecox." After meeting Jung in Amsterdam, Jelliffe apparently then had lunch with him later that month in Zurich, as he recalled in a letter to Freud from March 6, 1939 (1933, p. 323; Burnham, 1983, p. 281). (There is no mention in his writings or letters of having visited Jung's Burghölzli clinic in Zurich at this time.) Jelliffe was not to meet Freud until 1921 in Bad Gastein, Austria, "a fleeting contact" during which he presented Freud, who was about to depart, with a box of Cuban cigars at the train station (Jelliffe, 1933, p. 326). In Freud's last existing letter to Jelliffe, dated February 9, 1939, he recalls this moment and admits to shunning Jelliffe because he was talking to Wilhelm Stekel, one of Freud's original disciples who had parted ways with him over dissenting views: "I know you have been one of my sincerest and staunchest adherers through all these years. I now often laugh in remembrance of the bad reception I gave you at Gastein because I had first seen you in company of Stekel" (Burnham, 1983, p. 279). Although in 1907 Jelliffe had made this personal contact with Jung and was aware of Freud's ideas through his writings, he was not yet persuaded by the appeal of psychoanalysis.

In October 1908, Jelliffe went to Berlin for six months where he met Karl Abraham and worked with the German neurologist Hermann Oppenheim, who had opposed ideas about the traumatic origins of hysteria advanced by Jean-Martin Charcot, an approach to neuroses and the unconscious that had powerfully swayed Freud for a short time between 1895 and 1896 (Makari, 2008, pp. 27–30). He then spent six months in Paris exposing himself to the work of French neurologists, as he reports: "Here other types of psychotherapy were being practiced. I followed [Joseph Jules] Dejerine in his wards, became intrigued with his insistence on the emotional factors in medicine; listened to [Pierre] Janet's meticulous case history taking and his brilliant expositions; followed [Joseph] Babinski who was only just beginning his teachings on pithiatism" (1933, p. 323). However, Jelliffe was not convinced of the efficacy of any of the therapeutic approaches he had witnessed firsthand. In 1909, when Freud and Jung came to the United

States with Sandor Ferenczi to give their famous Clark University lectures on psychoanalysis, Jelliffe was away in Paris. However, at this time, Jelliffe admitted: "I was ready for a deeper and more vital understanding than any that had been offered me thus far" (1933, p. 324). In his eagerness for more experience, he began working that year as a visiting physician at the New York Neurological Institute. In 1910, A.A. Brill, already an established psychoanalyst, joined the staff at the Institute and through their association Jelliffe became a serious student of psychoanalysis.

Conversion to psychoanalysis

Brill remembers that when he first met Jelliffe in 1908, "he did not give me the impression that he knew or thought much of psychoanalysis" (1939, p. 531). However, two years later, Jelliffe converted to psychoanalysis, as he reports in "Glimpses of a Freudian Odyssey" (1933): "After our clinics, three times a week Brill and I walked homewards together through the park, and as formerly with Dr. White we argued and argued and he persisted and thus I became a convinced Freudian" (p. 325). These walks while talking about psychoanalysis are reminiscent of Brill's long walks with Freud in Vienna only a few years before. Brill reported his own version of these early discussions with Jelliffe, recalling their first conversation when his colleague "showed at that time definite resistances to psychoanalysis" (1947, p. 582). Brill then wrote of his successful plan to convert Jelliffe:

> I conceived his attitude towards psychoanalysis as a direct challenge and forthwith decided to change his mind. That I succeeded in my efforts is well-known....However, to give you a more intimate view of Jelliffe's conversion to Freud, let me read the following quotation from a letter which I received from him, April 2, 1943:...."Our walks through the park started something in me of inestimable value and I shall never be able to tell you what they did for me in the way of assembling and crystallizing a large background of general medical experience. I felt that bottom rock had been reached and we could then build with confidence. I had been reading Freud, but you made it vital and real for me. It was a 'forge' into which things could be plunged and then hammered out into shape. This you helped me do, and your help was generous and unstinted. Your genuine and intrinsic honesty, as well as your good sense, made me cleave to you as a brother I never really had and supplemented my contacts with White that have been so invaluable."
>
> (1947, p. 582)

Jelliffe had long been seeking a clear direction in his medical career and through Brill, his focus sharpened into an adherence to psychoanalysis.

Jelliffe soon began integrating psychoanalysis into his psychotherapy practice and his writings. As early as 1905 he mentioned Freud's theories in two book reviews for the *Journal of Nervous and Mental Disease*, and in 1913 he published his first article about psychoanalysis, "Some Notes on 'Transference,'" in the *Journal of Abnormal Psychology*, admitting: "I am aware of the somewhat simplistic nature of this my first psychoanalytic communication. I tender it as a slight earnest of my purpose to understand" (p. 309). In this paper, later read at a meeting of the American Psychopathological Association, he wrote about dreams and transference, revealing his experience with the psychoanalytic approach in his own work:

> I take it to be the experience of many here who have put the psycho-analytic methods to the test of experience that they soon commence to recognize themselves in the patient's dreams. At first the stereotypy struck me—it was only later, that I began to see how various might be the symbolizations which expressed the identification and the transfer-ence at the same time.
>
> For me to be a *policeman*, a *priest*, a *chauffeur*, is quite understandable to those of you who look at me now. As policeman I have "shielded from harm," have "kept away enemies," have "arrested impudent intruders," and "frightened away naughty boys"; as priest, confession has been ready and admonition invited, while as a chauffeur or engineer positive transference has permitted dangerous journeys over rough roads and in stormy weather, and even invited to flight and a new life.
>
> These are all every-day occurrences, I feel, to those of you at all inter-ested in psychoanalysis.
>
> (pp. 305–306)

Jelliffe went on to discuss a patient whose dreams exposed her feelings to-ward him: "This patient has shown the most marked ambivalence in her transferences—at times the rising barriers have threatened to drive her away, but with the subtle barometer of the dream-revealed transference, stormy scenes have been avoided, and the analysis has almost laid bare the entire contents of this Pandora's box" (p. 309). By this time, Jelliffe was fully immersed in the practice of psychoanalysis in New York.

Jelliffe's patients

Beyond the archival material from Mabel Dodge's psychoanalysis with Jelliffe, we know only a little about the identity and experiences of his other patients. Most of those who are known were associated with Dodge and often directed to him by her. At the beginning of her analysis with Jelliffe, she admitted in her memoir *Movers and Shakers* (1936): "I longed to draw others into the new world where I found myself: a world where things fitted into a set of definitions and terms that I had never even dreamt of" (p. 440). During a weekend visit in 1916 to Dodge's country home, Finney Farm, Jelliffe met a number of her friends who would soon come to him for analysis: Robert "Bobby" Edmond Jones, the Norwegian-American poet Bayard Boyeson, and the writer and critic Leo Stein. Dodge had also hoped that her lover, the artist Maurice Sterne, would be lured into analysis, but, alas, he prevailed in his refusal: "Palpably, Maurice had evaded Jelliffe's attempts to talk to him by always being in the room where the doctor was not" (p. 441).

Bobby Jones

Dodge reports that during Jelliffe's visit to Croton: "Before dinner he had found Bobby making sketches for a play, out on the dining-room table. These drawings decided him that Bobby, too, needed psychoanalysis, and before long I led him unresisting to Jelliffe's office" (1936, p. 441). No other documents exist to point to Jones in analysis with Jelliffe.

However, Dodge apparently urged Jones into treatment again, ten years later, this time with Jung in Zurich, as he acknowledged in a February 6, 1927 letter from Switzerland, "It was you who got me to come here." She partially funded his therapy through donations from their shared friends (Rudnick, 1984, p. 185). In a letter to Dodge circa summer 1926, he describes his analysis with Jung: "There is no trace of medicine or therapeutics in it. A subtle deep terrible mystical journey, torments, vigils, illuminations. I think we have a very good working combination.... Jung says that I have the most remarkable gift for animating other people that he has ever seen." On September 22, 1926, Jones writes again to Dodge, giving her Jung's address, apparently because she was interested in starting treatment with him herself. On October 4, 1926, he reports that Jung refused to treat someone named "Mary" and warns Dodge: "You better not be fractious or he won't take you." Dodge never did meet Jung, even though he visited Taos in 1925. She was in New York at the time.

Bayard Boyeson

In a letter to Dodge from August 1916, Bayard Boyeson referred to his analysis with Jelliffe, and she reveals in *Movers and Shakers* (1936) that Jelliffe shared with her some details of Boyeson's treatment:

> Dr. Jelliffe kept me *au courant* with his case, for he simply couldn't resist talking things over with someone who really took an intelligent interest, and his speculative mind flashed into the dark corners of life and lighted up many dark corners. It entertained him very much to find that Bayard had once raised three crops of alfalfa in one year on his fields in Athol, and had since that time completely lain back upon this achievement as

though he would let the knowledge of it support him in idleness for the rest of his life! Those three crops were forever coming up in his analysis! They constituted his justification and his doom. Jelliffe's duty was to remove this fantasy of accomplishment so that some activity might flow in him once more. So he started to amputate it from poor Bayard. The end of the first month came and Jelliffe was still prying it out of him. Then Bayard decided it was too expensive to continue. Jelliffe shook his head sadly but with a humorous twinkle in his eyes.

"It is the resistance," he told me. "He does not want to give up his neurosis and I am a danger to it."

(pp. 463–464)

On July 22, 1916, Dodge had written to Jelliffe about Boyeson: "Bayard went downhill so that I talked to him straight out & told him he had to go away. That he was using the place [Finney Farm] to go to pieces in & I wouldn't have it—that he hadn't done his share or helped me at all but had just taken & taken & such situation couldn't last & that he must go. It was the shock he needed....I am fond of him but I couldn't see him go to pieces under my eyes. I shall keep track of him." She and Jelliffe shared a deep concern for Boyeson and, in fact, the three of them appear together in several of Dodge's 1916 dreams.

Leo Stein

When Leo Stein consulted with Jelliffe, he wrote to Dodge at Croton, circa 1916: "I don't know when I'll be sufficiently footloose to get to Croton again. I see Jelliffe for the moment almost every day"; another letter, circa spring 1916, reads: "I have an engagement with Jelliffe for Wednesday at 5." Stein also wrote to Dodge, circa late 1916: "I saw Jelliffe a few days ago & told him the story of my recent life. When I had finished he asked me what I proposed to do & I told him that I thought I should try to work for a while & that if things did not prosper then I should resume the analysis. He quite agreed & so the matter stands." Stein was a strong believer in self-analysis of dreams and neuroses. He also wrote to Dodge, circa 1916, about consulting with Brill and then discontinuing, preferring Jelliffe: "My reasons for not going on... had to do largely with third persons and besides that S.E.J. has a mind & personality that interested me much more."

Mary Foote

The painter Mary Foote, who painted a portrait of Jelliffe in the late 1910s, and visited him at his Lake George summer home, was also very likely in treatment with him, as she suggests in a letter to Dodge circa 1916 or 1917:

"I'll undoubtedly hurl myself at Jelliffe—or the little dried up Jew [likely an offensive reference to Brill] of the same profession—sooner or later, but I must get a job first—can't face debt with my New England past—In the meantime do let me know when Jelliffe comes out again [to Croton]." Dodge had written to Jelliffe circa fall 1916: "I don't want to mix up in things which don't concern me much but I may as well tell you that Mary Foote is on tip toe with anxiety to begin analysis." In a later letter, dated December 4, circa 1916, Foote reports to Dodge: "I never see Jelliffe any more [sic]....Have you given up Brill & gone back to Jelliffe?"

Nina Bull

In 1916, while Dodge was in analysis with Jelliffe, she was also trying Divine Science treatment with her friend Nina Bull (see Interlude 7). Bull was considering therapy for her daughter Katherine, as she wrote to Dodge: "I've been pondering pretty deeply over the psychoanalysis idea for K—but don't feel ready to try it yet....That time I talked with Jelliffe in yr motor, I knew he couldn't do much for me, for while I realized there was a lot he knew which I didn't, I also realized that there was a lot I knew which he didn't! Brill impressed me more than Jelliffe." In the same letter she predicts: "I am doubtful if I shall ever be analyzed....I have yet to hear of the person who has been psychoanalyzed into a state of higher spiritual consciousness." However, Bull eventually entered analysis with Jelliffe, as she reports in an undated, circa 1935, letter to Dodge: "Psychoanalysis with Jelliffe gets more interesting and illuminating every day. Some times [sic] I wish I'd done it earlier—but on the whole I don[']t believe I was ready to take it in with all the far reaching implications—until now."

Max Eastman

Max Eastman was introduced to Jelliffe in 1914 by the Jungian analyst Beatrice Hinkle, who believed he should consult with a male psychoanalyst. As he recalled in his memoir: "Psychoanalysis was in those days a disreputable therapy struggling desperately for recognition. Dr. Jelliffe may have thought of me as potential help in the struggle; he may merely have found my case interesting. At any rate he agreed to psychoanalyze me for a fee that would be a song today, and I went to him four times a week for several months during the winter and spring of 1914" (1948, p. 491). During this treatment, Eastman became a student of Freud's teachings, reading all of his translated books, and then "rehearsing the doctrine point by point with its agile-minded apostle, and becoming once more a kind of amateur specialist in mental healing" (p. 491). This description of Eastman's interactions with Jelliffe closely follows Dodge's own reports of the intellectual stimulation of her sessions which ultimately left her with this assessment: "I am afraid I did not learn much about myself with Jelliffe, but I did get a very complete line on *him*...and I enjoyed my outings in his office" (Luhan, 1936, p. 454). Eastman, too, enjoyed his time with Jelliffe, but admitted "my problems, needless to say, were not solved by this feat of learning. I turned up no new memories of childhood and never appropriated emotionally any of the unconscious drives that seemed to appear in my dreams" (1948, p. 491). Eastman's list of the themes he considered with Jelliffe—"homo-sexuality, mother fixation, Oedipus, Electra and inferiority complexes, narcissism, exhibitionism, autoeroticism" (p. 491)—echo those that Dodge explored in her analysis with Jelliffe two years later. Eastman concluded, that, even though he felt "the peculiar affection toward Jelliffe which Freud calls 'transference,'" he did not agree with Freud's assessment of "this excited attachment of neurotics to their doctor-confidants as 'the most unshakable proof' that all neuroses have their origin in sex, a jump to conclusions which I regard as lacking in simple common sense. Jelliffe himself was full of these wild Freudian jumps, and my affection for him could not carry me along" (pp. 491–492). In considering reasons for ending her own treatment, Dodge might have written this same last phrase about Jelliffe: *my affection for him could not carry me along.*

Years after the end of his analysis, Eastman asked Jelliffe for his case notes, but he was not able to locate them, and instead sent a summary: "'You weren't quite aware of the Oedipus situation, the hostility to the father working itself out in prejudiced radicalism. You were tied up also in a complex situation with your sister which made relations with your wife uncomfortable. There was a sister-identification, and through that identi-fication a fundamental narcissistic cathexis or investment'" (1948, p. 492). Eastman commented on these jargon-filled statements: "Jelliffe was too glib with ideas to be of sure help among facts" (1948, p. 492).[1] Although such language initially appealed to Dodge in her quest to understand and, along the way, acquire new vocabulary, for her, too, Jelliffe's interpretations ulti-mately left her unsatisfied.

Elizabeth Severn

Elizabeth Severn, a self-taught psychoanalyst, revealed in a 1952 interview with Kurt Eissler that she had been in analysis first with Jelliffe, then Joseph Asch, "a very nice fellow," next Otto Rank in 1924, and finally Ferenczi. She was (now famously) Ferenczi's patient for eight years who appeared as "R.N." in his *Clinical Diary* (1932). Severn also reported in this interview that she found Jelliffe: "A very sadistic man. Very. Able man, intellectually, and I hear excellent things said of him, recently" (1952, p. 3). About her anal-ysis with him, she said: "I was extremely disappointed with my work with him. And also with Rank. Got absolutely nowhere. I learned their theory, but their application of them [*sic*] was most unsatisfactory and very one-sided" (p. 4). Severn had met with Freud in Vienna in 1925 and told him "about the men that I had tried to learn about psychoanalysis with in this country [America], and was very dissatisfied. And I don't think he was surprised. He didn't say so to me, but I understand that he was disappointed in the American attitude which, as you know, is quick and apt to be superficial" (p. 4). Severn explained to Eissler: "I came to the conclusion that the trouble was that the early students of Freud had not been thoroughly analyzed. They had been analyzed in an intellectual manner, and I don't think the transferences had been worked out fully" (p. 1). She had asked Freud about this concern and reported that "this limitation did not appear to Freud to be a limitation" and "he believed that they were prepared" (p. 3).

In Severn's *The Psychology of Behavior* (1917), she criticizes "the average present-day Psycho-analyst," certainly a reference to Jelliffe, as Peter Rudnytsky forcefully argues in his unpublished manuscript about Severn.[2] Here is what Severn scathingly writes:

> To perform this operation as it is done by the average present-day Psycho-analyst is like having a surgical process for the removal of a tumour without any succeeding medical care for the upbuilding of the weakened constitution. The mind is a delicate instrument and the application to it of the analytical process is more than likely to produce a mental shock of some kind, a reaction simple or violent according to the extent of the original damage. The Christian Scientists call it a "chemicalization" and all Mental Scientists know the symptoms even though unacquainted, as often happens, with the rationale of their treatment.
>
> (p. 258)

In an account of her own experiences in psychoanalysis, particularly with Ferenczi, *The Discovery of the Self: A Study in Psychological Cure* ([1933] 2017), Severn exposes what she considers to be limitations of analysis, some of which she likely experienced with Jelliffe. She writes: "The greatest objection to be made against psychoanalysis as such is, in my opinion, its *rigidity*. Being devised as a systemic and observational method, it lacks in flexibility and humanness in its application to sick people" (pp. 51–52). Echoing exactly Jelliffe's interpretation of resistance in Boyeson's decision not to continue therapy because of the expense, Severn observes that psychoanalysis is "inclined to regard every objection of the patient as an unwillingness or supposed 'resistance'" (p. 52). She also advises: "The analyst has to be very tactful in this process and listen to many arguments against admitting the new values and points of view that he recommends," and she asserts that the patient "needs also an opportunity to say when he thinks the analyst is in the wrong, since the person of the analyst represents of necessity an authority to him" (p. 52). Severn identifies here the potential dangers of the power imbalance in psychoanalysis, where an analyst's rigid adherence to his opinion or interpretation can leave little or no room for the patient's freedom to disagree.

Dodge could have meaningfully contributed to Severn's critique of the *"rigidity"* of psychoanalysis, since she herself named Jelliffe's "dogmatic" approach in a letter to him, circa May 1916 (see Interlude 15), challenging "some elements in your technique of analysis...I think your dogmatic trend halts me! I don't feel your right to prescribe a philosophy....I don't believe it comes within the realm of psychoanalysis to impose a formula for thinking." Dodge added: "But don't you think you could leave out some of your judgements [sic] (mentally as well as spoken—more than spoken in fact) and have a little more leeway for the conceptions of the patient without regarding them as fantasy,—& the present type of letter as regression!" Severn's warning about analysis is relevant here: "But unless the patient's objections are encouraged and treated seriously, and unless the analyst is prepared to admit that he may sometimes be in the wrong, even to the relinquishment of his most pet theories, no progress can be made and, indeed, great harm, may be done" (1933, p. 52). In Jelliffe's written reply to Dodge (see Interlude 16), he welcomed her letter and admitted his shortcomings: "I am sorry you feel I dogmatize: I myself am dogmatic that I have no right to do so. As a thorough-going sophist and pragmatist my own philosophy cannot and must not be imposed on another of different experience." He even offered: "I am glad you can formulate my dogmatism, as you have; it is one of my difficulties, more born of the desire to hurry people along than to make them conform. I am after all a wretched conformist myself and to be held up as a single pattern, machine maker of souls—although perhaps an hyperbolic way of taking your phrase—is a shock." Given her feelings about her analysis with him, Severn might have been surprised by Jelliffe's willingness to engage in a dialogue with Dodge that questioned his technique.

Psychoanalytic Review

In the fall of 1913, Jelliffe and White founded the *Psychoanalytic Review: A Journal Devoted to an Understanding of Human Conduct*, with the intention of presenting a broad range of articles and perspectives on psychology, with psychoanalysis providing the overall context. White evidently had invited Jung to contribute to the first issue, as he had been enthusiastic about the idea of an inclusive psychoanalytic journal when he visited with White in the fall of 1912, at the same time that Jung and Freud were in the midst of estrangement over their differences. Jung had been in New York in September 1912 at the invitation of Jelliffe to deliver lectures at Fordham University's International Extension Course in Medicine. In fact, he stayed with Jelliffe during this time, again at Jelliffe's invitation, as stated in a letter to Jelliffe dated May 13, 1912. After his lectures, Jung traveled to Washington, D.C. to visit White at St. Elizabeths Hospital (Burnham, 1983, pp. 189–190; SJA).

Jung's letter in the first issue of the *Review* praised Jelliffe and White for their endeavor:

> I welcome as a most opportune plan the idea of the editors to unite in their journal the contributions of competent specialists in the various fields. We need not only the work of medical psychologists, but also that of philologists, historians, archeologists, mythologists, folklore students, ethnologists, philosophers, theologians, pedagogues and biologists.
>
> I am free to admit that this enterprise is ambitious and highly creditable to the liberal and progressive spirit of America....I wish the best of success to this new venture.
>
> (pp. 117–118)

In a claim that may have rankled Freud, the founder of psychoanalysis, Jelliffe described the *Review* as the "only journal in English" that "aims to be catholic in its tendencies, a faithful mirror of the psychoanalytic movement, and to represent no schisms or schools but a free forum for all" (1913–1914, p. 444).

Freud had likely heard about or read Jung's letter in this first issue of the *Psychoanalytic Review*. White apparently had also invited Freud to contribute to the journal, but seemingly after Jung's piece was published in the fall of 1913. Freud had not yet met either White or Jelliffe when he wrote to White on July 7, 1914. Admitting that it "surprises me" to be asked, he refused to send a paper for a number of reasons: he cited hearing that "Jelliffe once refused to pay membership dues to the New York Society on the ground that he had no money for a foreign publisher. This, I feel, amounts to considering psychoanalysis from the standpoint of business rather than of science"; Freud found it "unseemly" that the *Review* used translations of articles as a way of making up for the fact that "it is still difficult to fill it with [original] worthwhile contributions"; he considered the *Review* as competition with the journal he currently edited, *Internationale Zeitschrift für ärztliche Psychoanalyse*, founded in January 1913; finally, in this letter to White, Freud objected to "Jelliffe's intimacy with Jung, who in spite of his presidency has never lifted a finger for the International Association" (Burnham, 1983, pp. 195–196). Freud may have been miffed that he was not invited to contribute at the outset, and certainly at this point did not want to be in the company of Jung, as they had severed their correspondence in January 1913. Years later, Jelliffe (1933) explained: "It was a bit of a misunderstanding that caused the *Psychoanalytic Review* to open with a contribution by Jung instead of one by

Freud, some of the reasons for which are still unknown to me. Freud's reply to our invitation was not very cordial" (p. 326). Although he asserted that he was then a "convinced Freudian" (p. 325), Jelliffe's personal relationship with Freud did not develop until after their meeting in 1921. In fact, Freud came to believe that Jelliffe was a loyal adherent to psychoanalysis, as Blanton (1971) quotes Freud as saying on September 2, 1938: "'Brill apparently is the only friend I have in the New York group—or perhaps I should include Dr. Jelliffe'" (p. 108).[3]

"Technique of Psychoanalysis" papers

Jelliffe contributed significantly to the *Psychoanalytic Review* with his many "Technique of Psychoanalysis" papers, four entries woven through each of the first four volumes (in 1917, only two entries), each continuing where the last had left off. In the first volume, he explained his intention: "The present series of articles is planned for the beginner in psychoanalysis....At the outset it seems desirable to give a general outline of what psychoanalysis is.... Psychoanalysis is primarily to be considered as a method. As such, it seeks to establish a knowledge of the development of human motives" (1913–1914, p. 65). Aiming to teach "the neophyte," Jelliffe started with the basics of psychoanalytic thinking and practice, and later elaborated on a wide range of topics, including Freud's concept of the libido, repression, and dream interpretation.

In his first "Technique" paper, Jelliffe begins with history-taking, where "one's attitude should be an absolutely impartial and uncritical one" and the analyst should be prepared to listen for stretches of time, not interrupting or asking leading questions (1913–1914, p. 73). He advises that after the first few sessions with a patient, "A complete physical examination is usually necessary....It must never be overlooked that physical disturbances may exist side by side with psychical ones" (p. 75). As much as he acknowledges the interconnectedness of emotional and physical symptoms, he also stresses the importance of determining whether any physical disorder exists. (It is not clear if he intends that the treating analyst should be the one to conduct the physical exam.)

Jelliffe describes the difficulty of analyzing the "well-to-do," since "the democratic attitude of psychoanalysis, its pragmatic and humanistic tendencies run counter to their aristocratic, rationalistic and individualistic mode of education. They are very indolent. Novel reading, drug taking, alcoholism and social fussing constitute their most frequently used pathways to escape from being bored to death." He considers that, for the wealthy, "auto-erotic fantasy, sexual tittle tattle, definite liaisons or perversions may be the sole excitements that apparently give any value to life" (p. 301).

For him, "the main object of a psychoanalytic cure" is "the making of the patient free and independent" (p. 305). Jelliffe asserts the importance of the analyst's self-monitoring: "Continual self[-]analysis is requisite during the course of analytic work. The analysis of a resistance always shows psychoanalytic scotomata on the part of the analyst....The would-be analyst should work resolutely with his own dreams, if possible with the aid of some one [sic] versed in psychoanalysis. A few passing remarks on a corner or at a chance meeting are worse than useless" (1915, p. 73).

Attention to transference is crucial: "It is worth while [sic] observing the dress of the patients, particularly of the woman. It is at times plainly indicative of positive transference and may be the first indication of too strong a transference" (1916, p. 254). He regrets self-disclosure: "I think sooner or later I have regretted every personal confidence given. It is particularly in the unloosing of the transference that this technical error shows up to the greatest disadvantage. Freud calls attention to this in several of his papers, and points out how for some patients the analysis of the analyst becomes more interesting than their own" (p. 258).

Jelliffe collected and revised these papers in 1917 and published them as a monograph, *The Technique of Psychoanalysis*, in the Nervous and Mental Disease series. Brill admitted that when he started reading Jelliffe's "Technique" papers, he was "at first more or less irritated by his mode of approach, but my temper changed as I continued reading. I noticed that Jelliffe accepted everything that Freud said, but utilized the psychoanalytic concepts in accordance with the expressions of his personality. Jelliffe was really a naturalist to start with; he was a botanist, a chemist, a hygienist, and above all, a deep and daring thinker to whom nothing difficult was an impossible task" (1939, p. 534). When Jelliffe further revised his monograph for a second edition in 1920, Brill wrote to him on May 1, 1921: "I assume that you realize that your whole mode of approach is more of the Jung Anschauung than Freud's. After all, it matters little, except that you give me this feeling and yr book certainly speaks the same" (SJA). In his biography of Jelliffe, Burnham (1983) admits, "It is extremely difficult to show exactly the extent to which Jelliffe was a Jungian, or, indeed, even the particular ways in which he was one" (p. 79). He then emphasizes that both were intensely focused on the concept of the libido—"the most important of Jelliffe's Jungianisms was... endowing libido with almost anthropomorphic characteristics"—, paid close attention to associations and symbolizations, and had similar styles and language (p. 79). Although Freud and Jung disagreed about the nature of libido and the unconscious, they had both already published significant, sometimes starkly divergent, contributions to psychoanalysis. With his lifelong capacity to integrate, Jelliffe's "Technique" papers combined elements from both Freud and Jung to advance psychoanalytic education in the United States at this time.

Diseases of the Nervous System

Jelliffe and White collaborated on a major textbook, *Diseases of the Nervous System: A Text-Book of Neurology and Psychiatry,* which was first published in 1915, reissued in a number of later editions, and was innovative in featuring a holistic view of the person and emphasizing psychological factors in physical symptoms. All editions were introduced by an essay that emphasized the crucial role of the unconscious in the functioning of the body. The preface to the first edition presents this unconventional approach: "The diseases of the nervous system are no longer compassed by a description of the gross lesions of the brain, spinal cord, cranial and peripheral nerves." The authors emphasize the increased medical knowledge in the sympathetic and autonomic nervous systems, as well as "the mechanisms that operate at the psychic or mental levels," emphasizing that these mental mechanisms are "intimately related to the vegetative levels where through the emotions they act unconsciously." Jelliffe and White explain the division of their book into three parts: "the vegetative, the sensori-motor, and the psychic levels, the reactions in all of which come to pass through the medium of the nervous system." They argue that a human being operates through all three levels: "For these reasons the treatise has been called primarily a work on the diseases of the nervous system rather than two books, one on neurology and one on psychiatry, which would perpetuate a distinction which the authors believe to be wholly artificial" (pp. iii—iv). This insistence on psychological factors bearing significantly on the diseases of the nervous system distinguished the radical approach of their textbook.

The second edition in 1917 includes an introduction greatly expanded (from two to five pages), where Jelliffe and White[4] are even bolder in both their writing and pronouncements. They observe that "the titles of our textbooks…set forth that they deal with nervous and mental diseases, inferring [sic] that these two groups have little relation, the one to the other, and, by the same token, fail to indicate that they either or both have any relation to the rest of the body" and then proclaim: "All this is wrong" (p. 17). They assert that "psychoanalysis is as important for the understanding of the construction of the psyche as dissection is for the understanding of the structure of the body" and declare: "The greatest deficiency in the psychology of the nineteenth century relative to the understanding of human conduct has been the neglect of the unconscious" (p. 20). Drawing upon the ideas of both Freud (a personal unconscious) and Jung (a more collective unconscious), they stress the rewards of acknowledging the unconscious and of paying attention to symbolization:

> So long as the unconscious failed to be recognized, just so long was the gap between so-called body and so-called mind too wide to be bridged, and so there arose the two concepts, body and mind, which gave origin to the necessity of defining their relations. Consciousness covered over and obscured the inner organs of the psyche just as the skin hides the inner organs of the body from vision. But just as a knowledge of the

body first became possible by the removal of the skin and the revealing of the structures that lay beneath, so a knowledge of the psyche first became possible when the outer covering of consciousness was penetrated and what lay at greater depth was revealed. As soon as this was done, the wonderful history of the psyche began to give up its secrets, and the distinction between body and mind began to dissolve, until now it has come to be considered that the psyche is the end-result in an orderly series of progressions in which the body has used successfully more complex tools to deal with the problem of integration and adjustment.

(p. 21)

This passage elegantly describes the process of considering the interplay of mind and body, and articulates how meaning can emanate from symptoms. In 1916, Jelliffe published (with his assistant Elida Evans) "Psoriasis as Hysterical Conversion Symbolization" in the *New York Medical Journal,* his preliminary claim to this innovative understanding of a chronic disease that considered "the dynamics of the skin reactions in terms of the hidden psychological factors of the individual life, the patient's thought fossils, to wit" (p. 5). Jelliffe's early work in psychosomatic medicine distinguished him as a psychoanalyst who keenly observed the body and its unconscious expressions.

Jelliffe communicated to his patients his revolutionary approach to the nervous system and its diseases. In her analysis with him, Dodge absorbed his teachings, explaining: "One of the most interesting speculations Jelliffe went in for was apparently a new field never worked much before—the set of symbols that compose all the parts of the body" (1936, p. 440):

Dr. Jelliffe told me his fascinating theories on disease and his belief that nearly all bodily illness is a failure of the spirit expressing itself at the physical level, just as disorders of the brain represent, at the symbolic level, the inabilities of the psyche....Tumors, cancers and so on, appeared to him to be manifestations in the flesh of one's unsublimated hatreds for people or situations outside oneself whom one regarded as parasites and whom one was unable to successfully deal with. Most of the insanities that were not of organic origin were, he thought, due to one's own inability to cope with oneself....The respiratory organs, he said, stood for human aspiration, the breath was no less than the breath of God. Failure in aspiration resulted in a breaking down of the lungs, the bronchial tubes, or the larynx. The creation, birth, and development of the soul could be reckoned in these parts, and they corresponded with the lower organs of sex where creation on another plane was effected. "As below, so above."

(pp. 20, 440)

Once familiar with Jelliffe's theories, Dodge applied them to herself toward better understanding, even reflecting back to the winter of 1912–1913 when she had her tonsils removed and concluding: "Certainly my throat was testimony either to some lack of aspiration or of failure to achieve. I was poisoned by it" (1936, p. 20).

It is also quite possible that Dodge, in her initial curiosity and enthusiasm for psychoanalysis, even before she started treatment herself, may have read Jelliffe's "Technique of Psychoanalysis" papers in the *Psychoanalytic Review*, thereby providing her with a glimpse of what happens in an analytic session.

Notes

1 Eastman later consulted with Brill and, "by way of experiment," asked him for "his impression of the ground of my emotional troubles": "People are always repeating some pattern from their childhood. You and I have not talked much, but from what I know of your history and your family, I think you have a strong mother-fixation. Your pattern is that you want to get away from your mother and yet be with her" (1948, p. 492). Even though Eastman complained that "Brill is no more convincing theoretically to me than Jelliffe was," he warmed to him differently: "He has an intuitive sensitivity towards people that makes him a master in the clinic" (1948, p. 492).

2 Rudnytsky, P.L. (forthcoming, Routledge, Relational Perspectives series), *Mutual Analysis: Ferenczi, Severn, and the Origins of Trauma Theory*. I am grateful to Peter Rudnytsky for introducing me to the writings of Elizabeth Severn, sharing with me both his findings about her time in analysis with Jelliffe and his unpublished writings.

3 I am also grateful to Peter Rudnytsky for calling my attention to this quotation.

4 As to the authorship of different parts of the textbook, Jelliffe once admitted: "White and I have written and published so many things together that I am not certain when I quote from one of them whether to say 'White and Jelliffe,' or 'Jelliffe and White'" (Lewis, 1966, p. 225).

Chapter 3

Mabel Dodge in psychoanalysis with Smith Ely Jelliffe

Jelliffe's "Technique" papers and Dodge's analysis

Jelliffe provided such specific and direct instructions to the beginning psychoanalyst in his "Technique" papers, that it becomes possible to imagine, perhaps quite accurately, Dodge's initial encounter and subsequent sessions with him, particularly when illuminated by his case notes and her descriptions of their work together.

He recommends that during the initial session that the patient's "'talk' may be hastily jotted down, or written in shorthand" (1913–1914, p. 73), a practice he clearly used with Dodge, as his notes seem to have been taken verbatim and are filled with many abbreviations and idiosyncratic symbols, such as "*Many* ♀ *interested in me # One I did get interested in*," "*Just part of* ☉ *temperament*," and "*This was in Italy: much* ♀-♀ *about*." "In a very short time," he observes, "the analyst experiences the pleasant sensation that the patient feels that someone is really trying to understand what is going on in their mind" and warns: "It is of the highest importance not to explain too much to the patient about his neurosis in the beginning" (p. 74). Jelliffe acknowledges the experiences of both patient and analyst here, grasping the importance of the analyst's restraint and focused attention while he listens to what the patient brings, and the patient's deep wish to be known, a central theme for Dodge, whose desperation to be noticed determined the pattern of her days.

Jelliffe writes at length about the crucial importance of this first session with the patient where the analyst "should observe every little sign....the very first sentence uttered by the patient contains the clue to their whole general situation. The analyst should also recall that he is under close scrutiny as well and should hold himself as impassive as possible, yet be appreciative, anxious to learn and genuinely receptive" (1915, pp. 73–74). Dodge's "first sentence" was delivered in a letter to Jelliffe, where she pronounced herself in possession of a "jealousy complex which has produced an anxiety neurosis," an idea expanded in her initial session. Jelliffe continues:

The patient will usually tell why he or she has come and what the symptoms are....The first hour should be wisely used to gain as much confidence as possible. Such confidence is gained largely through the patient observing that the analyst is really listening and understanding....

One may take the history systematically, guiding the patient along certain points, history of the family, etc., but it is preferable to say to the patient, "Tell me all about yourself, and I shall listen. If I am not quite clear as to what you mean I shall ask you in detail, but tell me everything that comes to your mind."

(pp. 74–75)

Jelliffe's suggestion to invite the patient to "tell me all about yourself" with the promise "I shall listen" must have reached Mabel Dodge at her core, for she was not accustomed, lonely, and unloved child that she was, to someone desiring details of her internal life. Even if Jelliffe did not say this exact sentence to Dodge, his dedication to careful and unhurried listening was undoubtedly communicated.

After determining that the patient is suitable for analysis, Jelliffe advises that one should begin at once to meet four or five times a week, without explaining to the patient "the general scheme, or what he is attempting to do, beyond asking the patient to do most of the talking, and entering into the proper unfolding of the unconscious only as it comes up" (1915, p. 79). In *Diseases of the Nervous System* (1915), Jelliffe and White proposed "at least three séances each week" (p. 77). Dodge did start her analysis with Jelliffe immediately after her intake session on January 3, 1916, meeting with him again three times that week (January 5, 6, and 7), and then with a frequency of between two and four weekly visits.

In his 1915 "Technique" paper, Jelliffe then encourages the analyst to be on the lookout for dreams: "It is frequently of service to get a dream or dreams which have been dreamed before coming for treatment and it is of much value in guiding one's self, to obtain the first dream that the patient has after starting treatment. No special stress should be laid upon these in the beginning, but they should be written down, and put aside for future reference" (p. 79). In fact, at some point, perhaps at Jelliffe's request, Dodge presented him with three typed dreams (#s 1, 2, & 3) from January 2, 1916, the day before her initial intake session with him. These dreams feature images of a house with many large and small rooms, a brother (Dodge had no siblings), a car driving on a bad road with other cars stuck in the mud, "very fat" people, a child who wanted to urinate, and a beautiful woman. Although Jelliffe did not record Dodge's corresponding associations, themes emerge suggesting choice (of room), forward movement (stuck cars), and over-indulgence, lack of control (fat people). Jelliffe emphasized the value of the first dream the patient has after beginning therapy. If Dodge dated her dreams by the day that preceded the night, then her dream from January 3

(# 4) would have followed her first meeting with him and likely have been of great interest: "I was expected to marry a very fat man who ate enormous quantities of food and after he ate let down his s--- first on one side then on the other to aid his digestion." Unfortunately, there is no mention of this dream in Jelliffe's notes, so Dodge's associations to it are unknown. She did, however, describe him as "a little paunchy" when she first met him (1936, p. 443), an initial observation that may have informed this dream. Even her developing transference—"expected to marry"—is hinted at here.

Jelliffe pays close attention to dreams when discussing transference in his 1916 "Technique" paper: "The first dream of the patient is extremely important. As Freud says[1] if this is neglected one may have to retrace one's steps very definitely in order to catch up the patient's interest" (p. 41). He then gives an amusing example:

> The following dream was that of a young woman of thirty-two who was suffering from a mild depression, a sense of unworthiness and of failure. *"I was in a room and on a balcony to my left was a man dressed in a Roman toga, talking Chinese, and preaching a Hebrew religion."* The ideas which free association brought out of this dream were very diverse but from them I learned, for myself at any rate, that her unconscious was commenting on the choice of my words and of my ideas. She had learned a little concerning the nationality of Freud and it was, as I evidently set forth too much in explanation, Chinese to her. The analysis of my own resistances taught me to come down from the balcony and try to understand her better.
>
> (p. 41)

Jelliffe shows some humility here, catching himself speaking to his new patient with too much jargon and too many words. Dodge reported that his language often included words such as "complex," "neurosis," and "unconscious," and that he sometimes offered ideas that did not resonate with her. For example, when she "confided to him my curious hankering to cut off my hair," he challenged: "'And who do you know who has long hair like rays? *Who* is it that you want to shear?'" When she replied she didn't know, he triumphantly announced, "'Phoebus Apollo!...The Sun!'" Dodge concluded these were "unfamiliar quirks of his mind" that amused her, but lost her interest (1936, p. 444).

Jelliffe credits Freud with having been the first to understand "how the use of the dream can help the analyst to watch the transference, the barometer of the patient's unconscious hopes and discouragements, his desire to get security, his disapproval if he thinks he fails" (1916, p. 41). Jelliffe appears often in Dodge's dreams, mostly as himself in his office, but also in one dream (# 23), as both a lawyer and an English bishop, and in one dream association (# 103) Dodge wonders if "Dr. J. & I" are "after my father & mother complexes." In a number of dreams, he is in the company of Bayard

Boyeson, a homosexual man. Dodge sees Jelliffe as an authority, or a collaborator, or someone whose attention she hopes to attract, perhaps erotically. In one dream (# 97) she seeks to elicit his concern by deliberately falling down the stairs. Even if not explicitly discernable in Jelliffe's case notes, it is highly probable that he and Dodge examined the transference implications of his presence in her dreams.

Jelliffe's approach to psychoanalysis and dream interpretation, as presented in *Diseases of the Nervous System*

In their 1915 textbook, Jelliffe and White included a section on psychoanalysis, "the method by which the human mind is, so to speak, dissected, and by means of which the hidden motives of conduct are sought" (p. 72), a part of the chapter on "Mental Examination Methods" that expanded in each subsequent edition. In 1917, they added an eloquent summary of the goal of this work:

> The object of psychoanalysis is not merely a dissection of the psyche and the discovery of the roots of the psychosis or neurosis, as the case may be, but is distinctly therapeutic. The physician tries to show the patient to himself as he really is. The patient is thus enabled to see how his symptoms are the results of hanging on to infantile ways of pleasure-seeking, self-indulgences, which are repulsive to his better self. When he has seen this the path is pointed along which he must go toward the effective sublimation, socialization, of his infantile tendencies in activities that are useful and which meet with conscious approval. The object of psychoanalysis then is to liberate the psychic energy which is bound up in infantile ways of pleasure-seeking and set it free for socially useful ends.
>
> (p. 98)

In his analytic practice, Jelliffe was an active participant in this process, making suggestions and interpretations, and pointing the patient toward sublimation and a more bearable way of being in the world. He acknowledged that he sometimes intervened too quickly, reporting that a patient's dream "gave me a sharp rap on the knuckles for going so fast" (1916, p. 42). He also pressed patients to "stand up to their tasks" (1915, p. 409) and "develop backbone" (1913–1914, p. 186). Nevertheless, in his work with Mabel Dodge, he did seem to try to reveal her to herself, aiming toward deeper understanding.

Jelliffe and White (1915) define what constitutes a complex: "a constellation of ideas, grouped about a central event that conditions a highly painful emotional state" that is then repressed into the unconscious and "gives origin to various symptoms" (p. 73). After describing the various ways that complexes can express themselves—through symbolism, displacement, conversion, or substitution—they turn to the topic of dreams and their interpretation: "The analysis of dreams is for the purpose of determining the presence and nature of complexes which are exercising a controlling effect upon the patient's conduct and feelings" (p. 74). They describe the process of free association in asking a patient to "take a certain element of the dream... and hold it in his mind, and then tell freely all of the ideas that come to him. He is told to tell all of the ideas without any effort on his part of selection, no matter whether the ideas appear to him to have any relationship with the portion of the dream that he has been told to keep in mind or not, and no matter whether they appear ridiculous" (p. 76). Although this approach to working with dreams was certainly common practice for psychoanalysts at this time, reading Jelliffe's own words and instructions informs our consideration of the sessions where he and Dodge explored her dream life.

Mabel Dodge in analysis with Jelliffe

In 1916, Mabel Dodge was 37 years old and the mother of a 14-year-old son, John Evans, and she had been separated for two years from Edwin Dodge. She suffered from chronic restlessness and depression for which she had long sought a variety of remedies, including Divine Science, New Thought, the rest cure and medicines advocated by doctors in Florence and New York, and treatment from the neurologist Dr. Bernard Sachs in New York who was decidedly against psychoanalysis (and had apparently told her, as Jelliffe noted on January 7, 1916, "to stop thinking about modern art"). She had survived at least four suicide attempts (as recorded in Jelliffe's notes from January 13, 1916: "*4 times I really have tried it*"), including taking a whole bottle of strychnine pills—either soon after her first marriage to Karl Evans in 1900 (Luhan, 1954, p. 12) or after Evans was killed in a hunting accident, her son was born, and she was despairing over her long affair with her physician John Parmenter (Luhan, "Intimate Memories, Vol. II.," n.d., p. 708)—, swallowing figs she had filled with ground-up glass in Florence around 1910 over a romantic obsession with her chauffeur, and then, when that failed, drinking a bottle of laudanum that she had gotten from her Italian doctor (Luhan 1935, p. 207; 1954, p. 31), and consuming an entire bottle of veronal pills sometime during her relationship with John Reed between 1913 and 1915 (Jelliffe's notes, January 13). In Jelliffe's notes from January 6, Dodge also admitted to an earlier fifth attempt—"*I tried to shoot self*"— during the scandal of her affair with Parmenter (that began soon before she became pregnant with her son, John, in 1901).

Dodge was living at her leased country home at Finney Farm in Croton-on-Hudson with the sculptor and painter Maurice Sterne (Figure 3.1), whom she had first met in the spring of 1915 at a dance recital given by

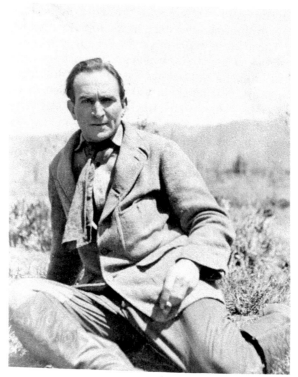

Figure 3.1 Maurice Sterne, circa 1917. Courtesy of the Beinecke Rare Book and Manuscript Library.

students from the Elizabeth Duncan School. As she describes in *Movers and Shakers* (1936), she had spotted him immediately in the crowd: "What I liked about him was his handsome look of suffering. A dark torture ennobled him and added a great deal of dignity to that countenance" (p. 350). They soon developed a tempestuous relationship over the summer in Provincetown—where they "continued to play with the idea of marriage in much the same way that one pokes at a snake with a stick. The idea was dangerous and revolting; yet we couldn't leave it alone" (p. 394)—and then returned to Finney Farm together. Sterne was a strong presence in her life and that unnerved her, as she was used to being the more forceful one. Dodge resented him even as she drew energy from him: "Whenever his life moved in him, I checked it because I could not let him be himself; I could not stand him as he was; I must raise him and make him different" (p. 428). Their relationship was characterized

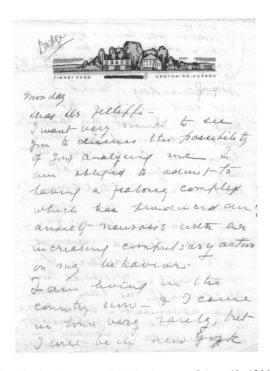

Figure 3.2 Mabel Dodge letter to Jelliffe, January [circa 1], 1916. Courtesy of the Beinecke Rare Book and Manuscript Library.

by extremes of passion, jealousy, destructiveness, and distance, as well as Dodge's intense and violent ambivalence.

In the thick of this volatility, she wrote to Jelliffe from Finney Farm on January [circa 1], 1916 (Figure 3.2):

> Dear Dr. Jelliffe,
> I want very much to see you to discuss the possibility of your analysing me. I am obliged to admit to having a jealousy complex which has produced an anxiety neurosis with an increasing compulsory action on my behavior. I am living in the country now, & come in town very rarely, but I will be in New York on Wednesday, and I will call up your house and try & get an appointment with you if you will have time to see me that day. If you are not there when I telephone—which will be near ten o'clock—will you please leave word with your secretary if I may see you & what time. Of course if we can make any agreement I will come in town to see you whenever it is necessary.
> Sincerely,
> Mabel Dodge

Dodge immediately began analysis with Jelliffe in his office at 64 West 56th Street (Figure 3.3), traveling there either from Finney Farm or from her apartment at 23 Fifth Avenue. His first case note is dated January 3, 1916, which was, in fact, a Monday. Jelliffe diagnosed Dodge with "psychoneurosis" in these handwritten notes (see Figure 3.4 and transcription) and, following the headings on the intake form, conducted an extensive inquiry into her family and childhood. She reported that her father, now dead, had gout and rheumatism, and was hospitalized in a sanatorium. She acknowledged the shock of her first husband's death and her state of "neurasthenia/ feel on edge/ Exhaustion." She outlined the sequence of marrying Karl Evans, giving birth to her son, John, 18 months later, then marrying Edwin Dodge

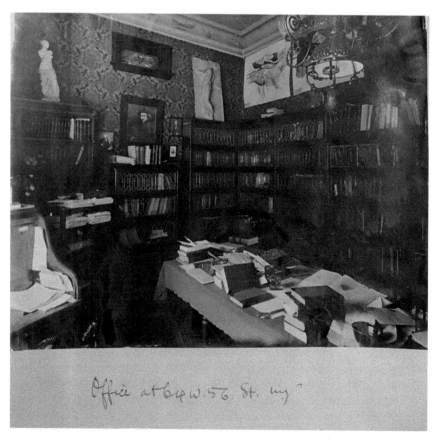

Figure 3.3 Smith Ely Jelliffe's office, 64 West 56 Street, New York, circa 1910s. Courtesy of the Library of Congress.

18 months after Evans was killed, and living with him until 1913. She mentioned Edwin's syphilis.

After indicating Mabel Dodge's answers to the standard intake questions, Jelliffe then recorded her own words to describe her history and current situation, beginning poignantly with: "An only child never in possession of my kingdom: Root of my character." Dodge presented herself to Jelliffe as tortured by the "poison" of jealousy that caused her to "Get yellow/ Blood flows out of my heart" (much as her father had been when observing her mother with other men) and compelled by a need to dominate and control the other (as she had done with both lovers and friends, including John Reed and Hutchins Hapgood) in her "Outraged sense of possession." She observed the relationship between her menstrual cycle and her feelings—"At menstrual period ++, resistance less: issues greater"—a linking of the physical with the emotional that Jelliffe certainly would have supported. In a driven manner, she urgently turned toward men and sex as ways to both nurture herself and secure a sense of identity: "Suffering intolerable: my only source of living. Contact c. life only through an individual: absorbed in or through some ♂." She revealed the vulnerability that resulted from her complete consumption of herself in the life of her romantic interest, and her subsequent loneliness and fear when not immersed: "Periods of blocking: Vacuum/ death." (As she had written to the Boston neurologist Morton Prince in 1914: "Thrown back upon myself I found there was nothing but a vacuum. Gazing out to the world for something to cling to I found only a vacuum.") She also reported her capacity to form some kind of internal protection: "I found it in self:/ nothing can hurt me." In these intake notes, Dodge reveals her fluency in self-observation and the complicated workings of intense emotions.

Dodge entered analysis with Jelliffe seeking relief from these empty and unbearable states and her terrible dependence on Sterne: "Come to Θ [i.e., "you," meaning Jelliffe] to learn how to do it." Although she admits that she has "not read much" psychoanalysis, she lists the sources of her knowledge so far, including Max Eastman, A.A. Brill, and Leo Stein, and perhaps her mention of "Interpretation of dreams" means that she has read Freud's 1900 work, which had first been translated into English by Brill in 1912. She entertained the idea that she was manic-depressive as a way of explaining her alternating moods, as she stated (only once) in her memoirs when she first consulted with Brill later in 1916: "'Do you believe a manic-depressive can cure herself?'" (1936, p. 506).

In a chapter devoted to Jelliffe in *Movers and Shakers* (1936), Dodge remembers him at their first meeting as "tall, in a black suit of smooth cloth, a little paunchy, his small, green eyes set rather close together" (p. 443), a description closely matching his own: "I myself am large and stout—5° 10',

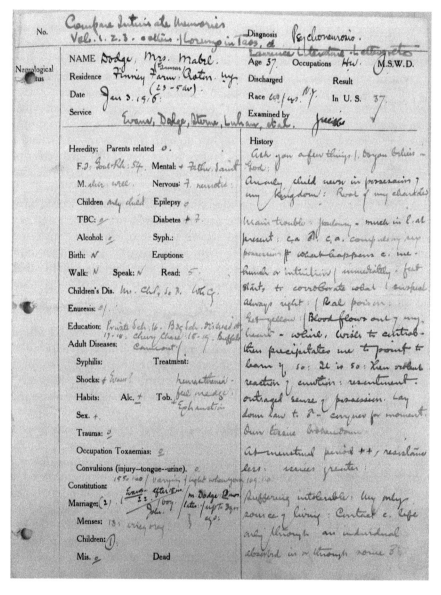

Figure 3.4 Smith Ely Jelliffe's intake of Mrs. Mabel Dodge, January 3, 1916. Courtesy of the Beinecke Rare Book and Manuscript Library.

Transcription of Jelliffe's January 3, 1916 intake notes:

[Added later by Jelliffe, likely in 1930s, as indicated by italics:]
*Compare Intimate Memories Vols. 1. 2. 3. & others./ Lorenzo in Taos, &
Lawrence Literature, Letters etc.*

		Diagnosis	Psychoneurosis
NAME	Dodge, Mrs. Mabel (Ganson)	**Age** 37 **Occupations** HW (M).S.W.D. [i.e., housewife]	
Residence	Finney Farm: Croton, NY (23–5 Av)	**Discharged**	**Result**
Date	Jan 3, 1916:	**Race** W/ US NY	**In U.S.** 37
Service		**Examined by** Jelliffe	

Evans, Dodge, Sterne, Luhan, et al.
Heredity: Parents related 0.
F. d: Gout & Rh: 54. **Mental:** + Father Sanit[arium]
[or "Sanatorium," as in Jelliffe's March 23 notes, dream 57]

M. alive: well	**Mental:** F. neurotic.
Children only child	**Epilepsy** 0
TBC: 0	**Diabetes** + F.
Alcohol: 0	**Syph.:**
Birth: N	**Eruptions:**
Walk: N **Speak:** N	**Read:** 5

Children's Dis. Ms. ChPx ScF WhCg
[i.e., measles or mumps; chicken pox; scarlet fever;
whooping cough]
Enuresis: 0
Education: Private Sch. 16 Bdg Sch. Disliked it.
        17–18. Chevy Chase 18–19. Buffalo
        came out
Adult Diseases:

Syphilis:	**Treatment:**
Shocks: + Evans?	Neurasthenia feel on edge Exhaustion
Habits: Alc. +	**Tob.** +

Sex. +
Trauma: 0
Occupational Toxaemias: 0
Convulsions (injury—tongue—urine). 0
Constitution: 155–160/ Varying/ light when young 109. 110
Marriage: (2) 1 <u>Evans</u> after 18 mos.   m. Dodge 18 mos.
        22   later./up to 3 yrs ago:
        1 boy.   } [i.e., syphilis]
        John.
Menses: 13: irreg reg
Children: 1
Mis. 0   **Dead**

History

Ask you a few things/. Do you believe in God:/
An only child never in possession of my kingdom: Root of my character.

Main trouble: Jealousy—much in l[ove]. at present: c. a ♂, c. a compul-
sory sex possession# What happens c. me—hunch or intuition/ immediately feel start to corroborate what I suspect always right:/ Real poison.
Get yellow/ Blood flows out of my heart—whirl. Wish to control—then
precipitates me to point to learn if so: It is so: then violent reaction of
emotion: resentment. Outraged sense of possession. Lay down law to
♂—Conquer for moment. Our tissue broken down.

At menstrual period ++, resistance less: issues greater:

Suffering intolerable: my only source of living. Contact c. life only
through an individual: absorbed in or through some ♂.

History—continued (page 2 of intake, not reproduced)

Self-preservation involved:/ Activated to life thereby +++ intensity.
Come to ⊙ [i.e., "you," meaning Jelliffe] to learn how to do it: Constructive, as others have all been destructive:#

Question of fidelity:/-

Periods of blocking: Vacuum/ death:/ Then some social constructive
work: or some ♂ agent to do the same thing.

Up to last Oct. amputation. Hades. Now safe, reached security: now
grown up. I found it in self:/ nothing can hurt me. Then another ♂:/
Seriously involved./

Touch of defense/.

Psa: Not read much: talked with ⊙/ Max E[astman]./ Dr Brill./ did
not care for him./ Leo Stein/ Interpretation of dreams./ Translations:
resistances./

200 pounds, clean shaven, with a roundish face" (1916, p. 162). She reports that he began:

> "Jung has taught us," he said, "that when one reaches an impasse, it is because he is unable to function in the way his own particular nature wishes. When we try to force ourselves to go in directions contrary to the psyche, she rebels. You do not like your present life. Why?"
>
> I launched into a description of my situation with Maurice. It was a great relief to talk, to tell it all...to tell how I hated things about him even while I loved him and was unable to live without him.
>
> (p. 439)

During this initial session when she shared details of her relationship with Sterne, Dodge experienced the release of unburdening in the attentive presence of her analyst. Jelliffe's reference to Jung's teachings to introduce his question to Dodge about her life indicates the strong influence that Jung had on his early practice, manifesting perhaps most in his inquiry into libido and his interpretations of associations and symbolizations. However, even though Dodge reports that Jelliffe cited Jung when asking about her life, his thinking and practice were also greatly shaped by Freud's theories. Jelliffe was an enthusiastic and consistent advocate for psychoanalysis who developed an eclectic approach incorporating Jung, Freud, and his own psychosomatic perspective on medicine.

Dodge then describes the process of her psychoanalysis with Jelliffe:

> I enjoyed my visits three times a week to Jelliffe's office. He had a speculative mind with an amusing intuition. As he turned my attention more and more upon the inner workings of my own nature, curious spiritual events began to occur, and my starved perceptions, that had been centered for months upon Maurice, reveled in the new direction of interest. It became an absorbing game to play with oneself, reading one's motives, and trying to understand the symbols by which the soul expressed itself.
>
> Psychoanalysis was apparently a kind of tattletaleing [sic]. I was able to tell, not only everything about myself, but all about Maurice. I grew calm and self-sufficient, and felt superior to him in the evening when, returning from New York, I found him still in the grip of his nervous fears and worries.
>
> I tried to tell him about the system and how it worked, but he hated it and said it all revolted him. When I told Jelliffe this, he exclaimed:
>
> "Ah, naturally! He has a resistance. Whenever people particularly need psychoanalysis, they have a great resistance to it."

....There was the Electra complex, and the Oedipus complex and there was the Libido with its manifold activities, seeking every chance for outlet, and then all that thing about Power and Money!

(pp. 439–440)

Dodge was empowered by the confidence she gained in her ability to name things, identify complexes, and use psychoanalytic language (as if uttering these phrases gave her authority or indicated understanding). One can imagine Jelliffe's triumphant pronouncements of complexes and Dodge's fascination with these ideas. The "superior" feeling she had over Sterne must have been welcome to someone who longed to return to a place of strength when she had felt so diminished by jealousy about his attraction to other women and his immersion in his art. For a time, Dodge was captivated by the playfulness of uncovering meaning in symbols, searching for unconscious motivations, and applying the concepts of psychoanalysis to herself and others.

Energized by these new ideas, Dodge became convinced that Sterne was at the root of her difficulties. She recalls: "It was customary during an analysis, Dr. Jelliffe told me, for the patient to be separated temporarily from the family, or from those nearest one, who were in some way involved with the compulsions and complexities of the case. I did not doubt now but that Maurice was the complete picture of whatever was the matter with me" (p. 446). She even believed that Jelliffe "had been trying to pry us apart, had been ready to accept, for me, anything that would take my attention off Maurice long enough for me to become independent and separate from him" (p. 456). When she temporarily banished Sterne from Croton in February 1916, reportedly with Jelliffe's instruction and blessing, Dodge remembers her feelings of relief:

For me it was exactly like a holiday, as though Maurice had been a tremendous job from which I was granted a vacation—and what was left of the strange grind that constituted our love affair, was the love without the strangeness or the strain. It seems to me I never loved him with any ease except when we were separated, and then tenderness and a kind of compassion entered into me. I felt relieved of him and wished I could give him the same relief that bathed me—that let my nerves spread out in the warm free atmosphere of Finney Farm when he was not there!

(pp. 447–448)

This pattern repeated itself throughout their tumultuous union. Away from Sterne, Dodge felt she could "allow my great craving for love to grow stronger—fastening more securely upon him for its satisfaction. While he was away, I had felt love in me and supposed it was for him" (p. 456). She then expressed her love in letters to him, thereby inspiring Sterne to return, at which point, "alas, his presence caused it to sink down in me again, leaving only the strain and the agony of wishing for a different and more adequate object for its fulfillment" (p. 456). Dodge writes despairingly of these early months of 1916: "We struggled on and on through the winter, through the spring" (1936, p. 457). She was determined to get Sterne into psychoanalysis, believing that it would ease their fraught situation.

As Dodge reports in *Movers and Shakers* (1936), in the spring of 1916, she invited Jelliffe to the country—"Jelliffe had been curious about the Finney Farm constellation and I had asked him for a week-end" (p. 441)—with the intention that he would observe firsthand Sterne's provocations and urge him into analysis. She wrote to Jelliffe: "you might be able to 'get' him now" (see Interlude 11). At her next session following this visit, she asked him if he had witnessed what she considered to be Sterne's suggestive and perverse behavior:

> "Why, no," Jelliffe said, "I didn't notice anything like that. I thought he seemed a little embarrassed, that is all."
>
> "Oh, he is too devious for any of you," I cried. "Devious and unfrank! When I accused him of it last night, do you know what he said? 'Mabel, I was just trying to do my part.'"
>
> "Maybe he was," said Jelliffe. "Certainly if he intended anything else, it was unconscious. Possibly your interpretation of it is colored by your own unconsciousness," he continued, looking at me searchingly. "You know we are always projecting ourselves. Often what we think we find in others is nothing but our own hidden life. What we need is the power to see in ourselves the traits and motives we imagine we detect in others! So long as we are merely subjective all our criticism is but self-criticism."
>
> Heavens! I thought. I must track down *the Maurice* in me now! Was the real Maurice quite other than I had pictured him to myself? Heavens!! Was I attached to *myself* instead of to him as I had supposed?
>
> (p. 443)

This exchange between them was disillusioning for Dodge, as she had hoped that Jelliffe would take her side and not point her toward unconscious mechanisms or theories of projection. She did not want to find in herself what she saw in Sterne. When invested in her own version of the truth, she lost faith in some fundamentals of analytic thinking and pressed forward with her agenda. Dodge's initial excitement about her work with Jelliffe faded after a while, perhaps hastened by this incident. When she wrote *Movers and Shakers* (1936), she reflected back on her analysis and concluded: "These were interesting, fascinating, new ideas. Unfortunately, they remained in the realm of ideas only and produced no change in my nature....Jelliffe couldn't really help me to understanding, and when the amusing speculations had gone on for a few months, they finally ceased to amuse, and the old fatigue and depression came back" (pp. 443, 467).

However, the actual ending of Dodge's analysis with Jelliffe was more complicated and caused by more than just the return of her fatigue and depression. In the first days of June 1916, Dodge likely ingested a substance to induce an abortion. Jelliffe knew of this pregnancy and Dodge's ambivalence about, but preference for, keeping the baby, as she indicated in two letters to him, circa May 24 and circa May 26 (see Interludes 17 & 18, also footnotes for dreams 130 & 134–142). He was also aware, as revealed in his session notes, about the loss of this baby. This overpowering disappointment certainly contributed to Dodge's mental distress and her urgent need for help at this time in June when Jelliffe was soon leaving for the summer. (Although her divorce from Edwin Dodge was final on June 8, 1916, it is highly doubtful that this was a cause of upset.) His lengthy absence from his practice was likely due to Jelliffe's own devastating and sudden loss of his wife in March 1916 to a cerebral hemorrhage. He wrote to Dodge on June 21, 1916: "For myself I am hoping for a good rest and for new scenes. The last three months have really been ghastly. Many thanks for your patience and forbearance." Dodge could not wait for Jelliffe to return.

Suffering and desperate for direction and support, Dodge reached out to Brill, as she recalls in *Movers and Shakers* (1936):

> I was alone: I had to have help and I thought of Dr. Brill. He had helped Andrew [Dasburg]...and others I knew of, and I could not go back to Jelliffe, for I didn't want to *talk*, now, I wanted to live.
>
> When I went to see Brill, he was taking his vacation and only coming to his office once a week. He saw me and told me he could not take me until later in the fall; but I told him I was badly in need of something, I didn't know what. I was frightened, for I felt I could not endure my terrible burden of melancholy. He said, oh, yes, I could, and he turned me away. I found he was right.
>
> (pp. 497–498)

As Brill predicted, Dodge found inner resources unknown to her and managed through the summer, sensing the return of her strength. She reports that she "lived looking forward to the analysis with the new doctor: this time it would be Freudian, instead of with Jung's method which Dr. Jelliffe purported to practice" (1936, p. 498).

In June 1916, Dodge wrote Jelliffe to explain why she had sought out Brill while he was away: "I went out of my head one night—then got hysteric pains—then chills & fever...& then I felt I was going <u>queer</u> & so I went to him. I didn't want to go to a woman & he seemed the best man....I feel badly to think you may be angry or something at me but I had to do something....I wish you had been here." She tries to reassure Jelliffe of her preference for him, had he been available. In her next letter, from July 1, 1916, Dodge describes more fully her defection to Brill, first referring to a lost letter in which she falsely reported she was doing fine and then twisting the truth about when she ended with Jelliffe:

> I wasn't quite honest with you when I last wrote you that I was feeling quite all well. I hadn't been very steady for a fortnight but I felt it was no use coming in to you since you were going away so soon. The last week or ten days got worse—& I began to have hysterical pain. But still I did nothing until two nights ago I completely lost consciousness & control of myself in a violent anger....The next day I was so ill nervously that I went to consult Brill. I told him I had unwisely stopped my analysis some time ago & asked if I could continue it with him. He said that was impossible—that he couldn't help me by continuing another man's analysis—that he couldn't take me as your patient—the way a general practitioner might do—temporarily.
>
> I said that naturally I would probably have gone back to you had you been on the spot—that all I want is to get well—that I want to do what is necessary for that & that I wanted to come to him for the summer—feeling I <u>must</u> do something. He said he would take me as a patient if I begin an analysis with him & continue it—& I told him I would. I don't want you to misunderstand—nor do I want to lose your friendship but I find myself in a state of nerves more difficult to control than if the analysis had not already accomplished its work of breaking up resistances [*sic*] & loosening energies & I <u>must</u> find the means of sublimation & freedom.
>
> Please write me that you understand all this.

Dodge's attempts again to convince Jelliffe of the circumstantial reasons for her turning to Brill, rather than a deliberate termination in order to enter treatment with a different analyst, contradict how she later described this moment in *Movers and Shakers* (1936), where she reflected that she "wanted to live" rather than "*talk*" (p. 498). She also seems to try to appease Jelliffe by acknowledging the positive effects of her work with him, and using the language of psychoanalysis.

Dodge again wrote to Jelliffe on July 22, 1916 to inform him that she is in Provincetown for the rest of the summer, at Brill's instruction, and had seen

Brill (even though he reportedly could not begin with her "until later in the fall") "six or eight times & it helped me a good deal, but I needed the change of air & company. I am still gibbering of course but not quite so much tension. The nervous depression is frightful." She then asks Jelliffe how he is, observes that his last letter "sounds cheerful & full of vitality" and, following up on his invitation, offers that she could come visit him at Lake George in late August or September.

The last documented session between Dodge and Jelliffe is recorded in his notes from October 23, 1916, when he had returned to New York and resumed his practice. As Jelliffe writes (with his voice in italics):

> Wanted to see you very much after you went on your vacation./ Brill./ can't wait. Bromides:/ Volcano opened and what to do. Take me for summer: Would not do that: Not fair to analysis: to me & him: No choice and so I did it....He would take me only if I promised not to come to S.E.J. I promised. *I told her that it was duress. I had no quarrel c. M.D. but I did not take it right in part of A.A.B. & would have nothing to do c. him. He had done the same thing for several patients & I was through c. him. I did not care to treat her either.*

Despite Jelliffe's tone in this final session and Dodge's own retroactive minimizing of the effects of her analysis when she described it in *Movers and Shakers* (1936), they maintained a correspondence until 1939, six years before his death. Their letters primarily concern shared intellectual interests, such as exchanges of their writing and comments on books they had read. Jelliffe remained a significant figure for Dodge years after her analysis with him, as she attests in a letter on February 18, 1924: "You continue to be for me one of the islands of interest of the past years—and when I have something that it seems would interest <u>you</u> I feel like sending it to you."

Postscript: In fact, on January 26, 1918, Dodge, now married to Maurice Sterne and living with him in Taos, New Mexico, wrote to Jelliffe and sent him a short article that she had written: "While observing them all [Sterne, Bobby Jones, and John Evans] play cards, an idea came to me which I am having my stenographer type & send to you. Perhaps you can use it in your P.A. Review. I hope so." Jelliffe did include "A Game of Cards—Hearts" by "M. Dodge" (even though by that time she was Mabel Sterne) in volume 5 of the 1918 *Psychoanalytic Review* (see Appendix B). She asks the question "What *is* 'playing cards'?" and proposes that the game may be a "substitute for the game of life" and is also "the game of love" where "every repression may seek its outlet, every thwarted instinct may have its release." She explores the meanings of the different cards, suggesting they are "symbols of characters who are eternally ourselves" (pp. 442–444). In this paper, Dodge applies her knowledge of psychoanalysis to the game of cards, and, in sending it to Jelliffe for his approval, was also continuing to seek his attention and admiration.

Mabel Dodge on dream interpretation

It is striking that not once in her narrative of her analysis with Jelliffe in *Movers and Shakers* (1936) does Dodge give any hint of the existence of her own active dream life or mention the role of dreams and their interpretations. This is an intriguing omission given the richness, depth, and highly specific content of her dreams. The only reference to dreams in her memoir is to those of Maurice Sterne, which he had included in his letters to Dodge, intended for Jelliffe's perusal. She dismissed these as "kindergarten dreams that he [Sterne] could scarcely fail to understand" (p. 454), a condescending comment that reveals her resentment of his continual refusal to enter into psychoanalytic treatment, and also her judgment of the lack of depth in his psyche.

Although not featured in any of her published memoirs, Dodge's understanding of the crucial role of dreams in psychoanalysis appears in an unpublished manuscript that she wrote in 1938, "On Human Relations: A Personal Interpretation." Written years after her analysis, this work reveals an appreciation of the power of working with dreams she had first developed in her treatment with Jelliffe. Dodge evaluates the significance of Freud's ideas about dreams: "Freud's great contribution is in his discovery that by examining dreams and correctly interpreting them, the origin of the conflict that is disturbing the patient can be uncovered. The stage where our unconscious, buried life plays itself out exists in the dream world" (1938a, p. 78). She then describes the process of dream interpretation:

> When the patient is persuaded to recite his dreams, the analyst follows up with the question:
> "What does that remind you of, with what do you associate that?"
> He may be referring to an intense scene the dreamer was engaged in over some trivial action that seems all out of proportion to the emotion that the actors projected into it. For what enormous significance is attached to trivial dream actions sometimes! Everyone has known this curious and seemingly senseless, topsy-turvy, juggling of feeling and the objects in a dream.
>
> (pp. 80–81)

Dodge sheds light on the moment when meaning emerges:

> Sometimes at the end of perhaps an hour a light breaks upon the recital of the seemingly irrational sequence of associations where one

anecdote has followed another, and where one emotion has passed into another and been expressed; all at once a realisation about himself may come to the patient, a realisation of something hidden in his unconscious whose existence he has never suspected. This realisation may be the recognition of a long[-]suppressed wish, a guilty wish, or a hateful inferior attitude that has been holding him back. The patient may feel himself flooded with a surprise that makes his blood leap and suffuses him with a shame he has never known. He reddens and squirms, then sometimes he tries to laugh it off. No matter how it takes him, all is well so long as he admits its truth.

(p. 82)

Dodge seems to write here from personal experience, of having known this feeling of recognition and sudden understanding. In her autobiographical "Psycho-Analysis with Dr. Brill" (1938b), Brill reminds her how to interpret her dream: "'You remember that one is all the actors in one's dream—the different aspects of the person. Well, what does this dream suggest to you?'" She responds reflexively: "'My goodness! Really! I don't think I feel like that. Maybe I do, though,' I added swallowing hard" (p. 4). Dodge knows the pain of acquiring insight, as she continues: "How describe the peculiar and infinitely variable course of a psychoanalytic ordeal? For ordeal it is and must be since all change is painful, and all organic growth means change; change of boundaries, measurements, attitudes, stubborn resistances, efforts to stay put" (p. 4). Dodge could be willful and immovable, determined to find evidence for her opinion of herself and others. But she also could challenge herself to consider change and make efforts toward deeper insight and compassion.

The Dreams of Mabel Dodge

Mabel Dodge's dreams provide an unusual form of entry into the history and culture of Greenwich Village in 1916, a community teeming with radical politics, torrid love affairs, surging creativity, heightened curiosity, and fervent experimentation with ideas and ways of living. Her dreams are populated by the movers and shakers of the moment: the writers and journalists Max Eastman, Walter Lippmann, and John Reed; the artists Andrew Dasburg, Marsden Hartley, and her lover, Maurice Sterne; critic and art collector Leo Stein; the poets Edwin Arlington Robinson and Bayard Boyeson; the dancer Isadora Duncan; the art dealer and photographer Alfred Stieglitz; and frequently her current analyst, Dr. Jelliffe. Dodge's own mother and father make many appearances in her dreams, as does her son, John Evans.

In Dodge's dreams, actual events are sometimes represented. Robert Edmond Jones almost dies from appendicitis. Dodge takes a female lover, an experience she repeated over the years, beginning with Violet and Beatrice when she was in boarding school and then with others during her time in Florence. A man has syphilis, as did Dodge's husband Edwin, as well as Maurice Sterne. Dodge's throat is blocked by phlegm, an image related to having had her tonsils removed soon after she moved into 23 Fifth Avenue. Isadora Duncan has a new baby, one who died soon after birth. Dodge goes to the seacoast to get her divorce, as she did, in fact, in Salem, Massachusetts.

In Dodge's dreams, a bed is covered by insects, a breast is exposed, and a black cat jumps. There are evocative colors: purple cloth, dark blue silk, a cold grey blue chair, bright lavender Valentines, green and violet ribbons, a blue and white sailor's costume, and dark red damask. She dreams more than once about impotence, the warmth of a lap, food, trains, boats and cars, horses, precipices, old women, and letters.

Following is the complete archive of dreams recorded by Dodge during her analysis with Jelliffe. This collection provides unprecedented access to one woman's dream life, as well as to the private process of psychoanalysis, where analyst and patient engage with dream and association to pursue the shared goal of a deeper grasp of the psyche. When considered together with Jelliffe's corresponding notes and exchanges of letters between them, these dreams reveal Dodge's dedication to uncovering symbolic meaning by delving into the past. They also illustrate her ardent efforts to comprehend the nature of her relationships and the effects of her lonely childhood upon her life, as well as obstacles to understanding.

Dodge was clearly eager to apply the language and concepts of psychoanalysis to her perceptions of herself and others. She enthusiastically used terms such as "father complex," "infantile perversion," "transfer," and "unconscious" in her dreams and associations, and in her letters to Jelliffe. Dodge embraced ideas such as the relation between excrement, gold, and power, and wholeheartedly believed in the existence and influence of the unconscious.

Freud's now-familiar ideas about the interpretation of dreams—with their manifest content providing a window through associations into latent content—clearly drive Jelliffe's inquiry, as illustrated by the format of his notes with their attention to numerous details of the dreams such as colors, locations, objects, and people. Jelliffe's approach to interpretation is illustrated in one of his "Technique of Psychoanalysis" papers where he presents the dream of a patient who had "hysterical conversion signs,

among them an intense acne around the mouth" and includes his analysis
in brackets:

> "*I am alone on a desert island* [wish for lack of conformity to social
> demands] *Hawaii, Honolulu, or what not* [wild infantile libido]. *I was told
> that I would meet every one* [sic] *I loved on the Island* [early wish source].
> *I met my mother* [first nutrition object and first determiner for mouth lo-
> cation of wish = acne] *and she was very sad* [identification of own state].
> *Her husband did not love her any more* [detachment of patient's own li-
> bido from husband—for nutritive and other defects]. *I met a cousin of
> mine with two lovely children* [own missed opportunities] *and she was
> very happy. She asked me why I was so sad, and I said because my father
> did not love my mother any more* [sic] *and she said* [sad self vs. happy self]:
> *if you believed in Yogi, as I do, you would be happy* [transfer symbol and
> wish for recovery].["]

(1916, p. 163)

Although Jelliffe did not insert his interpretations as above into his record
of Dodge's dreams, this example reveals his method of analysis, with emphasis on libido and childhood wishes. Burnham (1983) points out that
Jelliffe "spoke of how much he benefited from each rereading of Freud's *Interpretation of Dreams*" (p. 76). With this influence in mind, and in the context of the enthusiasm at this time for discovering hidden motives driven by
primitive or sexual desires as well as the embracing of dreams as conveyors
of meaning, Freud's interpretations of typical dreams and common dream
symbols are sometimes included in footnotes to Dodge's dreams. However,
Jelliffe certainly grasped that identification of meanings was not enough
for an analysis, explaining about one case: "This patient would have to be
analyzed as any other and no amount of *telling her what the symbols meant*
would cure her. That knowledge must come from the inside, otherwise why
all the conscious defence...? Thus the analyst comes to a knowledge of the
symbol values at the same time as the patient and only by patiently asking:
What comes to your mind? what then? what does that suggest?" (1917, p. 82).
While a contemporary perspective on dreams sees the interpretation itself
as a relational act, with the patient and analyst together creating meaning in
their examination of each dream, it remains possible for readers to connect
Dodge's dreams and their associations to her history and conflicts described
so voluminously in her memoirs.

"We found an inner room unknown to me." Dodge and Jelliffe must
have delighted together in this image from her dream (# 104) about visiting
Stieglitz. She valued Jelliffe as a guide through this new terrain and appealed to him in a letter, circa January 1916 (Interlude 2): "the only way out
is thro' suffering unless you can show me a way—Dr. Jelliffe." Although
she then warned him (incorrectly) that she "can't transfer," for a period

of almost six months Dodge relied on Jelliffe as an authoritative figure, leaving her treatment with a heightened awareness of her longings and inner torments, as well as a respect for the elements of play and discovery in psychoanalysis.

Note

1 Jelliffe cites his source as: "The Dynamics of Transference" (1912), although his ideas also seem to come from "The Handling of Dream-Interpretation in Psycho-Analysis" (1911).

Chapter 4

Cast of characters

Paul Ayrault

A Columbia University student who was John Evans's tutor at the Villa Curonia in Italy and became Mabel Dodge's lover in 1912. In *European Experiences* (1935), Dodge describes Ayrault and her attraction to him: "Paul was twenty-three or -four years old, and he was six feet tall with a beautiful body, a goodly shaped, small head, crinkly, curly, light hair, china-blue eyes, and a rather raw-boned nose and mouth. Unfinished. That was the conventional inevitability. I was interested now in the flavor of the blond and blue-eyed race that is fresh and cool and fragrant in its youth" (p. 310). This passionate relationship threatened to dissolve her marriage to Edwin Dodge.

Neith Boyce

A feminist novelist and playwright who was married to author and journalist Hutchins Hapgood, one of Mabel Dodge's closest friends. Boyce wrote a play entitled *Constancy*, based upon the love affair between Dodge and John Reed, that was performed in Provincetown, Massachusetts in July 1915 by actors of the emerging Provincetown Players.

In the context of their open marriage, Hapgood had an affair with Lucy Collier (John Collier's wife, see below) toward the end of 1915, continuing into the following year. In January 1916, Boyce wrote a number of letters to Dodge from Provincetown, explaining to her why she was wrong to interfere in their situation and accused her of inflaming it with false statements: "Didn't you do me a rather bad turn with Lucy?....I'm sure you put the idea into her head or at least gave her the phrase about my still 'having Hutch by the throat!' I know you did!" And: "I do wish you could have seen Hutch the last three weeks here—with two women making love to him—one by letter and one in presence—and how he liked it! He was perfectly darling! And he told me as he was leaving that these three weeks have been the happiest time of his life. And they were of mine, too. It was the sweetest time. You can't quite get that, can you? If you can, you won't feel bothered about us."

Hapgood wrote with extraordinary candor about his relationship with Boyce in *The Story of a Lover* (1919), a struggle to understand her aloofness, his loneliness, and their nonetheless deep connection. He remembers: "Much of the time she was so quiet and so unresponsive that there was no place for me in her presence. Often I went away from her, irritated by her very perfection; by her self-sufficiency and calm" (p. 41). He observes "the complete isolation in which her spirit dwells, and the kind of shrinking that my approach causes in her" (p. 54). Hapgood explains something about their open marriage: "I encouraged her to have intimate friendships with other men....And to have her know other men intimately, just as I continually wished to know other women intimately, was with me a genuine desire" (pp. 109, 111). He reports that "no matter how intimate I was" with other women, "the unconscious instinct, that deep uncontrollable imagination kept me bound to Her as a slave is bound to its master....I could not be free of her" (p. 187).

Bayard Boyeson
(Referred to in dreams as "B.")

Norwegian-American homosexual poet who lived and worked at times in one of the guest cottages at Dodge's Finney Farm, notably during a period when Maurice Sterne was absent. At Jelliffe's suggestion—as she explained: "he felt that my subjective feeling for Maurice made me sick and that I was mired in an unsuitable situation" (1936, p. 456)—Dodge sent Sterne away in January 1916 to paint landscapes. Boyeson was staying with Dodge at this time and, according to her, Jelliffe encouraged increasing contact with him and was interested when Boyeson appeared in her dreams. In *Movers and Shakers* (1936), Dodge describes their growing connection: "Bayard was beginning to be more alert where I was concerned, or rather I was growing more aware of him, perhaps, and I noted how he was flashing keen smiles from his northern blue eyes when he read his poems to me in the evenings by the fire" (p. 456). She developed an alliance with him over psychoanalysis: "Since I couldn't persuade Maurice to go and be psychoanalyzed, I made Bayard go to try to get over his drinking. He became as fascinated as I was, and this banded us together against Maurice, who felt decidedly out of things" (pp. 440–441).

Florence Bradley

American actress and painter whom Dodge first met on a boat returning to the United States from Italy. Bradley approached Dodge while they were both out taking a walk, as Dodge reports: "She spoke to me first as we passed and repassed on the deck, for I have never spoken first to anyone in my life....'You were the only interesting-looking person on the boat,' she told me, and I felt she too had something special about her that marked her out from the rest of the passengers" (1935, p. 429). In 1910, Bradley painted a portrait of Dodge, and, in 1913, they shared an interest in producing and publishing Gertrude Stein's plays.

Nina Bull (née Wilcox)

Dodge's close childhood friend from Buffalo, originally Nina Wilcox, who married Harry Bull. She was one of the bridesmaids at Dodge's wedding to Karl Evans in 1900. In *Background* (1933a), Dodge devotes the first section of her chapter "Books and Playmates" to Nina, recalling: "Nina was a sad child. She never had a smile on her face. She was pale and somber.... She was always grave, inhibited—maybe—from birth or maybe from her step-mother, who seemed to hate her." However, Dodge also reports: "I liked playing with Nina because I could make her do just as I liked. Quite early I won the upper hand over her, though of course that isn't saying much—the poor child!.... So I was the leader and Nina followed after wherever I went" (pp. 71, 73–74).

Nina Bull was a Divine Science practitioner in New York and was treating Dodge at this time, while Dodge was also in analysis with Jelliffe. Divine Science drew its inspiration from spiritualists who believed that problems such as Dodge's stemmed from an overreliance on consciousness and mental abilities, with "cure" coming from abandonment of the wish to acquire knowledge, a direction opposed to the emphasis on insight in psychoanalysis as practiced by Jelliffe and Brill.

Seward Cary

One of the six Cary sons, fifteen years older than Mabel, and one of Dodge's favored and adventurous companions from her teenage years in Buffalo. In *European Experiences* (1935), she describes his tremendous appeal and her early understanding of the complexities and nuances of attraction:

> Seward caught my imagination when I was seventeen or eighteen....
> He was lean and dark and he looked like pictures I had seen of Indians....
> When he rode in the polo games three times a week, I watched him—all my attention for him....After the game, when he walked past us to the shower upstairs in the clubhouse, I waited for his glance—all my willingness going out to him.
> And it did not take long for him to pick up the excitement in me and gather it to him for he was instinctive like an animal, and as clean and true in his responses, and as unfeeling, in his heartless way. Seward was

never troubled by the heart-love, nor did he waken it in women, but he gave them a lively feeling of themselves and an unreckoning love of dangerous living.

(p. 5)

She evaluates their connection: "The attraction between us was psychical rather than physical. I mean I was drawn by his magnetism, I was aroused and alive to him whenever he was near, but I wasn't longing for the consummation that grown-up men and women want....I never wanted him physically in my life. But I wanted terribly to be with him" (p. 7).

Seward Cary's mother, Julia, was the daughter of William Love from Batavia, a town about an hour from Buffalo that was also the birthplace of Mabel's maternal grandmother, Grandma Ganson. In *Background* (1933a), Dodge reports that Julia "was said to have been adopted into the Iroquois tribe when a girl and made a princess, whatever that means, because the Indians said she had their blood in her veins and was one of them. Surely she did look like an old Indian man—and she had their endurance and cheerfulness, and complete absence of made-up emotions. All her sons except Walter looked like Indians, dark-skinned and clear-cut" (p. 104). Grandma Ganson was also rumored to have Indian blood (see note 4 for dream 41).

John Collier

A social worker and anthropologist who was close friends with Mabel Dodge. In *Movers and Shakers* (1936), she describes his appearance: "He was a small, blond Southerner, intense, preoccupied, and always looking wind-blown on the quietest day. Because he could not seem to love his own kind of people, and as he was full of a reformer's enthusiasm for humanity, he turned to other races and worked for them" (p. 323). Collier worked at the People's Institute on Fifth Avenue and 13th Street, in a role explained by Dodge: "He still had that job of trying to preserve the flavors of other nationalities when they came to New York. Singly, he tried to stem the ponderous tide of Americanization. He worked indefatigably; with committees and sub-committees he strove by means of pageants, parades and prizes, to persuade Italians, Russians, Germans, and all the others, to keep their national dress, their customs, their diets, their religions, and all their folk ways" (p. 323). In a letter circa 1915, Collier wrote to Dodge: "You, Mabel Dodge, are one of the two most mentally stimulating people I know—in your case I don't fully understand the reasons as yet" (p. 313). In 1920, when Collier visited her in Taos, these reasons may have become very clear: she introduced him to the Native Americans at the Taos Pueblo and he immersed himself in learning their history and culture, eventually championing their cause and fighting to protect their lands. Collier was to become the Commissioner of Indian Affairs under Franklin Delano Roosevelt in 1933.

Lucy Collier

Writer and an advocate for children's health and education in New York, married to John Collier. At this time in 1916, she was having a passionate affair with the writer Hutchins Hapgood. Dodge was an important confidante for Hapgood, although he became angry with her meddling and her failure to keep confidences, as he expresses in a letter to her from Provincetown, circa January 1916:

> You now have a need, under your present fad of "analysis" to immolate yourself—and others, on the altar of self-sacrifice....You are so sure about everything! For instance, you are sure that Lucy needs me more than I do her. I am not sure of it....I never said to you or any living soul that "Lucy needs to have her body loved." That is a coarse and untrue report of anything I said and I forbid you ever to repeat that statement to anybody. If you do, I'll never speak to you again. You are simply an abominable reporter and you ought never to trust yourself to quote anybody—not even their meaning.

Edwin Dodge
(Referred to in dreams as "E." or "E.D.")

Mabel Dodge's second husband whom she met in July 1904 on a ship bound for France. He was a wealthy young man from Boston, recently graduated from the École des Beaux Arts in Paris where he trained as an architect. He tirelessly pursued her until she agreed to marry him in October of that same year. Soon discontented again with the confines of marriage, in 1905 Mabel Dodge redirected her energies toward purchasing and renovating the Villa Curonia outside of Florence, using Edwin's money and funds from her mother. For a number of years, they lavishly entertained guests at the villa. Acting as hostess to members of the artistic, literary, and political avant-garde, as well as the social elite in Florence, served a stimulating purpose for Mabel Dodge at this time.

Mabel dedicated *European Experiences* (1935) to him: "For Edwin,...long suffering and always so kind..." (p. x).

Elizabeth Duncan

Older sister of Isadora Duncan, and a dancer herself who had become for Dodge "one of the few great women friends I have had at intervals during my life" (1936, p. 336). With Dodge's financial help, Elizabeth Duncan established a dance school in Croton near Finney Farm in 1915, where Dodge soon enrolled her son.

Isadora Duncan

American dancer, widely acclaimed as the founder of modern interpretive dance. When Dodge first saw Isadora Duncan perform in January 1915, she initially felt a strong connection with her, as she describes in *Movers and Shakers* (1936): "I went to see Isadora dance with her young girls and the mass of little children she had brought from Russia. It seemed to me I recognized what she did in the dance, and that it was like my own daily, nightly return to the Source. Power rose in her from her Center and flowed vividly along her limbs" (pp. 319–320). Responding to Duncan's passionate appeal to her audience to find a location where she could teach dance to American children, Dodge arranged a meeting for Duncan with the mayor of New York, an afternoon that quickly deteriorated as Duncan verbally attacked the mayor for not releasing an imprisoned woman, refused to have the children perform a dance for him, and inadvertently exposed one of her breasts. After this failed effort, Dodge turned her creative attention and financial resources to assist Elizabeth Duncan in establishing a school in Croton. To Elizabeth, Isadora called Mabel Dodge "'A Double-faced Chinese cat!'" (pp. 325–331, 337).

Max Eastman

American author and editor of *The Masses*, a journal devoted to arts and politics. Eastman also contributed articles to other periodicals, such as *Everybody's Magazine*, where he published two articles on psychoanalysis in 1915. Like Dodge, Eastman consulted with both Jelliffe and Brill for psychoanalysis and also explored alternate approaches to mind cure such as New Thought, a movement he described as "a kind of practical-minded first cousin to Christian Science, a mixture of suggestive therapeutics, psychic phenomena, non-church religion, and a business of conquering the world through sheer sentiments of optimism" (1948, p. 240). Eastman was married to Ida Rauh and had a cottage near Finney Farm, impulsively purchased one afternoon in 1915 after a visit with Dodge in Croton during which she asked him pointedly, "'Max, why don't you arrange your life?'" (p. 537). He encouraged Dodge's writing and published some of her work in *The Masses*. In a letter from 1916, he wrote to her about one of her stories, a fictional account of her tumultuous relationship with Sterne: "You have a gift and energy of creation that ought to be more sacred to you than any personal thing....This is an intense and compelling work of art, and I hope you know it" (Luhan, 1936, p. 435).

John Evans

Mabel Dodge's only child, a son born in 1902 from her first marriage to Karl Evans in 1900, which ended when Evans was killed in a hunting accident.

As Dodge openly describes in *European Experiences* (1935), she was highly ambivalent about her pregnancy and felt tortured about the idea of having a child. In the moments soon after her son was born in January 1902, she looked at him and admitted: "In a flash…I saw the pathos and the pity of life and I thought, 'I don't like it,' and my heart shut up right then and there.…I didn't feel the baby. I didn't feel anything for it. I saw it was a nice baby, but it didn't seem to be mine. I felt sorry for myself and wounded all over my life.…It seemed to me I didn't want a baby after all" (p. 51). In her account of the days following John's birth in "Doctors: Fifty Years of Experience" (1954), Dodge instinctively wanted him out of her presence: "As I looked at him he raised his head and gave me a rather dirty look.…'You'd better take him away now,' I said nervously.…I had to stay in bed a few days because I had been torn from giving birth to that stranger. They kept bringing him into my room and putting him on the bed beside me but I'd never seem to know him, somehow. And he looked at me so oddly. Soon he caused a feeling of guilt rising in me, guilt that I had never felt before in my life" (p. 20).

Dodge's guilt and initial rejection of John Evans were likely related to questions about his paternity, as she had been having an affair with her physician Dr. John Parmenter when she got pregnant. As she lamented in "Doctors": "I hardly knew whose baby I was going to have" (p. 19). In fact, it was Parmenter who delivered her baby and whose first name John was given to her son. Around the time of her pregnancy and giving birth, Dodge considered Parmenter "the motivation and cause for living" (p. 17) and longed for him to divorce his wife as promised. In a strange twist, Dodge discovered that her mother was simultaneously having an affair with Parmenter, when she walked in on the two of them and her mother "hastily pulled down her skirts" (1954, p. 19). Clearly, Dodge's preoccupation with her feelings for Parmenter during the early days of her son's life must have added enormously to her distaste for motherhood. She writes that eventually: "My curious reluctance to see the baby dwindled away and though I had ceased to feel sadness, neither did I feel any love for him, and I felt sorry for us both on this account" (1935, p. 52).

In July 1904, John Evans, two years old, accompanied Dodge and two nurses, one for each of them due to Dodge's depression at being a widow and a new mother, on a ship to Europe. During the crossing, she met Edwin Dodge and months later agreed to marry him, reflecting that she consented "maybe for John" (1935, p. 77). John spent many childhood years at the Villa Curonia in Florence, taught by tutors, and then, when they returned to the United States in September 1911, enrolled at the Morristown School in New Jersey.

Constance Fletcher

Julia Constance Fletcher, the American-born novelist and playwright who used the pseudonym George Fleming and lived most of her life in Venice. She wrote her first novel, *Kismet* (1878), when she was only 18. As a playwright, she was most successful with *The Canary* (1900) and in her adaptation (1903) of Rudyard Kipling's *The Light That Failed* (1890). Fletcher was close friends with both Oscar Wilde and Henry James; the former dedicated his poem *Ravenna* (1878) to her, while the latter based the plot of his novella *The Aspern Papers* (1888) on her failed relationship with Lord Lovelace, Lord Byron's grandson. Her only meeting with Gertrude Stein, in 1911 at Dodge's Villa Curonia in Italy, resulted in Stein's word portrait, "Portrait of Constance Fletcher," published later in *Geography and Plays* in 1922. According to Alice B. Toklas, Stein's companion, in *What is Remembered* (1963), it was Fletcher who encouraged Dodge to have copies printed of Stein's 1912 "Portrait of Mabel Dodge at the Villa Curonia" (pp. 75–76).

Mary Foote

American painter who had studied art at the Yale Art School and in Paris, and who lived at 3 Washington Square, near 23 Fifth Avenue. After becoming an orphan at age 12, she was raised by Mark Twain's family. She developed close friendships with Twain as well as Henry James, and the painters John Singer Sargent and James McNeil Whistler. In *European Experiences* (1935), Dodge describes her during a visit to the Villa Curonia: "Mary Foote was as plain as a perch—yet a stylish perch, clear-cut and chic, and possessed of the kind of humor that defended her from the unusual by ridicule" (p. 310). While at the Villa in 1912, Foote met Paul Ayrault and became the recipient of both his and Dodge's confidences about their affair. Ayrault wrote to Dodge on October 24, 1912: "I called on Mary Foote this afternoon and she confessed that she knew that we love each other….I told Mary exactly how things stood….She advised waiting awhile longer but said we had her blessing if we went ahead now." In a letter to Dodge from the same time, Foote reported on her visit with Ayrault: "I didn't know <u>what</u> to say to the poor child—I <u>couldn't</u> be very enthusiastic & yet it was awful to pour cold water on things because there is nothing like one's sensations of course when one is in the state of mind he appears to be in….I suppose it may work out all right & my blessings be upon you whatever you do—but <u>do</u> pause!….<u>Why</u> did you do it?" In another letter, Foote admitted: "The more I think about you & Paul the more agitated I become. What <u>will</u> you do?….How can you give up that entirely satisfactory Edwin?—& go off with a Columbia boy in his junior year, even if he is the charming Paul?"

Foote supported herself through commissioned portraits. She painted a portrait of Mabel Dodge and her son around 1911 and then another of Dodge alone, around 1915 (Figure 4.1). Foote also painted an undated (circa late 1910s) portrait of Jelliffe, whom she had met through Dodge. In a July 16, 1916 letter to Dodge, Foote wrote from California, where she had seen Jelliffe: "I gave Jelliffe your note & he told me afterwards that he had written you that you'd better take one of his houses at Lake George for August & have me up with you to paint him which is such a strenuous program that I

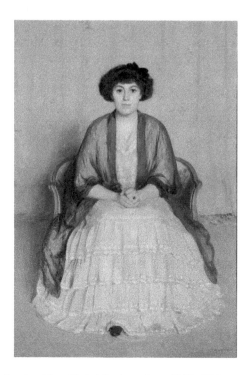

Figure 4.1 Mary Foote, *Mrs. Mabel Dodge*, circa 1915. This portrait was among 20 of Foote's paintings in an exhibition at M. Knoedler and Company in New York, May 1–13, 1916. Courtesy of the Beinecke Rare Book and Manuscript Library.

can't face it at all at present—I would much prefer to do him in N.Y." The same day, Jelliffe wrote to Dodge, reporting that he had seen Mary Foote and had received her letter. He offered: "Maybe a little later you could come up to Lake George and get a good rest and the portrait might be started." Dodge then wrote to Jelliffe on July 22, 1916, explaining that she would be in Provincetown for August, but "I would have liked to go up there with Mary if she went. Perhaps she & I could motor up & stay a bit in Aug. or Sept. Write me here—& we'l[l] see. Will you give her this letter." Foote most likely consulted with Jelliffe for analysis at some point in 1916 or 1917.

In 1917, Foote traveled to New Mexico to visit Dodge in Taos, where she painted Native Americans and pueblos.

Charles Ganson

Mabel Dodge's father, the son of a wealthy banker (Grandpa Ganson to Mabel) based in Buffalo, but never employed in any profession himself, despite training in the law. Charles Ganson was a severely moody man who suffered from gout and rheumatism and was often isolated in his study. In *Background* (1933a), she reports: "His irritable nature had spoiled his whole being. Even at a distance, there appeared to be an angriness about him. One saw it in all the outlines of his body and in every movement he made.... His empty life! The energy in him turned to poison, stagnating in his veins, and his only outlets were anxiety, jealousy, and querulousness" (pp. 26, 28). Even though she observed moments of his kindness to others, such as when he "always followed up an attack of swearing at Andy, the coachman, with a present of long black cigars" (p. 27), Dodge concluded: "I knew with all the prescience of a child that my father had no love for me at all. To him I was something that made a noise sometimes in the house and had to be told to get out of the way" (p. 26). While he was living his last days, miserable in his illness, Dodge reported that she felt "cold as ice"; when he died in November 1902, she described the funeral as "infinitely boring and rather disgusting to me. I had no other feelings" (1935, pp. 53, 54).

Sara Cook Ganson

Mabel Dodge's mother, the daughter of a prominent family descended from early settlers in Bath, New York, whose father (Grandpa Cook to Mabel) was the president of the bank in Bath until he moved to New York with her mother (Grandma Cook) and built a mansion on Fifth Avenue. In *Background* (1933a), Dodge describes her own mother who "like all her family, had real beauty" (p. 24) and was "a strong, energetic woman with ruddy hair and truly no words in her mouth....Always plump, in the later years she grew quite stout. She had no imagination and no fear and she seemed to live without love, though both my father and she loved their animals. They each had a dog...and they always had a tenderness for these" (p. 23). Dodge grew up excruciatingly aware of the unhappiness in her parents' marriage, observing that when her father "flew into a storming rage of jealousy and stamped and shouted and called her names," she watched her mother's "cold, merciless, expressionless contempt behind her book or newspaper" (p. 25). She bemoaned: "My mother had no mind. I mean it almost literally. She did not think about things....She was obstinate, repressed, and unloving. But she was courageous, inflexible, and independent, and at times very generous" (p. 24).

Hutchins Hapgood

Author and journalist married to Neith Boyce who was an active and crucial member of Mabel Dodge's early salons. Dodge described him as "the warmest, most sympathetic hound....He was one of the most attractive and lovable human beings I ever knew, and I soon became deeply attached to him and wanted to be with him all the time. I told him all about myself—everything—and oh! how he sympathized" (pp. 45, 47). When they met in 1912, as Hapgood reports in his autobiography, *A Victorian in the Modern World* (1939), Dodge was "completely innocent of the world of labor and of revolution in politics, art and industry. She lived in the purely conservative world, although her restless energy and her enormous temperamental instinct created frequent ructions in that world....My world excited Mabel; and she wanted to get into it....so she got me to bring to her apartment all kinds and conditions of men and women, so long as they were expressive" (p. 347). Through Hapgood, Dodge met many of the radicals and intellectuals in Greenwich Village. In *Movers and Shakers* (1936), she writes: "Oh, dear old Hutch! Writing of you brings back those days so clearly! How we talked and talked, and laughed withal! How eager we were, and how hopeful....Can I, I wonder, interpret now the contacts I had with all of these people as broadly and with as much understanding as you did years ago when you were my guide through the labyrinths of character and endeavor?" (p. 54). Hapgood writes at length in his memoir about Dodge and her emotionally barren upbringing:

> When I first met Mabel, she was young and very pretty. Hers was an unconventional prettiness; she looked like no other woman who was pretty. It was one of her side attractions, but yet, in spite of the fact that some men fell in love with her, I don't think it was the characteristic or usual response in men's imagination. The normal way of a male is to fall in love with a woman who is like a plant, with roots in the ground and with a possibility of eternal flowering....But one of the most striking things about Mabel was that she seemed to lack this root-like quality. I said once to Lincoln Steffens, who knew and liked Mabel, "She is like a cut flower." It seemed to him strikingly true; and to me it accounts for her never-ending movement; she continuously seeks the nourishment which some harsh fate has withheld from her, and which she can come in contact with only by the most violent effort.
>
> (p. 349)

Hapgood was one of the early founders of the Provincetown Players. In the summer of 1916, he and Boyce performed in *Enemies*, a play they co-wrote that presents the complicated negotiations of a married couple around issues of intimacy, jealousy, and betrayal, likely informed by the challenges in their open marriage and Hapgood's affair with Lucy Collier. Hapgood elegantly explored these themes in *The Story of a Lover* (1919), existing in manuscript form in 1916 but not yet published. His narrative of their marriage included this frustration: "I had an intense desire to satisfy longing. My deepest pleasure was to give pleasure....And the pain that almost drove me mad at times was that She had no need for me to satisfy! Other women had and how at times I strove to satisfy them!" (p. 188). Hapgood concluded: "Here I am at middle life living with the one woman I want to live with....and yet, in spite of it all, [she is] passionately unsatisfied! Passionately unsatisfied, and yet to me she is more beautiful, more wonderful than ever!" (p. 197).

Marsden Hartley

American painter represented by New York art dealer Alfred Stieglitz whose gallery 291 served as a central meeting place for avant-garde artists. It was there that Dodge met Hartley. She purchased his 1913 *Portrait of Berlin* (Collection of the Beinecke Rare Book and Manuscript Library, Yale University), an abstract portrait of a German officer that was included in an exhibition of Hartley's Berlin paintings at 291 in January 1914. The catalogue for the show included a foreword by Dodge and excerpts from a Gertrude Stein play in which Hartley is a character. After Hartley attended his first salon at 23 Fifth Avenue in 1913, he wrote to Dodge: "I want to tell you that I think we are going to have lots to say to each other....I do hope you don't go away for long while I am in New York because I feel the need of unusual lights in dark places and there seems so much of this there around you" (Luhan, 1936, p. 95). In March 1914, Hartley left for Europe, returning to New York in December 1915 from Berlin. In February 1916, Hartley spent some time at Finney Farm with Dodge. However, she became tired of his presence, perhaps as indicated in her dream association (for dream 23, Jelliffe's notes from January 20, 1916) that he was "still there": "There was something solitary and unassimilable about Marsden and it hurt me more to have him there than to write him he must go!" (Luhan, 1936, p. 460).

Robert "Bobby" Edmond Jones

American scenic designer who was a classmate of John Reed's at Harvard and had designed scenery for the Paterson Strike Pageant, where Dodge first met him. He accompanied Reed and Dodge to Europe in June 1913 after the Pageant. In 1915, he returned to the United States from Germany and lived in an apartment adjoining Dodge's home at 23 Fifth Avenue, an arrangement that eased her loneliness. As she describes in *Movers and Shakers* (1936), Bobby's "vitality bubbled up in ecstasy and enthusiasm. I had little of this at the moment so I borrowed his. In this way we are all vampires sometimes. I really dipped into Bobby's pool and drank. He attached himself to me and I became his mother" (p. 315).

Walter Lippmann
(Referred to in dreams as "W." or "W.L.")

American author, editor, and journalist who was one of Mabel Dodge's closest friends at this time. Lippmann regularly attended her salons at 23 Fifth Avenue and was reportedly responsible for bringing A.A. Brill one evening to talk about Freud (Green, 1988, p. 59). He was one of the founding editors of *The New Republic* in 1914, a magazine devoted to political and cultural commentary. In 1916, Lippmann began a romantic relationship with Faye Albertson, the daughter of the Boston minister and socialist Ralph Albertson, an involvement he initially kept hidden from most of his friends, except for a few, including Dodge. Lippmann married Faye in 1917 and in the same year briefly became Assistant Secretary of War under Woodrow Wilson.

John Reed

American journalist and poet who was on the staff of the magazine *The Masses* and a periodic lover of Dodge's from 1913 until 1915. Dodge first met Reed in the spring of 1913 at a gathering of radicals in Greenwich Village, a meeting that resulted in the birth of the Paterson Strike Pageant. Working together feverishly to organize this dramatization of the striking silk workers in Paterson, New Jersey, that was staged at Madison Square Garden in June 1913, Dodge and Reed developed an intense connection. They traveled together to Europe after the Pageant and began a passionate and tortured relationship, with Dodge's all-consuming desires soon proving destructive due to her easily triggered jealousy of Reed's many interests outside of her, as she recalls in *Movers and Shakers* (1936): "I hated to see him interested in Things. I wasn't, and didn't like to have him even *look* at churches and leave me out of his attention" (p. 217). Their relationship ended in March 1915, clearing the way for Dodge's involvement with Maurice Sterne.

In December 1915, Reed met the playwright and journalist Louise Bryant, whom he married in 1916. They both traveled to Russia and wrote about the Russian Revolution, remaining together until Reed died of typhus in Moscow in 1920. Reed's *Ten Days That Shook the World* (1919) described the 1917 Bolshevik-led October Revolution that he witnessed firsthand in St. Petersburg.

Lincoln Steffens

American journalist and editor who regularly attended Dodge's evenings at 23 Fifth Avenue and lived a floor below John Reed in Washington Square. Steffens proclaimed Dodge's salon "the only successful salon I have ever seen in America." He remembers: "It was there and thus that some of us first heard of psychoanalysis and the new psychology of Freud and Jung, which in several discussions, one led by Walter Lippmann, introduced us to the idea that the minds of men were distorted by unconscious suppressions.... There were no warmer, quieter, more intensely thoughtful conversations at Mabel Dodge's than those on Freud and his implications" (1931, v. II, pp. 655–656).

Gertrude Stein

American-born modernist writer who held popular salons at 27 rue de Fleurus in Paris, where she lived with her brother Leo (until 1912) and her companion Alice B. Toklas (from 1910 on) in an apartment hung floor to ceiling with works of art by such newly discovered painters as Picasso, Matisse, and Cézanne. She first met Mabel Dodge in the early spring of 1911 and entrusted her with a manuscript of her lengthy novel, *The Making of Americans* (1925), still in progress. Dodge expressed her unbridled praise for its revolutionary form in a letter to Stein circa April 1911: "To me it is one of the most remarkable things I have ever read. There are things hammered out of consciousness into black & white that have never been expressed before" (GLSC). Stein and Toklas visited Mabel and Edwin Dodge in Florence, most notably in the fall of 1912 when she wrote "Portrait of Mabel Dodge at the Villa Curonia," originally titled "Mabel little Mabel with her face against the pane," a comparatively accessible word portrait describing in both concrete and abstract language Stein's experience of the villa and her hostess.

Leo Stein
(Referred to in dreams as "L." or "L.S.")

Gertrude Stein's brother, a writer and art critic who maintained a long friendship and correspondence with Mabel Dodge. Dodge first met Leo Stein at 27 rue de Fleurus at the same time she met Gertrude. In *European Experiences* (1935), Dodge explained his role at the famous weekly gatherings there, where he positioned himself in front of the paintings: "Leo stood patiently night after night wrestling with the inertia of his guests, expounding, teaching, interpreting, always the advocate of tension in art!" (p. 322).

In their correspondence from this time, it is clear that Leo Stein and Dodge shared a deep interest in psychoanalysis, as their letters contain many references to Brill, Jelliffe, and the work of analysis. In 1915 and 1916, Stein consulted with first Brill and then Jelliffe for analysis. In his memoir, *Journey into the Self* (1950), Stein reprints his letter to Gertrude from February 15, 1916, reporting: "I see a good deal of Mabel Dodge, spending as much as possible of my week-ends at Croton, where Mabel has her farm....Everybody is occupied more or less with psychoanalysis" (pp. 71–72). However, at some point in 1916, Stein turned away from traditional analysis, explaining: "It was a terrific neurosis. I tried psychoanalysis with two well-known analysts, but analysis couldn't make a dent in it. Perhaps if I had tried it earlier something might have been effected but I had piled repression on repression and they could not be budged" (1950, p. 197). When he ended his work with Jelliffe, Stein developed a strong belief in self-analysis, writing to Dodge in 1916: "I have done a great deal for my cousin (psychoanalytically) and something for myself. Yesterday I analysed [*sic*] some dreams and identified and clarified the homosexual component, which I am inclined to think was part of the primitive repression and connected itself with my or rather our (since he was chiefly there for my brothers) tutor in Vienna. This elucidation has given further relief." In September 1916, Stein again wrote to Dodge about his solitary psychoanalytic work, insisting that he had reached clarity in his pursuits: "There are indeed no novel facts at all, merely a rearrangement of those already known to reveal the truth till now hidden even from the penetrating eye of A.A.B. & S.E.J. Great men all, but a little obsessed by their own peculiar insights....I really believe I have solved my p.a. [i.e., psychoanalytic] problem & now shall need nothing except the reorganization of my habits to match." In a letter to the psychiatrist Trigant Burrow in 1941, Stein (1950) reflected on why he believed his analyses were not helpful: "Submission of any kind was impossible except on the assumption of indifference. Therefore I couldn't cooperate. Either I did it or let the other person do it. This was also the reason why it was impossible for me to be analyzed, and why I had to develop a method for doing it myself. Whether the prestige of Freud would have been sufficient I cannot say. Certainly that of Brill and Jelliffe was not" (p. 215).

Stein held strongly negative opinions about the suitability of the match between Dodge and Maurice Sterne. In late 1916, Stein wrote to her about his visit with Sterne who "mentioned the fact that you had spoken to him of our talk concerning the marriage prospect and my disapproval" and asserted: "Now my dear Mabel, I really like you far too much to have any patience with your making an ass of yourself. Sterne doesn't want a mother except temporarily and unless you succeed in dominating him more or less completely—in which case he'd be of not much more use to you than a pussy cat—you'd find that after a while that mother was out of a job though there might be one for a housekeeper." He continued with even more candor and professed insight: "Now I don't believe that you're seriously interested in what Sterne is doing and what[']s more I don't believe that in any vital sense you understand the problems (artistic) that agitate him. Art is something vital to you, I believe, as an experience. I don't believe it's vital to you as a problem—at least not, & that is what I refer to, an aesthetic problem."

Maurice Sterne
(Referred to in dreams as "M." or "S." or "M.S.")

Dodge's lover at this time, a Latvian-born artist whom she had met in the spring of 1915. She was forcefully attracted to him, as she relates in *Movers and Shakers* (1936): "He was positively enveloped in a cloud of secrecy and caution. The man might have been in a jungle, so watchful was he, so studied every glance and motion. That interested me. I wondered what it was all about" (p. 350). She immediately purchased one of his drawings at Birnbaum Gallery in New York and hoped to see him again. At the time

Dodge met Sterne, he had recently spent two years in Bali, immersed in drawing and painting native life. In his memoir, *Shadow and Light* (1952), he described her initial appeal: "It was much more than sex that attracted me to her. I was amazed with Mabel. For the first time in my life I could relax, rest my will, and do what someone else decided was best. It was a period when my own self-confidence had shrunk to zero. I was tired and diffident, and I found relief in Mabel's super-confidence" (p. 111). Dodge sensed this malleability in Sterne and set out to push him toward sculpture over painting: "'The man is meant for a sculptor—what fun it would be to make him into one'" (1936, p. 361). Their relationship was never without struggle, and Dodge admitted: "I unhesitatingly did all I could to strengthen my influence over him, and to bind him to me" (p. 372). She invited him to Provincetown for the summer of 1915 and offered him one of her two rented houses to use as a studio. However, Sterne (1952) soon came to "resent being a chattel, and whenever I insisted upon my own ways, she was puzzled. Thus, we muddled into a misalliance for which I was as much to blame as anyone" (pp. 111–112).

Despite his conclusion, and the unstable and often destructive nature of their relationship, Mabel Dodge and Maurice Sterne were married on August 23, 1917, after she impulsively proposed marriage.

Alfred Stieglitz

American art dealer, photographer, and publisher whose gallery 291 was a gathering place for the avant-garde in New York. Dodge first visited 291 with Hapgood at the end of 1912 and was immediately drawn to its atmosphere, the art, and Stieglitz himself. In her frequent trips to the gallery, Dodge met many artists and was exposed to the often daring art that Stieglitz exhibited on his walls, including works by Marsden Hartley, Andrew Dasburg, John Marin, Arthur Dove, and Max Weber. Stieglitz edited and published an influential magazine, *Camera Work*, from 1903 to 1917, featuring reproductions of photographs, paintings, drawings, and sculpture, as well as theoretical articles, poetry, art criticism, and writing such as Gertrude Stein's word portraits of Picasso and Matisse. In the July 1914 issue, he printed a poem by Dodge, "The Mirror," which begins: "I am the mirror wherein man sees man,/ Whenever he looks deep into my eyes/ And looks for me alone, he there descries/ The human plan." The poem ends with: "I am the alternating peace and strife—/ I am the mirror of all man ever is—/ I am the sum of all that has been his—/ For I am life" (p. 9).

Alice B. Toklas

American-born homemaker (cook, gardener, stenographer) and lifelong companion to Gertrude Stein, who lived with her at 27 rue de Fleurus, and became a writer herself later in life. Toklas typed all of Stein's handwritten manuscripts, for years serving as Stein's love object as well as her social secretary, publisher, and agent. According to Dodge, Toklas was jealous of her intense connection with Stein and worked to dissolve it. In *European Experiences* (1935), she reports: "As Gertrude went on with 'The Portrait of Mabel Dodge,' writing her unconscious lines, she seemed to grow warmer to me, to which I responded in a sort of flirtatious way." At lunch one day at the Villa Curonia, Dodge explains that Gertrude "sent me such a strong look over the table that it seemed to cut across the air to me in a band of electrified steel—a smile traveling across on it—powerful—Heavens!" Toklas then hurried out of the room and immediately "began to separate Gertrude and me—*poco-poco*" (pp. 332–333).

Carl Van Vechten

American critic and writer who had expressed a strong interest in black culture from an early date and was to become a leading supporter of the Harlem Renaissance. After their first meeting in 1913, Dodge soon invited Van Vechten to visit her at 23 Fifth Avenue. He became one of her closest friends, and she claimed that he was "the first person who animated my lifeless rooms" (1936, p. 16). It is curious, given their closeness and how widely populated Dodge's dreams are by her friends and acquaintances, that Van Vechten does not appear once in her recorded dreams from this time.

Chapter 5

The Dreams of Mabel Dodge

A note on how to approach the dreams

To recapitulate my suggested guidelines in the preface, after having read about Dodge's closest friends and family in "Cast of Characters," now proceed to the dreams, presented in the following format: the dream itself; Dodge's associations (if any) *in black italics*; Jelliffe's relevant case notes (if any) *in grey italics*; notes then appear in two forms at the end of each dream: in regular non-italicized type to identify people, places, events, and images; ***in bold italics*** for interpretive comments and questions that seek to illuminate preoccupations and themes that emerge from the dreams, as well as for Freud's interpretations of dreams and symbols that were predominant in both popular and psychoanalytic conversations at the time. Interludes are interspersed between the dreams, providing additional context and elucidation.

1.
January 2, 1916 (1 of 3)[1]
[typed]

Renting a house from some Japanese family, a <u>very</u> large family, but as they pass in procession before us they do not all look Japanese.[2] The house seems to have a great many drawing rooms, large and small. My brother [3] seems to be the person who really is going to rent and pay for the house and he objects to the small dining room, whereupon they show him a <u>very</u> large one.[4]

Notes:

1 As noted earlier, these three dreams date from the day before Dodge's intake session with Jelliffe on January 3, 1916. It is certainly possible he requested that she bring in any dreams for their first meeting.
2 The significance of "Japanese" is unknown, ***but the focus on the family not appearing Japanese when they pass by may reflect Dodge's pained***

awareness that others saw her one way, as a wealthy and satisfied woman, without sensing her inner struggles: "I gave...an impression of successful living. I know this was quite a usual assumption among my friends. All they saw was an effect of rich and varied life....I thought they never knew the agonies and the doubts that were the almost continuous accompaniment of what may have looked like a triumphal progress. Only Jelliffe and Brill knew those and even they would never know the whole of it" (Luhan, 1936, p. 514). As a first dream presented to Jelliffe, this idea of people not ultimately being seen as they are initially perceived seems quite relevant.

3 Mabel Dodge was an only child, *"never in possession of my kingdom: Root of my character,"* as she reported to Jelliffe in her intake on January 3, 1916. In her unpublished memoir "Family Affairs" (1933b), she writes that during her psychoanalysis with A.A. Brill, "I suffered and actually lived again the barren experience of being an only and unloved child" (p. 1). In *Background* (1933a), Dodge describes the aftermath of a fiery and teary exchange that she witnessed between her parents in their home as her mother walked away from her father: "I got up and turned away into my room and as I did so my mother shut his door on him and walked down the hall to where her own room was. So there we were, the three of us, separated into our different modes of loneliness—a family" (p. 36). *Although Dodge's autobiographical writings do not contain references to any wish for a sibling, it is likely that the company of a brother would have eased the pain of her early isolation and boredom.*

4 *As the first of three dreams that Dodge reports to Jelliffe at the beginning of her analysis when she was tormented by jealousy and stuck in her patterns of relating to others, these many rooms—both drawing and dining, large and small—may suggest some hopefulness about the possibility of choice, about where to be, how to act, about spaciousness and options. The preference for a larger dining room may reveal the necessity of greater space to accommodate Dodge's enormous appetites and desires.*

δ

2.
January 2, 1916 (2 of 3)
[typed]

Travelling in an automobile along a very bad road, soft mud with many cars stuck in it. As there are only two of us [1] we think we won't be stuck but there appear a number of people, some very fat—that should be picked up, and we hesitate as they only prevent our progress.[2] One very fat woman in particular.[3]

Notes:

1 *Might this refer to the two of them at the outset of their work together, just Dodge and Jelliffe?*
2 *Is this a fear of Dodge's, that entering analysis will make her stuck in some way, even though they appear to be making progress on the bad road where many cars are stuck? If they invite others into their car, some who are "very fat," this will slow them down and "prevent our progress." Is Dodge feeling guilty about her anticipated progress that may leave others, specifically Maurice Sterne, behind?*
3 In this and the following two dreams, "fat" appears as a prominent descriptor of characters, raising the question of the significance of weight for Dodge. In *Background* (1933a), she describes her mother and her aunt Louise as "rather fat like my grandmother, but Aunt Marianna, the oldest, and Aunt Georgie, the youngest…were tall and long-limbed like Grandpa Cook, and they seemed very attractive" (pp. 119–120). *Given that Dodge referred to Jelliffe as "paunchy" (1936, p. 443), this may be her first recorded transference dream, leaning toward the maternal.*

δ

3.
January 2, 1916 (3 of 3)
[typed]

Islands up in the sound near S. Norfalk.[1] Mrs. Whitehouse [2]—some child who wanted to urinate [3] in the dishpan. A beautiful woman to whom I was much attached, preferred her to the very fat man.[4]

> Jelliffe's notes from January 6, 1916:
> *Bladder & irritation:/ Cook [i.e., her mother's family's] jealousy: all comes there.*[5]

Notes:

1 Unidentified location, perhaps a reference to South Norfolk, Virginia, then an independent city, now part of the city of Chesapeake.
2 Unidentified.
3 References to urination appear twice more in Dodge's dreams (#s 90 & 131) and more frequently in Jelliffe's notes from her analysis (March 16, April 17, May 16). In her sessions, she recalled a number of childhood memories linking bathrooms, urination, and the smell of urine with fascination and excitement (see Jelliffe's notes from March 16 for dream 57, and May 16 for dream 122). *Freud (1900), in a passage added in 1919, followed Otto Rank's consideration that "a great number of dreams with*

*a urinary stimulus have in fact been caused by a **sexual** stimulus which has made a first attempt to find satisfaction regressively in the infantile form of urethral erotism" (p. 403).*

4 This reference to "fat" is repeated from the previous dream (see note 3) and continues in the next dream, where a "very fat man" appears.

5 *In his notes, Jelliffe almost certainly records Dodge's own words: Already connecting the body and the mind, Dodge observes that the jealousy that runs in her family finds expression in painful urination.*

δ

4.

January 3, 1916

[typed]

I was expected to marry a <u>very fat</u> man [1] who ate <u>enormous</u> quantities of food [2] and after he ate let down his s---first on one side then on the other to aid his digestion.

Notes:

1 *This is likely the third in a series of Dodge's first recorded transference dreams, here leaning toward the paternal in featuring Jelliffe as a well-fed man whom she had to marry, perhaps against her wishes. She may have been familiar with, and resistant to, the idea of erotic transference, of her analyst playing many roles for her, including lover or husband. The image of this man defecating to "aid digestion"—perhaps in order to make room for more food, that is, more analytic material—may stem from Dodge's initial experience of relief as she told Jelliffe everything that was on her mind and watched as he absorbed it.*

2 *Dodge made desperate attempts to secure both sustenance and attachments in her life, a drive crucially determined by her Buffalo childhood, with its intense loneliness and the cold atmosphere of her home.*

δ

5.

[undated, circa early January 1916]

[typed]

House in Vt. Move barn up and join to house for garage. Barn is full of hay. I want it cleared out or sold for fear of fire. W.[1] seems to be trying to set fire to it. Try throwing matches from above on the house. He succeeds. I go for water and begin to put out fire.[2] Ask P.[3] to help me get it out. I do not see why W. won't help but he says it would burn his hand and hurt his nails. He is manicuring his nails.[4]

Notes:

1 This likely refers to Walter Lippmann.
2 *This is early on in Dodge's treatment with Jelliffe: could this suggest she feels out of control of what she has already revealed? That the fire (or the analysis) could get out of her control? Also, fire may be related to the mention of "urinate" in dream 3, a connection that Freud (1905a) made in his Dora case history. In her first dream, "'A house was on fire. My father was standing beside my bed and woke me up,'" an association to her history of bed-wetting: "'something might happen in the night so that it might be necessary to leave the room'" (pp. 64, 65). Freud explained to Dora "why children were forbidden to play with matches": "'The fear is that if they do they will wet their bed. The antithesis of "water" and "fire" must be at the bottom of this. Perhaps it is believed that they will dream of fire and then try and put it out with water'" (pp. 71–72).*
3 This may refer to Paul Ayrault.
4 *W. does not want to get his hands dirty. Perhaps Dodge fears that Jelliffe does not want to go deeper into her material.*

δ

6.
[undated, circa early January 1916]
[typed]

A woman going to a train—has been with me. I go to a store across the street to sell a piece of material—purple cloth. They will give me 60 cts. I say all right and run with the money to the R.R. station to find my friend. Then I look at the money, which is queer shaped and I understand it is German money.[1] I think I will take it back but seem to be travelling on a trolley—'way off to another place. Get off and think I will start back but do not know the way.[2] Getting dark. Think I will telephone home but we have no telephone. Mrs. B.[3] has. Ask policeman how to get across the road. He points to the left,[4] but I cannot cross for some distance.

Notes:

1 *These references to money may relate to the fee for analysis, and the mention of German money to World War I.*
2 *This image suggests an analytic journey "to another place," with doubts about how to return to the origin of the travel.*
3 Unidentified. Although likely indicating Nina Bull, this could also be another of Dodge's friends, including Mary Berenson, wife of art historian Bernard Berenson, whom Dodge knew in Florence and referred to as "Mrs. B.B.," or Lily Braggiotti, daughter of composer Sebastian Schlesinger, who had married Isador Braggiotti and lived in Florence.

4   *Is there some significance in this pointing Dodge to the left, and in the fact*
    that a policeman gives the direction? Freud (1900), in a passage added in
    1911, quoted Wilhelm Stekel's interpretations of right and left: "According to
    Stekel, 'right' and 'left' in dreams have an ethical sense. 'The right-hand path
    always means the path of righteousness and the left-hand one that of crime.
    Thus "left" may represent homosexuality, incest or perversion, and "right"
    may represent marriage, intercourse with a prostitute and so on, always
    looked at from the subject's individual moral standpoint'" (pp. 357–358).

δ

7.
[undated, circa early January 1916]
[typed]

I saw a bed and it was full of various insects, flies, etc. Some seemed to be
on me too.[1]

Note:

1   *What could this image suggest? Dodge finds insects on a bed and*
    herself—perhaps they are one and the same, the bed and her body? Does
    this connect to her erotic life with Sterne? Could it suggest her fears
    about contracting syphilis from him?

δ

8.
[undated, circa early January 1916]
[typed]

Seem to be expecting a baby. Have great pain, then a bowel movement.[1]
Do not understand why baby does not come. Count back to last period,
which dates to my birthday, Jan. 11.[2] Think enough time has not elapsed.
Nurse is engaged, waiting. Aunt Louise [3] is waiting and has to be told that
it cannot be yet—it is a mistake.[4]
    Seem to be thin and not pregnant.[5]

Notes:

1   *Freud (1908b) equated a baby with feces in "On the Sexual Theories of Chil-*
    dren": "If the baby grows in the mother's body and is then removed from it, this
    can only happen along the one possible pathway—the anal aperture. The baby
    must be evacuated like a piece of excrement" (p. 219). In Freud's case history

of Hans (1909), he explained: "according to the sexual theory of children a baby is a 'lumf' [i.e., feces]" (p. 74).

2 Dodge's birthday is, in fact, February 26, not January 11. Possible reasons for why her birthday would appear incorrectly in her dream are that her son was born in January (date unknown) 1902 and also, as recorded in Jelliffe's notes from January 6, 1916, Dodge recalled that she had intercourse with Parmenter in January 1901, possibly their first liaison, and perhaps January therefore had a certain meaning for her.

3 One of Dodge's mother's three sisters who married their father's lawyer, Judge Rumsey Miller, with whom she had four children. Louise raised her family in Bath, New York in the same house, named the Homestead, where Dodge's maternal grandparents, whom she called Grandpa and Grandma Cook, had lived for more than a generation.

4 *This idea of a "mistake" could relate to Dodge's ambivalence about both pregnancy and having a baby with Sterne.*

5 *This dream may reveal Dodge's desire, stated directly in letters to Jelliffe, circa May 24 and circa May 26, 1916 (see Interludes 17 & 18), to become pregnant, despite the increased challenge due to the fact that in 1906 she had one ovary removed in an operation in Italy, as recorded by Jelliffe in his notes from January 11, 1916.*

δ

9.
Sunday [undated, circa early January 1916]
[typed]

One night dreamed of desired coitus, and husband impotent.[1]

> Jelliffe's notes from January 6, 1916:
> *A few realizations:/ Lived c. Ed. many years: no ♂♀ [i.e., intercourse], terrible state: finally left him….tried to get interested in outside things/ Free things (Brill, everybody & general discussion,[2] talking, because (respiratory libido) your idea interested me[)]….Voice & statements. Dynamic voice matters:/ ["]Mrs. Dodge always in background."] One of my rules not to speak [3]:/ One of my troubles here.[4]/ Could [speak]with one at a time./ made use of my ideas./ Interesting parallel:/ dancing [at] 16:/ same impossibility in group c. talking./ Committee on Industrial Relations [5]: Got them together:/ Then I was through:# Have tried it, but left it all now./ To bring elements together.[6]/*

Notes:

1 Although not living with her at the time, Dodge's current husband was Edwin, who had been a disappointing romantic partner. As she recalls

in *European Experiences* (1935), when he asked her to marry him, she replied: "I told him I wasn't in love with him and I felt nothing for him except a desire for him to be about, to help me, and to enable me to make something new and beautiful" (p. 77). **Since Dodge sought connection through sex, her sexless marriage was distressing and left her alone with herself.** According to another section of Jelliffe's January 6 notes, she admitted: "*M[arried]. E.D. to get away from other troubles:/ End of severe & difficult love affair [with Dr. Parmenter].*" In an unpublished section of her memoirs, she referred to this affair—"I felt I was on rather uncertain ground—and that perhaps everyone would go back on me if I had another scandal" (1927, pp. 510–511)—and described her disgust for her husband: "It made me sick to let Edwin have my body. Little by little I effected a complete separation between us. I was irked by his desire that was always after me, but I could not bear to gratify it. He drank a little more year by year now....Drink made him shrivel and grow smaller" (p. 509). Dodge concluded: "I wanted of him nothing except to be a husband and make a part of the background, and I wanted it for John as well as myself. I did not want to face a divorce and all the talk that that would make, as well as my family's disapproval" (1935, p. 446).

2   This probably refers to the time around 1915 when Brill spoke about psychoanalysis at her 23 Fifth Avenue salon, as she reports: "Dr. Brill had begun his Freudian analysis before that time, and it was thought to be just as queer as all the other attempts people were making to achieve some kind of social adaptation. We had him come down and talk to us one of the Evenings and several guests got up and left, they were so incensed at his assertions about unconscious behavior and its give-aways" (1936, p. 142). In 1912, Brill had translated Freud's *Interpretation of Dreams* (1900) (New York: Macmillan) into English, thereby making it more generally available and accessible in the United States.

3   At her salons, Dodge's silences were legendary. Although Max Eastman complained that "for the most part she sits like a lump and says nothing" (1948, p. 523), Lincoln Steffens observed: "Mabel Dodge managed her evenings, and no one felt that they were managed. She sat quietly in a great armchair and rarely said a word; her guests did the talking" (1931, v. II, p. 655). The English actor Robert de la Condamine inscribed in a book he gave to Dodge: "'To Mabel Dodge, who has the courage to sit still and the wisdom to keep silent'" (Luhan, 1935, p. 267).

4   *Does she mean that in psychoanalysis with Jelliffe she is going against her rule of "not to speak"?*

5   Although Dodge may be referring to the Committee on Industrial Relations that was formed by Congress in 1912 to evaluate labor law and

conditions, she could also mean the Industrial Workers of the World, an international labor union whose members, "the Wobblies" (among them her lover at the time John Reed), she hosted at her salons.

6 Dodge was a master at gathering different kinds of people at her salons beginning in 1913, but she lost interest in hosting after a few years.

δ

10.
Monday [undated, circa early January 1916]
[typed]

Living with husband as brother and sister.[1]

Note:

1 *This seems a direct reference to the impotence from the previous dream, with her association to the absence of sex in her marriage, and connects to the first dream where Dodge has a brother. This dream adds material to the developing theme of ambiguous family ties, where there is a blurring of boundaries with others: a husband can be a brother or sister.*

δ

11.
[undated, circa early January 1916]
[typed]

Seem to be going to see Aunt Louise in Bernardsville, N.Y.[1] Going with me are two boys about 10–12 years old. I am waiting for them to wash their clothes before we start. Also tell them to look up a train. Don't know where Aunt L. lives but find her, only it seems to be a shop and I am buying some dress material.

Find myself in a R.R. station. Seem to be coming out of one of those lapses I have. I then realize that I have not been home for some time longer than a day and think W.[2] will be worried. Have some idea of sending message. Think to myself, Now I will be myself—I have come out of this state of mind.

Notes:

1 There is no town listed by this name in New York, although Dodge could be referring to Brainardsville, a town at the very northern edge of the Adirondack Park, near the Canadian border.

2 This most likely refers to Walter Lippmann.

δ

12.
[undated, circa early January 1916]
[typed]

Traveling in some Indian vicinity.[1] Have two valuable presents—set with precious stones, one large, one small. Large one worth $2500. I want to present these to same two Indian people, young men, brothers. One he will accept, the little one I think. The other he turns over and shows me some mark on the back, which he says his tribe will see and object to.

Hazy picture of a naked woman receiving something as a gift. Children around.

Assoc. of woman— S[terne]. in s.[2] act.

Notes:

1   The appearance of an Indian location in this dream dates long before Dodge's move to New Mexico in December 1917. After she married Sterne in August 1917, she quickly tired of the relationship and dispatched him to New Mexico, as she explains in *Movers and Shakers* (1936): "'It's no use, Maurice. We can't make a go of it here. One of us must leave. And *I* want to stay here. I'm going to send you out to the Southwest. I've heard there are wonderful things to paint. Indians.'" After Sterne settled in Santa Fe, he wrote to her: "Do you want an object in life? Save the Indians, their art—culture—reveal it to the world! I hear astonishing things about the insensitiveness of our Indian office....That which...others are doing for the Negroes, you could, if you wanted to, do for the Indians, for you have energy and are the most sensitive little girl in the world—and, above all, there is somehow a strange relationship between yourself and the Indians" (pp. 532, 534–535). *This dream image also connects to rumors that her paternal grandmother, Grandma Ganson, had Indian blood and to Dodge's identification and fascination with her (see note 4 for dream 41).*

2   i.e., sex. Dodge was tormented by jealousy about Sterne's constant attraction to other women.

δ

13.
January 5, 1916

Some woman—I think it is Mrs. [Lucy] Collier [1]—has twins. She says: "See I have adopted two more." She lays them alongside the others in rows, about two years old.[2] They look maturely intelligent, with cynically amused smiles, tho' heavy & inanimate.

Soon after I am driving a pair of big horses.[3] One is too lively. I don't show my doubt of controlling him.[4] A girl by my side, Helen [5]—whom I haven't known since I was 16 or 17 & of whom I was jealous once [6]—& who used to be smug & self[-]righteous—a madonna type of sweet girl—leans forward & lifts the big horse off the ground without effort—by putting her arms about his body from behind. She laughs as she lifts him quite easily. Then she sets him down again. He hangs his head & smiles in an overcome amused way, & looks a little mortified.[7] I drive them on.

Jelliffe's notes from January 5, 1916:
16 yr old girl:/ Smug. Self[-]righteous-madonna like/ Opposite of self[.]
    I was wild & strong willed: rows, queer at home…/ F[ather]. & M[other].
at house—unpleasant atmosphere [8]/ *c. horses a great deal/ driving.*

Notes:

1 At this time, Hutchins Hapgood (in an open marriage with Neith Boyce) and Lucy Collier were deeply immersed in an affair. He wrote to Dodge circa early January 1916: "There is one thing I will tell you now—which please do not tell to anybody—I do not think that Lucy loves me or needs me more than I do her. She loves me and needs me but she loves Love more and what I cannot give she will get from others—as you did [with Paul Ayrault]! I do not think I shall hurt her….And I love her very much and am much in love….And Lucy loves John. And I love Neith."

2 *What might this suggest, this sequence of pairs? A woman has twins, adopts two more who are two years old, then Dodge drives a pair of horses. Perhaps this reveals her chronic loneliness and wish for a constant companion to ease her isolation.*

3 Dodge was comfortable with horses from a young age, as she reports in *Background* (1933a) that she often rode horses and ponies in Buffalo and at her various family summer homes, including riding plow horses bareback in Bath, near Buffalo (p. 155), and wildly engaging her pony Cupid in her antics in Lenox, Massachusetts when she placed her terrier Pearl on the back of the pony and herself in the cart behind: "It was fun to run all over the hills in the swaying cart and I loved to walk Cupid up a long hill…and then, standing up in the seat of the lurching small chariot, Pearl balancing perilously with back-blowing curls, simply tear down into the village at a full gallop" (p. 171).
   Perhaps most thrillingly and expertly, she rode unbroken horses with her adventurous friend from Buffalo, Seward Cary, who "would put me on one of those green animals and send me to the fence. The nervous horse—picked by Seward for his speed and his high nervous tension—would leap forward as I urged him, galloping to the fence. But, uneducated, he would pull up short at the obstacle and I would fly off into

the air and land on the ground with a thump....Falling came to mean nothing to me except to show Seward I wasn't afraid and that I would do anything he said. And by force of acting as though I were not afraid, I lost my fear" (Luhan, 1935, p. 6).

4   This focus on control may be an association to a terrible horse accident that occurred during Dodge's childhood. As she reports in *Background* (1933a), her parents were in a horse-drawn coupé on a Saturday night heading out for dinner when "the horses began to run away. The driver was bounced off the reeling carriage, and just as it was going over, my father managed to open the carriage door on his side and leap bravely out into the night. At that instant the whole thing tipped over and the horses continued to run, dragging it along on its side, my mother within! When they came to a standstill...my mother was almost unconscious inside, one velvet slipper sticking out of one window and the other out of the opposite window" (p. 41). *Control over others is a crucial motivation for Dodge, so she must hide her fear of not having control.*

5   Unidentified, not mentioned in *Background* (1933a). It is likely that Helen was one of Dodge's classmates at St. Margaret's in Buffalo, where she was enrolled until she was 16 years old, or at Miss Graham's School, a boarding school in New York City that she then attended for one semester, or at the Chevy Chase School in Maryland where she boarded for her final year of high school. *"Helen" is almost "Helena," the name of Jelliffe's wife, who could certainly already be figuring into Dodge's transference to him, a doubling of roles as she wonders if she is Jelliffe's patient or his wife.*

6   *Could this suggest Dodge's jealousy toward Helena Jelliffe?*

7   *The male horse has been easily lifted by a girl and then is "mortified," perhaps by how little effort it took to control him. This image may relate to Dodge's own sense of power over men and her disrespect for men who are manipulated too easily. This could also connect to her feelings about Jelliffe, whom she saw as "commanding" and "sure of himself, and not to be moved" (Luhan, 1936, p. 444).*

8   Dodge's home never felt pleasant, as it was filled with her father's unhappiness, her mother's lack of affection, and a constant threat of tears, shouting, or violence.

δ

14.
January 6, 1916

I am in a large dark room, in a big house. I am afraid. There is some menace. The wind shakes the house & makes strange knockings overhead. Something unknown is to be frightened at. I am crouching on the wooden floor.

[Bayard] Boyeson [1] is near me in the dark. He knows there is something to be afraid of but it is he who trys [*sic*] to reassure me & protect me. He trys [*sic*] to draw the covers over me closer. I repeatedly ask him what it is that is going to happen. I move nearer him. My hand brushes against his organs. I realize the lack of that personal relation between us & am glad. There are continued sounds.[2]

Jelliffe's notes from January 7, 1916:
B[ayard].B[oyeson].:/ J[elliffe]. either genius or madman/ My idea of what you will do to him.[3] Last night dreamed all night:/ Jealous breath/ Father like him./ Breath antisocial/ Sense of smell:/

Notes:

1   Boyeson is a frequent presence in Dodge's dreams from this time, resulting in the following exchange in her analysis, as she reports in *Movers and Shakers* (1936):

> Seeing Jelliffe welcome Bayard's appearance in my dreams, I asked him slyly:
> "Do you really think that flirtation is a form of sublimation—a suitable outlet?"
> "Surely," he replied. "At times it may become the necessary and constructive tool that one requires."
> "For an amputation, you mean?" I asked him quickly. For I had never admitted to him that Maurice was detrimental to me. I never admitted it. I was never really disloyal to the relationship that I clung to, I only wanted it fixed up so that we could be happy....He smiled at me:
> "Come! Come!" he murmured, reassuringly. "I do not want anything for you that you do not want for yourself. This is your affair. You yourself have that in you which will decide what is best. Your judgment, not mine, will solve your problem." (pp. 456–457)

2   *The fear and repeating knocking sounds in this dream, together with the reference to touching Boyeson's organs and her observation in her associations that her father was "like him," suggest an awareness of her father's sexual life, or perhaps fears of incest or hearing her parents having sex (primal scene).*

3   *This comment could be connected to Dodge's thinking about what Jelliffe should address when Boyeson comes to him for analysis. It may also hint at her awareness of Boyeson's homosexuality and wondering how that would play out in his treatment.*

δ

15.
[circa January 7, 1916] (1 of 2)
[written in red in Jelliffe's notes from January 7, 1916]

On a void space. In ground, little bunch of rice from which steam was rising, peculiar smell.[1] A voice said that is knowledge of evil.

> Jelliffe's notes from January 7, 1916:
> *Earliest dream I ever had:*
>> *Before I began to menstruate:*[2]
>>> *8–9: some little girl & I began to talk re babies….Began to think of one,/ Then I thought of it in my stomach which began to swell up—Began to be afraid:/ Shame,*[3] *humiliation, agony—did not dare to go to parties./ no relation c. mo./ Then I had to tell her—"I am going to have baby"—"I have thought myself into having it"*[4]—*She explained.*

Notes:

1 ***Given the content of her associations to pregnancy, this could be a disguised image of ejaculate, from which a strange smell emanated. This dream, then, may connect to the possible primal scene action in the previous dream. As revealed in Jelliffe's case notes from March 23, 1916 (see dreams 57 & 58), Dodge's father was sent to a sanatorium for "self-abuse," i.e., masturbation, soon after his marriage.*** One of Dodge's earliest memories is of visiting him there. This could be the "Insane Asylum" that she describes in Background (1933a) as a "darkened mass" where "we all knew there were people inside that we had seen among us. And we knew that any one [*sic*] might go there….It was one of the monstrous terrors that we almost knew and harbored" (p. 6).

2 Jelliffe's intake of Mabel Dodge (see Figure 3.4) records that she began menses at age 13, therefore dating this recalled dream from before 1892.

3 Dodge writes in *Background* (1933a) about an early experience of shame when she was staying in a New York hotel with her mother. An unfamiliar man greeted her mother in the lobby and she told him she would put Mabel to bed and then return to see him. Her mother instructed her to "go right to sleep" and then left her in the room alone and terrified: "Where was my mother and what was she doing? I felt it was secret and strange and shameful. How could a child have had any such knowledge of shame? Was it shame?" (p. 64).

4 At this very early age, Dodge had already experienced the power of her mind to create a dramatic effect upon her body, as she reports in an unpublished section of her memoirs where she and two friends wonder where babies come from:

> I don't know how this first idea of the power of thought came to me—I said: "You think and think of a baby until you think one for yourself

and it begins to grow in your stomach." And this notion took hold of me....I struggled to forget it—this Frankenstein of my thirteen years—but it would not leave me. All day long I thought about how babies came by thinking—and I grew more and more frightened and terribly ashamed. Pretty soon I saw that it was so, for my little belly began to swell, to grow large under my anxious hands....In an agony I went to my distant mother one hot summer day. She was always distant and unaware. When I, suffocating, managed to tell her my fear, she looked at me in cold amusement...."Nonsense, don't talk so. You can't have a baby without a <u>man</u>."....

"A man!" I thought, groping in my imagination for a clue to this. "How a man?" and at that moment the terror of thought gave place to the terror of the male. "Oh mama! How a man? Could a man have done this to me without my knowing it? Or when I was asleep? Oh <u>tell</u> me?" I begged. For the first time in my life I begged my mother. ("Intimate Memories, Vol. II," n.d., pp. 404–406)

Pregnancy appears as a frequent theme in Dodge's dreams, speaking to her need for maternal love in her inversely related effort to fill herself up with a baby. She stated in a letter to Jelliffe, circa May 24 (Interlude 17), that she "started life wanting fifteen children."

δ

16.
[circa January 7, 1916] (2 of 2)
[written in red in Jelliffe's notes from January 7, 1916]

Another repeating dream, terrible, nightmare, scream, bilious. Began very early 1–2 years old.

Indescribable. False values, something coming towards me.[1] I towards it. A world of unfamiliarities, as ceasing.

Jelliffe's notes from January 7, 1916:
tactile sense—vivid—hands get very large. Can feel self clasping self—all large.

Note:

1 *The palpable fear in this dream—"self clasping self"—connects to the two previous dreams, with loud noises, shame, and suggestions of sex. Could this be another dream containing fears of incest or another kind of threatening sexual activity?*

δ

17.
January 10, 1916

At one moment I saw I had on Mrs. [Constance] Fletcher's coat.[1] I don't know how I knew it was hers. It was furlined on the inside & on the outside had dark blue silk with small sprigs of flowers on it.[2] I looked on the inside & found it was lined with a patchwork quilting of different colored silks.

> Jelliffe's notes from January 10, 1916:
> *Flash: Mrs. Fletcher's coat:/ lots of other things last night....*
> *Fetichis [sic]:/ Woman's breast:/ squirted milk across room: Surprise shock:/ strange mode of retaliation./ one answers this with slight fright— (4–5).[3]*
> *Another occasion: Swedish nurse. asleep. mauling breast violent & gentle at the same time—(4–5).[4]*
> *Island of memory:/ self in bed: next another servant, to another, operation for cancer of breast: Wondered if I had hurt her/.[5]*

Notes:

1 The image of this coat may relate to a story about the meeting of Fletcher and Alice B. Toklas in 1911. Dodge had asked Toklas to meet Fletcher's train, as Toklas recalls in *What is Remembered* (1963): "You will know her, said Mabel, because she is deaf and will be wearing a purple robe. When I got to the railroad station Miss Fletcher came up to me. She was wearing not a purple robe but a bright green one, she was not deaf but nearly blind and peered through her lorgnons" (p. 66). *The fur inside this coat could serve to provide comfort and holding that Dodge might seek after the three previous dreams filled with fear and sexual overtones.*
2 If embroidered, these flowers may be a reference to Constance Fletcher's talent with thread.
3 In *Background* (1933a), Dodge tells the story of spying on the "girls" in the kitchen of her Buffalo home and witnessing an amazing spectacle: "They had a visitor, a fat gay female...I saw her rip open the front of her dress and drag her great breast out from the shelving corset that supported it. With a quick pressure she directed a stream of pale milk right across the room on to [sic] the three squawking servant girls, who hid their faces from this shower....I couldn't get the picture out of my mind. Continually I saw again the fine stream of grayish milk striking across the room, and I longed to see it again in actuality" (p. 30).
4 Dodge (1933a) reports that she attempted to recreate this scene of the milk-spurting breast with a Swedish servant girl named Elsa. One night while her mother was away in New York, Dodge convinced Elsa to sleep in her bed after pleading that she was scared to be alone:

I had no plan, no thought, of what I wanted—I just wanted.

I waited, quiet, until I knew she was asleep and then I drew nearer to her....With a great firmness, I leaned over her and seized her big warm breast in both hands. It was a large, ballooning, billowing breast, firm and resilient and with a stout, springing nipple. I leaned to it and fondled it. I felt my blood enliven me all over and I longed to approach the whole of my body to her bosom, to cover her completely by my entire surface and have the bounding breast touch me at every point. I rolled it ecstatically from side to side and slathered it with my dripping lips. As my sudden new, delicious pleasure increased, I grew rougher. I longed now to hurt it and wring something from it. I wanted to pound it and burst it. Suddenly I remembered that other breast seen long ago in the kitchen, and I wanted to force from this one the same steely stream of milk that I felt within it, resisting me....I and that breast were alone in the night and that was what I wanted. (pp. 30–31)

5 Dodge describes hearing about Elsa's cancer from a neighbor's servant, who reported: "'She had to have a cancer cut out of one breast. She never knew anything until one day she felt a lump there as big as an egg—and hard. And she's in the hospital now, poor thing! Who would have thought a big healthy girl like that would get such a thing?'" (1933a, pp. 32–33).

δ

18.
January 14, 1916

Morning. Light & feeling better in morning usually the reverse, also this morning crazy energetic. Yesterday: old me good thing: School[.]

A girl joins us *(2–3 people)*. She comes from abroad. She seems to be Maurie Box [1] whom *(adopted girl)* I used to know as sad. She is self[-]assured & laughing & dressed in smart attractive clothes. She has legs & shoes of an 1830 shape. *(certain pictures—no heel shoes [)]* I refer them to an 1830 dress *dress I saw in window day before* I saw in a window yesterday. I see her shoes are made of fur.[2] When she shows her soles they are like the bottom of an animal[']s feet & the toes are seperated [*sic*]. She joins us & leaves us & is happy & detached.

I join a funeral procession a large open space, a covered box in the centre, the coffin unseen.[3] Three motionless shapes stand to follow it all veiled in chiffon, no faces to be seen, colors crushed strawberry, grey blue & white.[4] We move on, the girl too.

Later I am in the South in the negro [5] portion of a town tho['] I don't see any negro[e]s. I am driving a pony [6] up a slippery hill. He slides sideways & falls thro' a crevice in a rock & swings down into a cave—he dangles at the end of the reins which I hold. I am down there & have to seize him in my arms & pull him down out of the air where he swings—then we go on.

Jelliffe's notes from January 15, 1916:
Always had a horror of being adopted: John often asks me if he's not adopted:/ One thing: recall—nurse to chambermaid my little shoes: father[']s shape = she'll never be able to deny her father: no/ Mother[']s family no relationship [7]:/

Notes:

1 Unidentified.
2 ***This image of fur connects to the furlined coat in the previous dream, continuing the feeling of comfort.***
3 It is unknown whether this dream is in response to an actual funeral, but a week later, Dodge has a related dream (# 26) when she sees crepe, a symbol of death, at a friend's house. Death was certainly in the headlines with daily reports of casualties from World War I. Or, this image could link to her father's funeral in 1902, as her associations frequently recall him.
4 These colors of red, white, and blue also appear in dream 44, as colors of the American flag, and perhaps are associations to the war.
5 This is the first of many references to "negro" people in Dodge's dreams. At this time in New York, during what came to be called the Great Migration, hundreds of thousands of black people from the South were migrating to urban areas in the North. Many settled in Harlem, eventually giving rise to the Harlem Renaissance that celebrated the music, literature, art, and culture of African-Americans. Dodge would very likely have seen the show of "Negro Art" in November 1914 at Stieglitz's 291 gallery, a crucial display of "statuary in wood by African Savages. This was the first time in the history of exhibitions, either in this country or elsewhere, that Negro statuary was shown solely from the point of view of art" (*Camera Work*, October 1916, p. 7). See note 5 about Van Vechten for dream 19.
6 As discussed in note 3 for dream 13, Dodge owned ponies when she was a child, including one named Cupid.
7 Dodge remembers hearing a nurse say that she was clearly related to her father because she has his shape, but does not take after her mother's appearance in any way. Therefore, she concludes, she could not possibly be adopted. ***However, could this adoption theme link to the lack of parental love that she suffered?*** Sometime in 1914, during the tumult of her relationship with John Reed, Dodge searched for a baby to adopt so that she could find an outlet for newly emerging maternal feelings. After

visiting many orphanages, she discovered no healthy babies available, but an eight-year-old girl, Elizabeth, had been returned to the orphanage because she wasn't successful in her studies. Dodge took her home for a trial and ended up not adopting her, but cared for her and paid for her education, sending her to the Elizabeth Duncan School with her son. John's question about being adopted may stem from his observations of the detached way his mother treated little Elizabeth during these years, like a doll she could clothe and bathe, as Dodge herself reported: "As I look back on it now, I think all I wanted was to make a picture of her. The raw human blood instinct for a baby had been defeated, for I still had nothing in my arms. I was still without the warm lump to hold and to relax with. Elizabeth was too big. But it was fun to dress her in her white muslins and her pink and blue ribbons" (Luhan, 1936, pp. 310–311). In addition, John likely sensed his mother's profound preoccupation during his early years that interfered with their initial attachment. As Dodge admitted, "All through the first years of his babyhood, it was as though I had been away from him, though he was always right there. I never knew John as a baby. This thought comes back over and over and tightens upon my heart like a hand" (1936, p. 308). Perhaps most relevant to John's frequent inquiry about being adopted is the question about his paternity, as Dodge was not certain about whether Dr. John Parmenter (whom John was named after) or her husband Karl Evans fathered her son. John may have sensed early on the looming presence of this family secret.

δ

19.
Saturday [circa January] 15, 1916 (1 of 2)

A man dashes by me & up the stairs of the elevated. I want to see if he will catch his train so I rush after him up 3 or 4 stairs at a time,[1] two or three flights. I lose him at the top but I find I am very high up, several flights higher than I was at the bottom. I go down. In a large darkish room—it is night—someone & I have someone sick [who] is young to take care of—a negro is a dark animal.[2] I don't know—we find there isn't a bit of <u>feed</u> left. I feel in the box, there are only a few <u>black</u> oats there—& someone else besides needs food.[3] I reprimand the other person & send them out to get it—perhaps I cry—perhaps someone else crys [sic]—it is all sad and worrisome. I have a baby in my arms.[4] I have a sensual feeling about it & it has a meaning[ful] look on its face. I rub its buttocks with my hand.

Jelliffe's notes from January 17, 1916:
Here is a note—...Advertisement in negro literature: (1913).[5] Always wanted to be a transmitter.[6]/....It may be I have never loved a.o. in my

life: possibly all only narcissistic [7]:/ *in the ♂ act I don't find I get any direct reaction. Extra stimuli: no feeling in vagina* [8]:/ *Better physical relation/ Rect[al] ♂ / 2 painful & repugnant. No other than that./ Colitis & hemorrhoids.*[9]

Notes:

1 This image recalls Freud's dream of mounting a flight of stairs: "I was going up three steps at a time and was delighted at my agility." In his analysis, he observed: "I usually go upstairs two or three steps at a time; and this was recognized in the dream itself as a wish-fulfilment: the ease with which I achieved it reassured me as to the functioning of my heart. Further, this method of going upstairs was an effective contrast to the inhibition in the second half of the dream" (Freud, 1900, p. 238). In general, but not in this particular dream, Freud connected this sense of movement to the arousal of sexual feelings (Freud, 1900, p. 272). *This movement up the stairs could indicate sexual content, as the dream ends with a "sensual feeling" about a baby at the same time that people are crying and the situation is "sad and worrisome."*

2 A reference to "negro" appeared in the previous dream. *Dodge's description here of "a negro" as a "dark animal" indicates her more primitive response, perhaps an association to the "darkish room."*

3 *There is not enough food—in fact, the only food is "black" and seems spoiled—to care for the sick person and "someone else," a situation Dodge herself never faced literally but certainly symbolically, as she painfully experienced lack of nurturance at home.*

4 *Dodge has longed for this very moment, a baby in her arms, an outlet for her maternal instincts. However, her report of a "sensual feeling" and the rubbing of the baby's buttocks cause the scene to turn toward the sexual, perhaps suggesting a confusion between caregiving and sexual intimacy?*

5 This advertisement is very likely the following one written by Dodge and intended for circulation among her friends and acquaintances: "A number of us feel that a new literature will be coming from the colored people, & this advertisement is to ask anyone who reads it to send any manuscripts that they may have—stories, poetry or plays or anything for a sympathetic reading to the name & address below. Mabel Dodge, 23 Fifth Avenue. New York." This note appears in the Jelliffe papers at MDLC and is dated 1914, not 1913, in what appears to be Jelliffe's handwriting. Dodge had most likely learned about "negro literature" through her close friendship with Carl Van Vechten. At one of Dodge's first salons, he had introduced two black performers, as she recalls: "The first Evening I can remember was engineered by Carl, who wanted to bring a pair of Negro entertainers he had seen somewhere who, he said, were marvelous. Carl's interest in Negroes began as far back as that, then" (1936, p. 79).

6 Through her salons at the Villa Curonia and 23 Fifth Avenue, Dodge was a transmitter, devoting herself to creating a lively atmosphere thrumming with the exchange of new ideas, debate, and the formation of new connections between people.

7 *Dodge offers this powerful interpretation: an awareness of the narcissistic gratification she often, or maybe exclusively, seeks in love relationships.*

8 Dodge speaks very directly to Jelliffe about her sexual feelings and how she could not locate her orgasm in her vagina. Freud (1905b) believed that the vaginal orgasm was superior to the clitoral orgasm (p. 221), and it is likely that Jelliffe's interest in the topic was informed by this idea, as supported by Dodge's admission in a letter to Jelliffe circa May 24 (see Interlude 17): "the orgasm took place in the vagina because that has occurred more or less since the analysis directed it there."

9 These reports of anal intercourse, colitis, and hemorrhoids are perhaps related and notably appear in her associations following a dream about rubbing the buttocks of a baby.

δ

20.
Saturday [circa January] 15, 1916 (2 of 2)

Later in a society—in the evening. I see Mrs. W.[1] from some distance from the side. I particularly notice her breast which I see hangs down. I can see it because she has a long open cloak on. I move so I can see it again.[2]

Notes:

1 Unidentified. This could refer to either Mrs. [first name unknown] Wolcott, a woman from Buffalo who also saw Mabel Dodge in Florence, or the unidentified Mrs. Whitehouse referred to in note 2 for dream 3, or, most likely, to Mrs. Wilcox, the stepmother of Dodge's friend Nina Wilcox in Buffalo. Nina's own mother had died in childbirth and her father soon married her mother's sister, Grace Rumsey.

2 *This drive to see the breast relates to Dodge's associations about the spurting milk in dream 17 and reveals her urgent hunger for nurturance.*

δ

21.
Monday, January 16, 1916 [1]

A large open space, like a market place. I see a lot of boxes [2] made of wooden framework with sides & top of chicken wire. I think it will be a good idea to fill one with apples & take into the house. Very far off I make out Leo Stein walking with some woman.[3]

Jelliffe's notes from January 17, 1916:
*Emotion of dream/ Baffling: peering: hard to get hold of. <u>Curing</u>: <u>Oranges,</u>
<u>apples</u> I mean into the house.*

   Chicken wire: sides & top/ suggests nothing/ cage of this dream [4] *gets
worse as I think.*

   *Stein/ Walking off in distance:/ some other people:/ Very apt to dream
of baby in arms* [5]:/

Notes:

1 Monday was January 17 in 1916. Dodge likely meant Sunday night, thus
January 16 as indicated.
2 *According to Freud (1900), boxes are symbols of the uterus (p. 354) and
here Dodge is wanting to "fill one with apples," perhaps a reference to getting pregnant.*
3 Stein's appearance with a woman may be related to current rumors
about his intention to marry Nina Auzius (whom he eventually married in 1921). He confided in Dodge about his intimate relationships,
as revealed in one letter to her, circa late 1916, where he accuses her of
leaking information: "I...wanted to bust somebody's head and this is
the sad part of it that your head had the preference. It all came about
because some one [*sic*] asked me whether it was true that I was going
to marry Nina. Now as this person had heard the thing from somebody anonymous and as my private affairs didn't seem to me to be
Greenwich Village's public business, I felt very much like taking it out
on you." He continues: "There is another matter in some ways more
important in all ways more private. What I told you about Gertrude &
myself. I hope you have not told that to others." As he admits in his
memoir, *Journey into the Self* (1950): "Those earliest experiences with
women led to a terrific fear of them and the refusal to admit that fear
led to an incapacity for the slightest submission. I was utterly incapable of the romantic chivalrous attitude of subordination...and could
hardly be polite to them. I had girl and women friends at all times but
my attitude toward them was simply comradely. All sex expression toward them was rigorously suppressed and was reserved in later years
for prostitutes" (p. 198). He wrote to Dodge circa late 1916 concerning
the prospect of her marrying Maurice Sterne: "Of course as you know,
I know very few women, especially of the kind that radiate, as one
might say, both tentacles and influence, and your dynamic breed may
have more representatives than I suspect. Nonetheless I cherish you as
my only specimen, and don't want to see you clipped either as to tentacles or wings."
4 *This association to the box (that she first wanted to fill with apples) as
a cage might betray Dodge's feelings of being trapped in her difficult*

relationship with Sterne: at the same time that she wants to have a baby, she is constrained by the fact she is in relationship with him.

5 *Dodge's longing for nurturance led her toward wanting a baby to love her, not for her to love.* She had dreamed of a baby in her arms in dream 19.

δ

22.
January 17–18, 1916

Neith [Boyce] [1] was showing me the house where she used to live—old fashioned & quaint. She shows me the dining room & says: "You see this was some woman's room. She wanted this piece of mahogany furniture turned around like this so she just put it so."

Associated with Neith, in the dream I see a picture of a beautiful motionless dark eastern—I cannot see whether it is a man or woman—it may be a Buddha.[2] In the background are heads of natives.[3] I remember I said yesterday "Neith is a primitive."[4]

Later by the sea I see some ducks & waterfowl. I tell Bayard [Boyeson] we must order some for the farm.

Notes:

1 At the time of this dream, Boyce and Hapgood were struggling to navigate the terms of their open marriage, mutually agreed upon, but problematic in the details, particularly of Hapgood's current affair with Lucy Collier. Both Boyce and Hapgood wrote to Dodge during this time. On January 13, 1916, Hapgood wrote to Dodge from Provincetown: "How I love you! With such an undisturbed, deep love, one that never varies….My feeling for you is one of the realist things in my life…. My life is wonderful—just now. Neith is more than wonderful." Only days later, he accused Dodge of being "so sure about everything!" as she had charged him with "Unselfishness! Egotism!" while betraying his trust: "You are always harsh and one-sided because you see only abstractions of people and never people." He signed this letter: "One of your past experiences." Boyce also wrote to Dodge in January 1916, trying to correct Dodge's assessment of the situation with Lucy Collier: "And you picture her and me fighting over Hutch's body? How enchanting! But I really think you're wrong there. I don't care so much about the sexual act as you think—it's not of primary importance! If she wants that with him she can have it, naturally….Mabel, you've taken a very primitive view of the situation—of what started out as to be a very civilized arrangement! (I think you do take a very primitive view of the love-relation anyway.)" Boyce and Hapgood's negotiations around

jealousy and the primary sexual relationship are in stark contrast to Dodge's fierce possessiveness of her lover Sterne.

2 This image of a Buddha or an "eastern" figure indicates Dodge's awareness of Eastern philosophy and religion, and her openness to other ways of thinking. When she first met Sterne in 1915, she observed that he had "'Oriental charm'" (1936, p. 351).

3 Sterne had painted native people during his years living in Bali from 1912 to 1914, and, soon after she met him, Dodge bought a drawing of a native priest from his exhibition at Birnbaum's gallery in New York.

4 This is the first appearance of the word primitive in Dodge's dreams: "Jelliffe had taught me to use that word: primitive" (Luhan, 1936, p. 455). See note 3 for dream 117.

δ

23.
January 19–20, 1916

I was trying to get something done in the law and also marry someone. Dr. Jelliffe was my lawyer & also an english bishop.[1] He was very wise & kind & reassuring. I drove around the public square in Rome in a carriage & then went to find Dr. Jelliffe. The person I was going to marry couldn't get away that evening so I said to Condamine [2] he would come. (He is h.s.[3]) So we went & met Dr. J. I said ["]'So & so' couldn't come so I brought Condamine." They both laughed at the farfetched joke. Then Dr. J. & I left him & we went on to make further preparations. We had to down-down (into the unconscious?) [4] a sort of ladder [5] in the air from the world above—down to his club. I went ahead lying back to the ladder & he coming after me. But the ladder proved to be only pieces of wood laid across each other. It was like a lot of loose matches. I held it together with my feet & hands & went on. I felt him nervous behind me & called out: "Come on—it's all right."[6] Suddenly he whispered "Look out—there's a message waiting for me."[7] I saw at the bottom of the ladder at the club—a black face [8] waiting. I knew he had a wire or a letter or a phone message. Then I woke up.

In another part of same dream I was in the huge over[-]burdened house of E.A.[9] Lots of people were coming to an afternoon party of some kind. I had written the sketch of an address for her [10] to make. She read it over & said it was splendid. Everyone including her were [sic] overdressed.[11] I felt bored & superior.[12]

Jelliffe's notes from January 20, 1916:
While in bed, suddenly Maurice [Sterne] stood in front of me, black, evil expression. Opaque, warm & heavy & thick—air up & down beyond me. struggle. shudder & horror, tried to get through it…[Marsden] Hartley

still there: no conversation up to yesterday: He said why Mabel do I always think of negroes: Maybe my face is getting a shade darker than I saw 2 yrs. ago. Jews & negroes.[13] *Jewish liver almost always a sick liver!...Hartley—spoke of pigment & liver:# Stern[e] said going to negro quarter# Then I commenced to think/ the negro. This explains M[arsden]. to me: factory boy, came up from gutter* [14]...

Robinson: poet: Walking in Boston: noted peculiar quality of brick, black faces in window: rub off on things./[15]

Another thing I put down...he [Hartley] does not talk./ 2–3 times facing. Whole face changed, "black & evil"[16] *saw things.*

Notes:

1 *Dodge sees her analyst as both a lawyer and a bishop, indications of her transference to him as an authority with power.*

2 Robert de la Condamine, nicknamed Robin, whom Dodge knew from Florence and whose homosexuality and efforts at celibacy were commonly known. As Dodge writes in *European Experiences* (1935), Condamine was "a strange, wonderful fellow" who was "uninhibited, happy, intelligent, and industrious. Very different, indeed, from the types who came to Italy to live and safely practice their tragic habit, safe because the Italian government had repealed the old law against that practice.... Robin's celibacy was deliberately philosophical, and chosen by him for the sake of the higher consciousness he could reach through continence. He wrote one of the most curious books in the world about various states of celibate being and experience" (pp. 264, 265–266).

3 i.e., homosexual.

4 *Dodge's interpretation here of going deeper, as signaling her belief in the unconscious, shows her as a good student and / or patient of Jelliffe's and worthy of his admiration.*

5 *Freud (1900) wrote: "Steps, ladders or staircases, or, as the case may be, walking up or down them, are representations of the sexual act" (p. 355). In fact, Dodge had her own erotic associations to a ladder. In her restoration of the Villa Curonia, she included a fanciful touch in her bedroom—a silk ladder coming from a trap door in the ceiling, intended for impulsive romantic visits from Edwin, whose room was directly above. "But," Dodge bemoaned, "Edwin never hastened down it except once to see if it would work, and it did, perfectly" (1935, 159).*

6 *This passage in the dream suggests Dodge's erotic transference to Jelliffe, encouraging him as they descended into the unconscious or her fantasy of sexual union with him. The ladder itself was fragile, however, not as strong as it appeared, and Dodge "held it together" as Jelliffe was "nervous behind me."*

7 *Could this message be a communication to Jelliffe from Dodge's unconscious?*

8 This black face connects to the mention of "negro" in dreams 18 and 19.

9 i.e., Edwin Arlington Robinson, American poet who was to win three Pulitzer Prizes. At this time, he had been living for a number of years at La Tourette, a brick mansion (reportedly haunted) in Staten Island that was owned by Clarissa Davidge, who, according to Dodge, "collected old furniture and promising artists" and "furnished her house with spinning wheels, Cape Cod china, four-post bedsteads, a painter and a poet" (1936, p. 123). After being introduced to each other by Davidge, Robinson and Dodge became friends, an unlikely occurrence according to Dodge's initial impressions of him, as she offers in *Movers and Shakers* (1936): "He was without doubt the most inarticulate man I have ever known. He usually couldn't or anyway didn't say a word....How I ever made friends with him, wrote him letters, got answers, consulted him about things, told him everything, in fact, and heard, in turn, his opinions of everyone and everything, is amazing to think of now, as I remember the hermetic exterior he presented" (pp. 129–130). However, they did connect, deeply, at a later meeting, as Dodge relates: "E.A. and I, in a reciprocal flicker of the utmost brevity, met, exchanged a certain essential knowledge of each other, realized each other, and for so long as we lasted, I knew, would be cronies, pals, comrades, friends, affinities, or whatever; too much *en rapport* to be lovers, too sympathetic, perhaps, to be lovers" (1936, p. 127). Dodge reports the following conversation between them that took place during a lunch together around this time:

> "Do you know they have doctors now to cure the *soul*?" he said.
> "Yes, and I'm going to be *done* some day," I laughed. "Just to find out about it."
> "Dangerous business, perhaps. Maybe the cure is worse than the disease."
> "Well, I'll let you know." (1936, p. 444)

Dodge then writes: "I was not finding it at all dangerous. It was interesting to watch my soul provide exciting subjects to discuss with Jelliffe. Whenever things got dull, something would turn up from down below to keep the ball rolling—and he and I chased it about" (1936, p. 445).

10 This almost certainly refers to Clarissa Davidge.

11 Dodge reported that Davidge "always dressed like the doll of any little girl of ten who has had recourse to the family ragbag and secured bits of gay silk, fur, and lace" (1936, p. 123).

12 These are familiar feelings for Dodge from her childhood and beyond.

13 It is unknown whether this preoccupation of Hartley's with "Jews & negroes" has any basis in fact, but the increasing appearance in Dodge's dreams of images of darker skin and black people may reflect her growing

exposure to black culture through Carl Van Vechten and the beginnings of the Harlem Renaissance. See note 5 for dream 19 and note 3 for dream 81.

14 Hartley grew up poor and once worked in a shoe factory in Maine (Hartley, 1997, p. 55).

15 Dodge provides the story behind her association to Robinson:

> ....And he told me an experience he had had in Boston one time. He said he liked to take long walks, not noticing his surroundings particularly. He liked to walk in long, uninterrupted rhythm while he worked things out.
>
> "That's why I like to go uptown [in New York] and walk round and round the reservoir," he continued. "When one walks on any of the avenues one is interrupted at every corner and one loses the rhythm. I liked to walk in Boston because there is less traffic there. Well, one day I started out among the red brick buildings of Boston and I walked and walked, not noticing much where I was going. After a while I came to myself. I was still among the red brick houses, but I noticed they were different. Different in quality from those I had come away from. Not different in shape or color, but different in quality. I couldn't make out what that difference was at first. Finally I noticed a Negro, then another. I saw I was in the Negro quarter. The Negroes made the red brick houses different. They were coming through...." (1936, p. 135)

16 *This classic association between black and evil may indicate Dodge's unconscious beliefs about "negro" people in her dreams, despite her professed openness to "negro literature" and having black entertainers at her salon (see note 3 for dream 81).*

δ

24.
[circa January 20, 1916]
[written in red in Jelliffe's notes from January 20, 1916]

Big omnibus: candy—driver asks if gritty powder—yes lived it—war [1] in air, smoke, parachutes, now drop, parachutes, one woman nearly drowned a lot of excitement: I was looking at it:

> Jelliffe's notes from January 20, 1916:
> *"One woman almost drowned."*
>   *Striking thing? Seeing aeroplane get on fire, put out parachute. They all on fire.*
>   *Emotional / Felt horror, heart beating, danger they were in; just something happening;/ pleasurable excitement.*

Note:

1 News about World War I was in the headlines of *The New York Times* every day, with reports of drownings ("260 Lost on Brindisi" when an Italian steamship sank after striking a mine in the Adriatic Sea) and warfare ("French Gun Fire Wrecks 2 Zeppelins") (January 19, 1916, p. 1). Reports of airplanes in battle were frequent: "Raid of French Aeroplanes Causes Great Panic in Bulgarian Capital" (January 11, 1916, p. 1) and "Allied Aviators in Many Fights…19 Air Duels in One Day" (January 20, 1916, p. 2).

δ

25.
Thursday night [undated, circa January 20, 1916]

I kept dreaming of tables spread with food & drink which would disappear or I would wake up before I could take anything. And flowers to pick which would disappear before I could get them.[1] Then Walter Lippmann [2] came along & took my thoughts off them. He was very near & affectionate & somehow consoling. I remembered on awakening how a cerebrally excited interest in him last time had helped me over the bad time with [John] Reed. [3] No sex attraction but mental attraction.

Notes:

1 *This theme of nurturance or beauty (flowers) disappearing speaks to Dodge's continual hunger for comfort and sustenance, and also perhaps to a fear that good things do not last.*
2 Lippmann appears a number of times in Dodge's dreams from this period. She turned to him for honest and direct advice on her relationships with Reed and Sterne. In *Movers and Shakers* (1936), Dodge writes movingly of his internal presence for her: "I don't think Walter ever knew how strongly he figured in my fantasies….The fact is, like most real women, all my life I had needed and longed for the strong man who would take the responsibility for me and my decisions. I wanted to lie back and float on the dominating decisive current of an all-knowing, all-understanding man….Walter seemed to be the only person I knew that I could really look up to, which I did in my imagination. It was a small private image and it helped me along" (p. 310).
3 It is interesting that Reed and Lippmann appear in the same dream, as they graduated in the same class from Harvard, and Lippmann, as mentioned above, often served as Dodge's consultant for her tumultuous union with Reed, a relationship that ended and resumed a number of times, with each of them entertaining other lovers, until Reed returned from

Europe in the fall of 1915 to find Dodge living with Sterne and no longer enamored with him. Reed then met journalist Louise Bryant in December 1915 and married her in November of the following year. This dream may have been stimulated in part by Dodge's awareness that Reed and Bryant began living together in January 1916 at 43 Washington Square South (Watson, 1991, p. 409).

δ

INTERLUDE 1.

During these early weeks of her analysis with Jelliffe, Dodge writes to him from Finney Farm with an idea for his participation in an issue of Alfred Stieglitz's journal *Camera Work*.

[circa January 1916]

Dear Dr. Jelliffe,

I have just been conspiring with myself & have written Stieglitz—to the effect that this number of Camera Work containing you & Brill should be devoted to a free discussion of Modern Art—& I told him that added to you & Brill, (whose article, I believe, is "The value of artistic expression in the Sane & the Insane"—) we should have Leo Stein write a critique of Modern Art defending the object & nature & his rival [Willard Huntington] Wright [1] write one defending the abstract—thus we have the two most able art critics, then two artists should write one defending the abstract & the other the concrete school in modern art, & then two gallery men, such as [Stephan] Bourgeois & [Newman Emerson] Montross,[2] to tell us the picture dealers['] point of view & attitudes towards it—(& from them we get the Public's point of view—!)—and altogether we would get up a fine balanced ambivalent symposium composed of pairs of opposites!

I wish you would do one called "The Psycho-Genetics of Modern Art"— because these pictures are the bodies of these artists—sick or well—& a true index to their souls & of what ails them. Just keep this as a note. I wrote it lest I forget to talk of it to you.

Ever yrs—
Mabel Dodge

Stieglitz had written to Dodge on January 20, 1916, about a meeting that she had maybe suggested, and with ideas for this issue that never appeared:

I was certainly sorry not to be able to be with you and Dr. J. I am sure we would have had a live[ly] time of it....
I spent an evening with Brill. It wasn't quite what I had been lead [*sic*] to expect, but it was nevertheless of importance. I had hoped

that he would have sufficient drawings etc., to make an exhibition. But he had in mind an article for Camera Work, illustrated with a few things—very extraordinary things—done by a certain patient of his, and other things done by children. The whole was to be published in Camera Work. I told him to go ahead and get his idea into form, and to give me the material....I see a great possibility of bringing out an interesting number devoted to the question that you, Dr. J., Brill, myself, as well as some others seem to be especially interest[ed] in just at present.

Notes:

1 New York art critic who praised the form of abstraction practiced by his brother, the Synchromist painter Stanton MacDonald-Wright.
2 Both New York art dealers.

δ

26.
Friday night [undated, circa January 21, 1916] (1 of 3)

I saw crape [1] on the door of the Cary [2] house in Buffalo tho' there were lots of people apparently living there, going in & out happily.

Notes:

1 Crape, or crepe, is a material sometimes used as a sign of mourning, such as when tied around a sleeve or hat.
2 Further down Delaware Avenue from Dodge's house, Dr. Walter Cary and his wife Julia (née Love) owned a grand mansion, described by Dodge in *Background* (1933a):

> Their house was a tall mass, towerlike and ending in a cupola. It stood near the street and was covered with ivy....it attracted me from the first time I saw it, and I knew that it was distinguished and alive. The *feeling* there was of a gracious, well-bred, appreciative family life where every one [*sic*] was unfolding his scroll as God had written it. The bitter irony and caustic, stinging, tonic wit that went on in that house were good for me from the first day I ever entered there.
>
> I was hardened and shaped a good deal by that house and the people in it in later years....
>
> This Cary house was exceptional because, though there were other fine old houses in Buffalo that remained the same to a dignified old age and did not change with new tastes, ...the real life would be dead and the house no longer a functioning organism....But at the Carys',

there was the family—the big, amusing family with all its color and variety living there...in the same faded elegance, the rather shabby and distinguished milieu. (pp. 16–17)

This atmosphere of liveliness that Dodge recalls at the Cary house, contrasted with both the sameness of the building's appearance and its aging, relates to the comparison in her dream between the presence of crepe, a symbol of death, and the joy of the house's inhabitants. During her adolescence, Dodge preferred the exciting company of Seward, one of the six Cary sons, over most of her companions.

δ

27.
Friday night [undated, circa January 21, 1916] (2 of 3)

Then Mrs. Untermeyer [1] & I gave a party together & I provided the food which I ordered served in a <u>drugstore</u> some distance away, & which consisted of big healthy but coarse sandwiches & bottles of beer.[2] I saw <u>she</u> thought them not very delicate but I felt I was in the right because they were so essentially wholesome & good even if rather gross in appearance & being served down in that shop!

Jelliffe's notes written at the end of the dream:
Mrs. S. Untermeyer: Money for [Elizabeth] Duncan School. Asks me to do things:/ He is a big corporation lawyer, white haired & pretty./ She gave me $1000./...John Collier & I started it.[3]

Notes:

1   Minnie Untermyer, who was married to Samuel Untermyer, a powerful and wealthy corporate lawyer and businessman in New York. Their name was often misspelled as "Untermeyer," as done here by both Dodge and Jelliffe. Minnie Untermyer was involved in philanthropic support for the arts, such as the New York Philharmonic, and wrote a number of letters to Mabel Dodge at this time, enclosing concert tickets for her and her friends.
2   This party atmosphere differs dramatically from the elaborate and sophisticated one offered by Dodge at her 23 Fifth Avenue salon: "Pinch-bottles and Curtis Cigarettes, poured by the hundreds from their neat pine boxes into white bowls, trays of Virginia ham and white Gorgonzola sandwiches, pale Italian boys in aprons" (Van Vechten, 1927, p. 122). *The frequent appearance of food in Dodge's dreams suggests her large appetite for satisfaction and pleasure.*
3   In *Movers and Shakers* (1936), Dodge recalls a moment in 1915 when she was deeply affected by seeing a performance directed by

Elizabeth Duncan that featured her young female dancers: "Here was something to work for, I thought. If people can be developed like these children, then we must have a school in America where Elizabeth can make American children dance like these little nymphs. It was Collier's idea and he began to plan" (p. 341). Dodge donated $1,000 toward purchasing a building for the school and others soon followed her lead.

δ

INTERLUDE 2.

At this place in Jelliffe's case notes, the following fragment of a letter from Dodge to him appears:

In these days just before being unwell everything gets more insecure. Everything is more doubtful & more fearful.

The other night when I got home from Dr. J[elliffe].'s—(it was the end of the first day that Maurice was away) the craving for him began like a terrible restlessness in my blood. I thought of him never coming back—of it stopping right there and I couldn't stand it. I tried to get him on the telephone and couldn't—the feeling rose all thro' my body in every cell like a madness of wanting him back. Nothing seemed real in the place without him. Nothing had its significance. No one seemed to be there for me—but they [are] like shadows. Maurice is the bridge between me & reality. When he is not there I am seperated [sic] from it by a bottomless gulf. I don't care for anything or anybody. Ideas don't interest me.

The next day I got him on the telephone. I asked him if he would come back. He said he didn't know. I asked him to come—& he finally said he would come in the afternoon. That didn't do me any good during the day. The day was dead for me. Besides I was afraid that perhaps he would not come & that made me feel desperate as tho' I were sinking in deep water. I thought of the days & months I would have to suffer that feeling if he doesn't come back. I could not do any act all day. I lay on my bed & read a book. The craving for him was in my solar plexus & abdomen—not in the sex centre. It felt as tho' all the nerves involuntarily stretched themselves tight towards the centre. The muscles contracted automatically—pulling in to the centre. The desperate feeling became more & more intense flooding my whole body in waves. I cared only for one thing. To be near Maurice. No thought did any good. No thought of psychoanalysis as a refuge—or God—or anything. I knew my relief could come from the cause of my disturbance. I saw I was like Bayard in as much as I am in the grip of a passion or desire which has become too strong—but unlike him in being unable to fight it. I don't see how I can fight it unless I have to. I realized it as an appetite—and yet as my only source of being alive. I can't live on ideas. I want a warm human relationship. And yet I saw this one as having been turned into a neurosis because of its masturbatory character. I believe that it has been that for me. And that the sex relation has always had that character and that that is why in every case it has turned into a neurasthenic weakening thing. I lay weakly on the bed all the afternoon. I thought if he didn't come I would have to go to New York & look for him.

Finally he came. I had a terrific rise in vitality & flung myself into his arms weeping. He was surprised & quiet. He didn't feel anything that I did. He hadn't been unhappy—to speak of! He had been thinking but not craving. We talked. He said he <u>must</u> work. He's feeling it's me—our relation that takes away his impulse—his energy. I know it must but why can't we organize our sex life? He says that even if he isn't thinking of it that when he is near me it is automatic now & the desire rises of itself & floods him. And he cannot restrain himself, but gives himself at the moment every reason why he should go ahead & do it. And then he makes me want it—& we do it. And afterwards we argue & say we <u>must</u> organize it better.

We have done this so much lately—this arguing. You see we have had this sex life so constantly—practically every night—of course some exceptions—for eight months. So that now it, so to speak, operates itself. He cannot be near me without it rising in him & if it does he arouses it in me. It has ceased to be an expression of love but is an expression of pleasure.

Last night even after our talk when we both knew that it is <u>that</u> that will seperate [*sic*] us—we had to do it before we could sleep. His first question this morning was to ask me how long it would take me to get over my unhappiness if he should go away. This nearly killed me. I feel as tho' I couldn't face the struggle that it will be for my nerves & my emotions. And besides that I <u>love him</u>. There is no doubt about that. I love his massive qualities & he is interesting to me & more worth while [*sic*] than many—richer in personality. And yet he says that here he cannot find his own centre—that he feels only a part of himself—that in New York or away he feels more complete & whole—& that here my personality absorbs <u>his</u>. I dread a falling to pieces such as I have gone thro' before. Months of melancholy & depression & suicidal mania—usually ending in some organic illness. This time it will be worse than ever. I hardly know how I think that but I feel it is so. I had hoped so desperately that we could learn to handle this situation & make something of it & our life together. I see that the thing may be impossible. He said this morning he <u>must</u> work—he must work—that in the end he cares for nothing else. That he would not suffer as I would is plain because he would throw himself into something else—perhaps his work. I <u>want</u> him to work but I want him too. He will go to New York if he can find a studio, he says.

I know that all my feelings are aggravated by my appro[a]ching un-wellness & that that is why I am tearful all the time—but I know, too, that just as before, whenever a relation has become too sex-centered &

masturbatory in itself, I have found myself in an impasse unable to go forward or back—so now the only way out is thro' suffering unless you can show me a way—Dr. Jelliffe. But I can't transfer because, you see, I'm conscious of that as a process & it wouldn't work.

δ

28.
Friday night [undated, circa January 21, 1916] (3 of 3)

Later I was in my nightgown in my room & I had a nosebleed & covered myself & the bed with blood—as well from being un-well as from the nose-bleed.[1]

Note:

1   The presence of blood in this dream relates to Dodge's menstrual pe-riod, as indicated by her reference to "being unwell" in her previous letter fragment to Jelliffe (Interlude 2). *What could this mean, Dodge's covering herself and the bed with blood from her nose and uterus? Is there abandon here, relief?*

δ

29.
Sunday, January 23, 1916 (1 of 2)

I dreamed I got back home & someone told me Bobby [Jones] had been taken to the hospital to be operated again for appendicitis.[1] They said it was pretty serious—I understood <u>fatal</u>. I went to the hospital & looked for him. I saw some sick men ranged down a staircase apparently. One of them looked up at me standing at the top of the staircase & said something, laughingly, & made a gesture with his hand to "shoo" a big black cat [2] which jumped down the stairs away from him & disappeared. I turned to look for Bobby.

I had other dreams but can't catch them.

Jelliffe's notes from January 24, 1916:
Repetition of coming home/ Bobby Jones: ...Child / one of my children, responsible/ Friend of [John] Reed[']s, gifted & starving...
   All others re Bobby/ Add to theater/ only thing cares for/ Extremely ambitious/ Vanity. Exhibitionism./ Very successful c. Bobby. Moral responsibility.
   Why Bobby die/ Jealous c. M[aurice]./ if he will do his work...

Notes:

1 Jones had undergone emergency surgery for appendicitis in 1915, following a severely worsening condition that arose while he and Dodge were staying with Hapgood and Boyce in Dobbs Ferry, New York. According to Dodge, Jones woke her in the middle of the night, complaining of excruciating stomach pain and she dismissed him with: "'Well, go and tie a wet towel around it!'" (1936, p. 317). They returned to New York in the morning by car, with Jones vomiting. Dodge's doctor met them at 23 Fifth Avenue and sent Jones to the hospital by ambulance. While Jones was in surgery, Dodge stayed home, agonizing over her delay in responding, and fearful for his life:

> I closed my eyes and with all my power I sent my life to Bobby to save him....With complete concentration I lodged myself, my force, my living spark, in him to reinforce him.
>   I felt myself sitting on the chair in my room with my energy streaming out of me. Like ribbons of fire it rushed from me with terrific velocity—a flow unchained and undiminished by flowing. I felt it going directly to Bobby and entering him for about fifteen minutes. Then it ceased and I knew it was all right with him. This was a strange new experience, and very real.
>   I drove to the hospital, but he was still under the anesthetic. Dr. Lorber said: "At first I thought we had lost him, but he rallied."
>   I waited until he was conscious and they let me go in to see him....
>   "I thought I was dying," he said, "and I didn't want to. Then I felt you coming to me. I felt you streaming into me like strong ribbons of energy, helping me. And that saved me." (1936, p. 317)

When Jones was strong enough to leave the hospital, he recovered at 23 Fifth Avenue. Dodge reports that they both were "filled with wonder" at his survival: "He said I had created him, that I was his real mother; and there seemed to be, truly, a psychic bond between us" (1936, p. 318).

2 The appearance of this common symbol for bad luck may relate to how close to death Jones was during his operation. However, it may also be a reference to the black cat named Scuro, who lived at Finney Farm, and the intense jealousy that Sterne's affection for this cat triggered in Dodge, as she relates at length in *Movers and Shakers* (1936):

> I will never forget the feeling that went through me one evening when I caught sight of Maurice stroking Scuro. The black cat arched his back with pleasure and half closed his peculiar eyes. Maurice's large hand rubbed him over and over rhythmically and Scuro turned about backwards and forwards....He purred loudly like a little palpitating engine and closed his eyes ecstatically. Now I could almost see the exchange between those two, Maurice pouring his hot magnetism into the cat,

the cat passing his electricity up to Maurice. It seemed terribly dark and evil. Perhaps this is "bestiality," I thought.

Maurice suddenly caught sight of my horror and laughed slyly and silently. "Scuro is a nice cat," he said, persisting in his ministrations. Scuro throbbed. At the continued revolt in my face, perhaps, Maurice giggled....His expression was rather foolish and mixed with fear, more innocent than his laugh, more innocent than his hand. It was as though he were doing something he was almost, though not quite, aware of. (pp. 427–428)

δ

30.
[circa January 23, 1916] (2 of 2)
[written in red in Jelliffe's notes from January 24, 1916]

Dream of F[ather]. & m[e]. Boat. off together: Cabin together, I insisted. I will take upper, he lower. I insisted: Luggage, he can[']t get it all in [1] .../ Suddenly changed into M[aurice].

Jelliffe's notes from January 24, 1916:
Started up at night incest idea c. M.[2]/ Today—distraught: I feel I am going crazy: nonsense of you & me.[3]

Notes:

1 This dream—certainly unsettling and unbearable for Dodge who was often repelled by her father— suggests incest in the passage about the luggage and how her father cannot "get it all in," as well as in Dodge's insistence on the shared cabin and the image of her on the upper berth and her father below.
2 This reference to incest probably refers to the possibility of Sterne loving his niece Ida (see notes 1 and 2 for dream 42).
3 *Is this "nonsense" a reference to an erotic transference toward Jelliffe and competition Sterne might feel with both Jelliffe and the analysis?* Dodge reported to Jelliffe on January 13: "*Sterne getting mean re analysis....He sees possibly a loss for him/. Have talked c. him quite frankly: Possibly I would get over being in l. c. him./ Other ♂.*"

δ

31.
January 24, 1916

I dreamed of sitting at the table & having food passed me.

δ

32.
January 25, 1916 (1 of 2)

Cannot remember any dreams distinctly.

In one I ran out of a house somewhere, ran away, jumped on a trolley car...there was some old man, Emmanuel Reicher [1] I think, who was impotent, somewhere in this dream. I got off the car, the conductor held me from behind & I slid down his legs, somehow they were on each side of me behind [2]....

Notes:

1 German actor, playwright, and director whose name is associated with Yiddish theater and who founded a theater organization in New York called the Modern Stage.
2 *This erotic image of a man holding Dodge from behind and her sliding down his legs that also straddled her starts off as somewhat parental—the way a father might use his legs as a slide for his child—and then twists into her being in between his legs. This image connects with the incest image from the previous dream.*

δ

33.
January 25, 1916 (2 of 2)

Another dream I was going to school. I missed a day & couldn't see which my class was...the children didn't look familiar. They sat there reciting. I asked if that was my class. I think they said no.

I had been away downstairs [1] or someplace having a love affair with a woman.[2] She was or reminded me of Miss Blood [3]...

This dream was all mixed & unsatisfactory at each moment.

Jelliffe's notes from January 26, 1916:
Awful headache, 3 day ℂ [4], usually that way: Gnawing fatigue: Wrote it out:/ When alone ↓....I have always believed that unhappiness earthbound: used to tease my father a great deal:/ 9 yr. old letter re mother & he/ Cracked ice.# Guilty [5] secret: which I don't know:/ Perhaps they would find it out/ in private room—possibly one may think I had read their letters [6]: (wait dream)
   School./ missed day:/ children: my classes:/ downstairs all mixed up....
   My interpretation: School & children. I skipped my work. Left, downstairs. Class & children—autoerotic.[7] Then when I went back, did not know me:
   Miss Blood: Florence: Princess Ghika [8] ♀♀?/ big dogs & cats & animals, mysterious. Little dried up old maid. Much $: all hidden./ used to

come to see me: I was always so healthy & blooming. I told her sun & sunbaths.

Why miss class! As in r.r. train: people in dog carts, waiting: for me no interest & no pleasure: uninteresting & indifferent..../ don't feel like other girls:/ just looked at them. once in a while attracted to teacher [9] *& forgot:/*

An apparent diary entry in Dodge's handwriting appears here after the dream:

Jan. 25
   There is something disturbing me all the time & I don't know what it is. I have felt it off & on all my life. It is something that I know but which I can't remember.[10]
   When I am with Sterne I don't feel it. I just feel light & natural. When he is away from here this thing keeps at me—whether I am reading or talking—& it nags me & disturbs me..& gives me a sinking feeling in my stomach. I feel all right when Sterne is here even if I'm unhappy—about some conscious thing at least I feel natural then.

Notes:

1 In dream 23, Dodge associates going "down-down" with entering the unconscious. ***This absence of hers, while being downstairs, may suggest an immersion in unconscious sexual fantasy.***

2 When Dodge was in boarding schools, she began erotic explorations with several of her female classmates, as she wrote about in *Background* (1933a), with Beatrice and, most explicitly, with Violet: "I reached out my hand and laid it shyly upon her left breast, cupping it with my palm. Instantly it was attuned to a music of the finest vibration....This response we made to each other at the contact of our flesh ran from hand to breast along the shining passages of our blood until in every cell we felt each other's presence" (p. 264). In France in 1904, she was enamored by Marcelle (Luhan, 1935, pp. 74–79), and in Italy she pursued several sexual relationships with women, revealed more explicitly in an unpublished part of *European Experiences*, "Making a Life, Part II" (1927) after only hinting at their allure in *European Experiences* (1935), including the English historian Maud Cruttwell and the American sculptor Janet Scudder. Cruttwell, "with teeth stained brown from the long, dark cigars she smoked continually" (1935, p. 282), waited for Dodge "adoringly" and lured her to her room: "She drew me onto her bed....She had a complete faith in her impulses. In her loves. No doubt of their validity ever entered her. So in that way she was pure. But I was not pure, returning to her after the distaste I had felt for her—and felt again. Out of idleness and ennui I went in there" (1927, pp. 317–318). With Scudder,

Dodge seemed less ambivalent, welcoming the feelings that emerged "in Paris that spring when Janet and I became focused upon each other": "The dissatisfaction and sadness I usually carried in my breast dissolved when this little fire grew between us and soon I was very happy because of Janet" (1927, pp. 323, 324). Dodge invited Scudder to Florence for the summer, and they traveled there together in a shared compartment on a night train, talking openly: "She and I had a long, strange conversation about love and fidelity, for I had to explain to her that one thing I had said to Edwin when I married him—that I would always be 'faithful' to him. She tried to convince me that that only applied to men, and that men were all that Edwin would mind in unfaithfulness. After she persuaded me, I should have wondered once [and] for all just where the line between men and women can be drawn—what makes a woman more a woman than a man, what makes a man more a man than woman, for her body was a strange anomaly" (1927, p. 324). In his notes from January 11, 1916, Jelliffe records her reported attraction to women: "*after m[arried]. Ed[win]. interested in ♀. Governess for John. Semi flirtation... no overt acts:/ deeply interested for a while/ This was in Italy: much ♀-♀ about./ Many ♀ interested in me # One I did get interested in./ Own satisfact[ion] # One day c. this ♀/ Manual m[asturbation]. Seducing them/ interested me...no personal satisf[action]# gradually worked up to a more complete ♀-♀/ necessity—lazy life in Italy.*" This last woman is likely Janet Scudder.

3 Florence Blood, an American philanthropist who founded and directed a hospital for wounded soldiers in France during World War I. She was friends with Gertrude Stein and lived openly as a lesbian at the Villa Gamberaia in Settignano, a village on a hill above Florence. In 1913, Stein wrote an abstract word portrait of Blood entitled "A Portrait of F. B.," similar in style to "A Portrait of Mabel Dodge at the Villa Curonia." After reading Dodge's portrait by Stein, Blood had written to Mabel: "I can't believe it in any way represents you—for if it did you would be man also & you are not surely?!" Whether Blood and Dodge had an affair is unknown.

4 Although the meaning of this symbol is unknown, it very possibly refers to masturbation, as suggested by the context here and in Jelliffe's notes for dream 48.

5 This is an alternative reading of a word that Rudnick (2012) quotes as "family." Rudnick cites Dodge's admission of a "family secret: which I don't know," then wonders if this "secret" could be that her father had syphilis or was homosexual (pp. 30–31). Reading the passage as *"guilty secret"* has different implications, as discussed in note 6 below.

6 If the symbol above means masturbation, that could be the *"guilty secret"* that Dodge mentions. An undated diary note in Dodge's hand states: "Tell Jelliffe...about having a guilty secret" (see Interlude 5). Or,

if the guilty secret is not hers, this passage could suggest a secret revealed in the *"letter re mother & he,"* possibly a secret concerning her mother's attraction to other men, as stated in Jelliffe's notes from January 15: *"She did look at people. M[other]. robust, red hair, natural, possibly affairs"* (see note 4 for dream 42 for more about Dodge's mother's secret life).

7 Dodge's use of this word speaks to her embracing of psychoanalytic terms (perhaps to please her analyst) and her openness with Jelliffe in discussing masturbation and her sexual behavior.

8 Florence Blood's romantic partner who shared and owned the villa with her. She is mentioned twice in Alice B. Toklas's *What is Remembered* (1963, pp. 49, 55). Born Anne-Marie Chassaigne, she was a famous courtesan and Folies Bergère dancer in Paris, had male and female lovers, changed her name to Liane de Pougy and then wrote a novel, *Idylle Saphique* (1901), about her lesbian relationship with American writer Natalie Clifford Barney. Princess Ghika acquired her title by marrying Prince George Ghika in 1910.

9 In *Background* (1933a), Dodge recalls her attraction to Miss Moore at St. Margaret's who was "alluring": "I had what the girls called a 'crush' on her. My thoughts went to her constantly and I memorized her, the tones in her dusky rolls of hair and the unfathomable, nameless exchange that I felt passing between us as she wore the rose I had brought to her." She also remembers the French teacher at the Chevy Chase School who "intrigued me....She had a certain attraction for me and I for her": "She also grew confidential under my continual attention. I knew I could always win people to me if I could be near them often enough and demand, by endless silent maneuvers, their interest or affection or whatever it was I wanted of them. She grew demonstrative with me and pressed me to her and gave me tender looks with her pale, brown, dilated eyes. Our attention upon each other established a current that ran between us—a current of magnetism, fascinating and exciting and enlivening" (pp. 213, 216, 275–276). As early as her teenage years, Dodge had learned how to urge others toward her with her attention and at times obsessive focus on them. In Jelliffe's notes from January 11, 1916, he recorded: *"Breasts/ Interest c. teachers, desire to dominate them, always took initiation."*

10 This passage certainly suggests an early disturbance in Dodge's life. ***Whatever the disturbing event or fact, Dodge observes that when Sterne is around—that is, when she feels preoccupied with a love object—she is not haunted by the disturbance. This admission illuminates the intensity with which Dodge constantly sought nurturance and attention from others, most often men, likely searching for something to quell her troubled feelings.***

δ

34.
January 26, 1916

Hackett [1] was reading out loud his article about Isadora [Duncan] in the New Republic [2] & I had a child with me. I held it up & said: "But look— this is Colette,[3] the littlest one that used to be with Isadora." She staid [*sic*] with me all thro' the dream. Everyone was very busy & happy. My father & mother were harmoniously arranging some meal.[4] Walter Lippmann [5] was working in the next room trying to make up some back work. I carried him a cup of coffee & put it down at his hand. He made a note on a crowded engagement pad—& said "That is Walter's holiday" & I smiled. I was very happy at this because I knew it meant he would spend it with me.

A very pleasant cheerful dream all through.

Jelliffe's notes from January 29, 1916:
Colette (4–5 yrs old, W.L. in next room./ Cooperative.)
    Hackett./ Don't care for his writing: He writes theater:…Book Rev:/ I say he never experiences, just happy phrase….
    Resemble: Little delicate faced person/ I like him as a person: not as a critic…. Whole New Republic Group: W. Lippmann: [Hackett] never made any impression on me one way or another:/ Recalls re S[terne]. & he could not trust me, a little girl then proud of honesty. 7–8, big farm, candy on shelf, somebody ate it. Aunt [Louise']s attitude, her children could not have done it.[6] Gr[eat]. discomfort: S[.]'s attitude the same.
    Colette/ not attractive. Isadora said she was a little genius: scrawny little thing 4–5: I had her. Holding up to H[ackett]. Here you see, his attitude negation, criticism.

Notes:

1 Francis Hackett, an Irish-born writer and literary critic who wrote novels, biographies, and plays. At this time, he and Walter Lippmann were both editors at *The New Republic*.
2 In the May 1, 1915 issue of *The New Republic*, Hackett mentions Duncan in his article "The Movies," arguing for consideration of the "possibilities of the moving picture": "That an art can lie submerged in mankind, as the Gothic cathedrals lay submerged in the unchiseled rocks of France, is one of the facts which give life its value. It is only of recent years, we may as well remember, that through the genius of Isadora Duncan we became again aware of the possibilities of dancing" (p. 329). No article by him devoted exclusively to Duncan appears in *The New Republic* from this time.
3 One of Isadora Duncan's youngest dancers who had studied at her school at Bellevue in Paris and then, along with a number of other children,

came to New York to continue dancing with her teacher (Kurth, 2001, pp. 323–324). She was singled out by the writer and editor Mary Fanton Roberts: "'Colette, in her wisp of a blue Greek tunic, literally did dance like Isadora. Day by day, she had watched the great dancer, until without a single practical lesson, she gave a miraculous imitation, missing none of Isadora's grace or subtle detail of gesture....The child's body was plastic, and Isadora had transcended all preliminaries of teaching and reached the child's receptive spirit'" (quoted in Terry, 1963, p. 140). Colette's last name is not given. Duncan regularly brought children with her from overseas and they often adopted her last name.

4   *This highly unlikely scene, given the estrangement and sometimes violent emotions between Dodge's parents, is an example of dream as wish fulfillment.*

5   Lippmann had accompanied Dodge to the ill-fated meeting between Duncan and the mayor of New York and was "utterly disgusted" by Duncan's behavior (Luhan, 1936, p. 331).

6   Dodge is recalling a painful incident from her childhood when she was not believed. During a visit to Aunt Louise's home, a cherished box of caramels received as a gift from Grandma Cook was kept on a high shelf in a closet. After the midday meal, Louise would give one caramel each to Mabel and her four cousins. As Dodge relates in *Background* (1933a): "We used to eat them slowly, each of us trying to make our own last the longest....The caramels were the greatest joy we had during my visit there one summer. Then something happened" (p. 157). One day, Aunt Louise discovered one of the caramels missing and accused Mabel of the theft after one of her own children reported that she had been in that room during the day to get some thread. Mabel vehemently denied taking the candy, but the event created a rift between her and her cousins: "All that day the other children and I were shy of each other, and it was as though we didn't know each other, though we had played together every year since we were babies. The unseen barrier had risen into our consciousness—the barrier of our difference" (p. 160). Perhaps most wounding was that Dodge's own mother did not believe her: "She didn't see how terribly important the whole thing was to me and how I was suffering from the unjust accusation. She was even more obtuse, more blind to her child, than any of them" (p. 159).

δ

35.
Sunday, January 30, 1916

I dreamed we were in the ocean & it was rough & we were watching a sailor (down in water somewhere) with a beard in another boat drop from a height with the water & land on his back & float & he did it so well that he hardly wetted himself—only his back—then he would get up & suddenly be back in place doing it over.[1] *Full of wonderment re new knowledge: (Mast.)* [2]

Later we were at the sea in some foreign place. Some people were going out in one little boat ahead & I had another little boat with three or four ♂♀ people in it & I was pulling it along the sand out to deeper water—it was getting darker & beginning to be rough & a pinkish light over things. The other boat was ahead & they were rowing. I finally got into our boat & sat down but found there were no oars or oarlocks.[3] And then someone said—it seems to me it was a fisherman or a native of the place *did not see him*—that it was going to be stormy & rain. So we pulled the boat & people back to shore again.

Then we were all sitting in the house on the shore. It was a kind of fisherman's ruin, I think. I feel as tho' my family had been along tho' not with the unpleasant sinking death like feeling that would usually give me.[4] There were quite a lot of people there, sitting around the wall on benches. The walls of the room were cement like the italian houses—& painted a nice pinkish color. A woman was leaning forward talking vociferously. I knew it was Baroness de Cassin [5] yet I saw she looked like Mrs. Chamberlain.[6]

This seaside place sounds like the place the Bramleys [7] told me about abroad where the de Cassins & they used to go long ago.

When I woke up & tried to recall this dream & tell it over to myself—when I got this far I found myself saying: "and it tasted like a death bed.." but with no unpleasant feeling as I said it, just descriptive....

Later in the same dream we were at another place and my father had had a room with something supernatural in it. He told about it laughingly [8] (the evening before John [Evans] & the MacKaye children [9] had been tipping tables here.) I said to my father "When we get to the Villa you must have the haunted rooms["][10]...& we were arranging who would have different rooms.

Then I motored Sterne over to see a view I had heard of. We got to a steep precipice in the car & Albert [11] stopped, there was a long abrupt drop & then out of the chasm arose some marvellous [*sic*] great pyramid shaped mountains of coal—all in little pieces & glittering & having colors in them. Behind was a splendid background of great walls of stone in strange square patterns. Sterne was enthusiastic over it.

Jelliffe's notes from January 31, 1916:
Saturday M. had gone to Pottsville [12]: Percy M[a]cKaye urged him to come back. I was in mood of his having gone [13]/ Last night: no stage:/ farewell/ once already/ S[ex]. all day...Goodbye in office/ never to see you again:/ Build life in privacy:/ Just started a divorce [14]/ He does not care particularly/ Since midday yesterday feeling better...

Dreamed Sat. night...ocean, rough & uneven: Sailor rough c. a beard: Tasted like a death bed—not unpleasant thought./

Notes:

1 *Freud (1900) might consider this a birth dream: "A large number of dreams, often accompanied by anxiety and having as their content such subjects as passing through narrow spaces or being in water, are based upon phantasies of intra-uterine life, of existence in the womb and of the act of birth" (p. 399). Or, with the observation that he "hardly wetted himself," it could be a dream about repeated sexual activity, something frequently engaged in by Dodge and Sterne, as she reports in her associations to this dream: "S[ex]. all day."*

2 *This could refer to Dodge's awe about her experiences in psychoanalysis and all she is learning about her unconscious and the workings of her mind, in addition to learning about her own sexual pleasure, as indicated by Jelliffe's clear abbreviation for masturbation.*

3 *Here Dodge initially discovers that she does not have any way to propel her boat, perhaps revealing her lack of control and agency in the face of turmoil. However, she heeds the warning about the storm and succeeds in bringing the boat back to shore, reasserting her effectiveness. This could symbolize the ups and downs in her relationship with Sterne and, at this time, as she reports in her associations, she had sent her lover away to paint.* In a related passage in her memoirs, Dodge writes: "I myself was that small boat and difficult enough I was finding navigation, never having been trained for it" (1936, p. 479).

4 In *Background* (1933a), Dodge refers often to the atmosphere of deadness in her home and surrounding her family: "Our house was a lifeless place"; "There never was a sense of life in our house. No one cared to be in it. Really no one *lived* in it, you might say. My father was in it the most of any of us, but he was usually up in his room"; the parlor was "a deathly place" (pp. 48, 49, 50).

5 A Baroness de Cassin is identified in Duke de Stacpoole's *Irish and Other Memories* (1922) as "a French lady" who was "a life-long friend" of the author's and hosted small gatherings in Paris "which were very cosmopolitan and exceedingly pleasant" (pp. 288–289).

6 Unidentified.

7 This likely refers to the Bramleys, mentioned in *European Experiences* (1935) among a list of guests to the Villa Curonia (p. 173).

8 An unlikely image in real life from a man whom Dodge recalls as communicating to her only "dark looks and angry sound" and "whose years passed in an increasing torment and whose temper grew worse with these years" (1933a, p. 23).

9 The three children of Marion and the poet and playwright Percy MacKaye, friends of Dodge's. Dodge described Percy as "gaunt, with long, unruly hair," a man who was "always excited, not, one realized, in his blood, but in his brain. Enthusiasm galvanized him. He continually

saw things were *wonderful, marvelous!*" (1936, p. 322). During a weekend visit to Finney Farm on March 28, 1916, MacKaye had written a poem, "Mabel: A Sketch," which begins: "What Mabel is she makes to be/ The heart of hospitality:/ A mute, unconscious artistry/ Of friendship" (Luhan, 1936, p. 462).

10 The Villa Curonia had a room apparently haunted by the ghost of Marguerite Michel, a resident of the villa when Dodge purchased it, who had tutored the previous owner's children. Dodge retained Marguerite to continue in her role as teacher to her own son. However, Marguerite was enfeebled by a cardiac ailment that interfered with her ability to work and, instead, she focused her energy on developing a ferociously jealous love for Mabel Dodge that continued until she left the villa for a hospital before she died. As Dodge reports in *European Experiences* (1935), at her departure, Marguerite warned: "'I am going now…but I love this house very much and I will come back to it no matter what happens'" (p. 281). Marguerite's room became the guest room, where visitors passed many fitful nights of sleep. One guest, Janet Scudder, complained: "'There's something the matter with that room….I just had a queer disturbed night—as though something were keeping me from sleeping….And when I woke up, I felt a long, cold foot pushing against me, as though trying to force me out of the bed'" (pp. 288–289). Dodge herself was thrilled with the presence of a ghost and seemed to take pleasure from the fearful experiences of her guests. Only Constance Fletcher had a joyous night in the company of Marguerite's ghost, awakening happy and initiating a conversation with her during which she offered to rouse Dodge. Marguerite replied: "'*Non, non, Mabella dorme, dorme cose bene! Mene vado—mene vado!*'" (p. 300).

11 Dodge's chauffeur while she lived in New York, whom she described as "smug" (1936, p. 36).

12 A town in Pennsylvania where Dodge had sent Sterne away to paint. He returned around March 2, 1916.

13 While Sterne was absent, Dodge experienced tender and compassionate feelings toward him that she could not feel in his presence.

14 Mabel was currently in the process of divorcing Edwin Dodge. In an undated letter, he writes to her:

> I have been thinking a good deal about Divorce lately. I spoke to your mother about it…in October; but she did not take to the idea at all kindly for incompatibility or desertion.
>
>   It has always seemed to me more dignified to get a divorce when the marriage is finished, rather than to wait until another is contemplated. I at least have no one in mind but of course I don[']t know what you have in mind. I saw Hutch [Hapgood] yesterday and he led me to think that you are considering it. Of course here in New York

there is only one ground and that isn't pretty, and my family don't [*sic*] see any reason for me to lay myself open to it. Residence in Paris is I think easy and divorce can be got. From something Hutch said, I came to the conclusion that you are thinking of it. I hope you will; and I hope you will be happy.

Their divorce was final on June 8, 1916. The cause listed was, in fact, "desertion," with Mabel identified as the "libellant" and Edwin as the "libellee" ("Certificate of Divorce," MDLC). (Edwin graciously wrote to her in 1917: "I hate to think as bitterly of you as your actions regarding the Divorce have made me; but perhaps reports coming through a third person have given me a wrong impression.")

δ

36.
Wednesday, February 2, 1916

Very hard to remember. Can't remember consecutively.

There was a boat out on the ocean I wanted—about 25 ft[.] long—dark red shaped like this ⌐▬▬. I wanted it so much I got it [1]—I don't know how—it came in shore to me & I got in & then saw it belonged to two ladies who were in it. I began to apologize but the older one smiled that "nothing matters" new thought school smile & said it was all right & we went to the other side of the island where they lived in one of those colonies. *"New Thought Colony"*[2]

   Max [Eastman] was there [3]—at table I was drawing for him & someone else was too. A design for a costume for Ida [Rauh] [4]…he was smiling foolishly. I drew a dress like this 👗, which he liked….

   I was at a new opera. I didn't care for it & wandered out. The audience was thin & not very good. I saw an italian peasant smoking a cigarette. I met Maurice outside & we walked along. Maurice reprimanded two men for speaking such a crude tongue. I thought it was german but it was Hungarian he said. He scolded them.

   Dr. J. & Bayard [5] asked me triumphantly if I knew Maurice was drunk all the time. I said I knew when he drank.

   Jelliffe's notes from February 2, 1916:
   Dream last night:
      Boat, dark red: Wanted it very much./ Got in belonged to 2♀. Nothing matters, new thought smile./ I began to apol[ogize]: older one said ok. new thought Colonies:# Max. E. at table….He smiling:/ He not geared up, loose not geared up smile./ foolish sort of a smile/ No skeleton:/ He liked this ballet dress/.# New Opera: did not care I wandered around…
      Red: this color; which I like, shawl, saw it other day…

Notes:

1 *Even though Dodge could be willful and demanding in her relationships, the ease of this wish fulfillment—with the boat appearing when she wanted it, without her explicit effort—is powerful. The acceptance of her by the two women who owned the boat also has an ease that must have been welcome.*

2 New Thought was a school of mind cure popular at the time that stressed optimism and the goodness of human beings, in contrast to, as explained by one of its leaders Horatio Dresser (1919), the "old thought," which was "undeniably pessimistic; it dwelt on sin, emphasized the darkness and misery of the world, the distress and the suffering. The new dwelt on life and light pointing the way to the mastery of all sorrow and suffering" (p. 160). The "new thought school smile" may be connected to the idea of the "law of attraction," as explained by Dresser: "To change or improve one's conditions, one must then change the inner centre, adopt a different attitude, make other and different affirmations, look out on life with more optimistic expectations" (pp. 160–161).

3 In fact, Eastman had sought treatment at a New Thought sanatorium in 1906, in Kingston, New York, for symptoms of fatigue and mysterious back pain. In his memoir, he devoted a chapter to his experience there, and sheds light on the "new thought school smile": He tells of the "cheerful, almost amused greeting" he received at breakfast his first morning and how he "felt like a new toy arriving in a happy nursery"; the optimistic atmosphere was heightened for him by the "loving-kindly radiance" of Rosanna, the dining-room supervisor, who radiated "the New Thought sweetness" (1948, pp. 242–243, 245, 246).

4 Actress and poet who married Eastman in 1911, credited by him for the initial impetus behind the founding of the Washington Square Players in New York. Rauh acted in the first productions of both the Washington Square Players and the Provincetown Players.

5 This is the first of three dreams within two weeks where Jelliffe and Boyeson appear with Dodge.

δ

INTERLUDE 3.

In an undated note to Jelliffe from this time, Dodge writes:

P.S. I am aghast at the mystery of Psycho-Analysis! No wonder it's called a major operation! You can hardly know more than your patients what will come out of an analysis! Do you realize—in Bayard's case—it has brought his latent homosexuality to the surface—so that I feel him becoming more & more one now? Have you noticed it? That is why he must go on with the analysis, I think. I don't know where he will end if he doesn't go on & pass out of the homosexual.

δ

37.
[circa February 5, 1916]
[written in red in Jelliffe's notes from February 5, 1916]

Eating something: Agreeable: don't recall taste, a spot in the night.

> Jelliffe's notes from February 5, 1916:
> *Can't even recall the dream feeling.*
> *Eating/. I'll tell you something else:/ I wanted to talk re E[dwin Dodge].*
> *I think the ☿ relation since E. a complex & caused me to be on the edge*
> *of a neurosis.[1]/ To know that clit[oral]. frigation [sic] [2] will not fix it.#*
> *Let[']s therefore take E. Sense of atonement.*

Notes:

1 Dodge's use of language here indicates how she and Jelliffe spoke in
   analysis about her troubles. As mentioned earlier, she suffered from the
   lack of intercourse in her marriage with Edwin. *Without a constant love
   interest and the reassurance siphoned off from a sexual relationship, Dodge
   experienced herself as unmoored, although she also came to understand the
   compulsive and maladaptive elements in her unrelenting search for sexual
   contact.*
2 Frig means to copulate or masturbate. Frigation is likely a word invented by
   Dodge.

δ

38.
Sunday [undated, circa early February 1916] (1 of 2)

I was playing the piano. Dr. Jelliffe & Bayard were talking. I was wondering
if Dr. J. was noticing me.[1] Hartley came up & said he would play something
for me. He sat down & played. I stood by him—I arranged my dress to fall
gracefully in good folds. I listened to Hartley & noticed Bayard & Dr. J.
talking. I wondered if they noticed me & how I was standing with my dress
so gracefully arranged.[2] I thought to myself Dr. J. is much more interested
in Bayard than in me.[3]

Notes:

1 *Dodge's dream reveals her strong paternal, and sometimes erotic, transference to Jelliffe, whose attention she craves. She received no such glances
   from either of her parents, who were lost in their own separate worlds, not
   noticing their daughter in her painful loneliness and desperate need for
   even the merest trace of recognition.*

2 Dodge was aware from a young age of the preparations women make to draw the attention of men. In *Background* (1933a), she reports seeing her mother dance at a party at their home: "I saw my mother flash past dressed in her white satin Empire gown that made her skin look so blond and her hair so burnished, and that I had watched her put on hours earlier" (p. 33). In *European Experiences* (1935), Dodge describes her mother as "blooming in light silk dresses with black velvet and paste buttons twinkling under lace ruffles" at the time she visited her daughter in France and "grew flirtatious" toward Edwin Dodge (p. 89).

3 This is the second time this month that Jelliffe and Boyeson appear together in Dodge's dreams, perhaps because, due to Dodge's influence, Boyeson was currently also in treatment with Jelliffe. They may have been joined in her mind as men she wanted attention from. In her dream, there is a suggestion of a homoerotic attraction between the two men, which would leave Dodge left out, an early and familiar feeling.

δ

39.
Sunday [circa early February 1916] (2 of 2)

I was in a lovely country in the spring, like Italy. I motored along & going down around a corner came on someone's house & grounds *not a love affair as you imagine*. Very beautiful, three grassy terraces leading down to a sort of centre, the house high up on a slope. I went on by it and saw some other places. I came to a beautiful empty house. I forget what I was going there for but I had some reason. I found myself going through the garden. I noticed a green bronze statue in a fountain pool. I was in the house....I had been thro' it & was going down the servants['] stairs. They were white like the walls & with blue & white stripes on the sides, then pink & white stripes. It was a circular staircase. I finally got downstairs to a hall. There was someone there. There was a sense of secrecy & agitation. I mean the kind of agitation & reserve there is when there is some royal person in a hotel who wants to get in & out & not be bothered—an important feeling. Someone told me it was Dr. J.'s patient that he spoke to me of.[1] She was tall & dark & somewhat pointed & thin. There were two little girls & a maid. They finally succeeded in getting out & away. Someone—<u>She</u> I think told me she had taken the beautiful place I had seen on my way there—to live in to do her analysis. It seemed she could live there & no one would find her because it was a far off out of the way beautiful place where she, like a royal person, could put off the world & just attend to this thing.[2]

I went into the garden again & noticed that the bronze figure was moving. It turned out to be a mechanical statue of green bronze, of a young girl.[3] It would take some steps & bend over & do something in the water, then get up & go back, & keep this up. But soon I noticed that it was really Percy

MacKaye's boy Robin,[4] tho' he <u>was</u> dark green! He went away out of the pool when I saw who it was.

Later I was with a lot of people on a small round hill. There was a top & it sloped quickly & suddenly away on all sides. Ida [Rauh] was there & a number of others. And there were trees. We acted, as it seems to me now, like children playing at recess out of doors. It was some game of hide & seek, or something like that. Ida was directing me....

Association: I came out on the train last night with Mr. Howe [5] & he told me Max & Ida had gone to California for a couple of months. He said he thought Max wanted to live there & write his books, 'cause his philosophy has gone to pieces.[6].

Is it because americains [sic] are fecal erotics [7] that there are so many patent medicines—& is it because they don't assimilate all they take in—& can't eliminate fast enough?

Notes:

1 Jelliffe did speak with Dodge at times about some of his other patients. See Interlude 4.
2 In the previous dream where Dodge wants to be noticed by Jelliffe, her competition is Boyeson, whereas in this dream, she meets a "royal" person who can afford to "put off the world" to live in a "far off out of the way beautiful place" to focus primarily on her analysis. *Dodge's competitive nature in her transference to Jelliffe seems revealed here, as she meets another of Jelliffe's patients who is more privileged and perhaps even more "important."*
3 This image of a sculpture coming to life recalls the famous Greek myth of Pygmalion and Galatea, in which the sculptor Pygmalion carves the figure of Galatea out of ivory and then falls in love with her. He prays to the goddess Aphrodite for a wife as beautiful as his creation, and she then grants his wish by bringing the sculpture to life. *Dodge may feel she is brought to life or enlivened through her analysis with Jelliffe.*
4 He also appeared in dream 35.
5 Frederick Howe, Commissioner of Immigration at Ellis Island in New York, who was friends with Dodge.
6 In his autobiography, *Enjoyment of Living* (1948), Eastman reports that he and Ida embarked upon "a two-months' lecture and money-raising tour across the country to San Diego" and that in 1916, he published "a book on the war and the socialist policy, another called *Journalism versus Art*" and, in *The Masses*, three installments to comprise his book, *Towards Liberty, The Method of Progress*, a work he intended to write that year. This may be what he was working on in California, as he mentions that one of his ambitions had been "to publish...my still unwritten book" (p. 538).

7 In *Movers and Shakers* (1936), Dodge writes: "I had observed the relationship between our money-making fixation and the great signs advertising all kinds of laxatives that decorated the billboards of our country and the back pages of magazines. No other nation bought and sold physic like Americans, that was obvious" (p. 516). Around this time, Dodge consulted only once with a Dr. [first name unknown] Bernard whose questionable, and later raided, practice focused on elimination and subsequent pleasure. As she reports: "Dr. Bernard was one of the shrewdest opportunists I ever met. He had thought things out and had settled himself in New York to exploit one of our national weaknesses: constipation! He determined that the constipation of American women should win him a fortune" (p. 516). His program included glass dilators for the rectum (sold resting on purple velvet in a mahogany box) and "the art of reversion" where the patient stands on her head wearing "Bernard Bloomers." Dr. Bernard explained to Dodge his "Dilation Treatment" and the eventually expected erotic experience: "'The rectum of the average American is abnormally small and has in many cases lost its elasticity. The intestines cannot evacuate through the American rectum. Now we begin with these and gradually increase the size until the rectal muscles become readjusted....You will shortly realize that evacuation as I induce it is a pleasure with which none other can compare! *None* other!'" (pp. 516–517). Freud certainly linked money and feces in "Character and Anal Erotism" (1908a), and discussed sublimation of the erotic impulses aroused by anal stimulation. See note 3 for dream 82 for a discussion of Jelliffe and Zenia X—'s 1914 article about urinary and fecal fantasies and their connection to primitive cultures.

δ

INTERLUDE 4.

Both Jelliffe and Brill talked with Dodge about their patients, sometimes even by name, revealing an apparently more casual approach to confidentiality that existed toward the beginning of psychoanalysis in the United States. As a physician, Jelliffe would have been expected to adhere to the Hippocratic Oath, which includes the passage: "What I may see or hear in the course of the treatment or even outside of the treatment in regard to the life of men, which on no account one must spread abroad, I will keep to myself holding such things shameful to be spoken about" (Edelstein, 1943, p. 3). In *Movers and Shakers* (1936), Dodge relates an instance when Jelliffe told her about a patient, a "grave, sweet-looking" woman Dodge regularly noticed when she arrived at his office: "He told me she was an old patient of his and of particular interest. 'She has cured herself of manic-depression,' he said, regarding me with an intent gaze. 'I have written up her case for the [*Psychoanalytic*] *Review*. You must read it.[1] You know that she is my proof that by understanding and hard work these manic-depressives may free themselves'" (p. 440). As discussed earlier, Dodge also revealed that Jelliffe talked with her about his analysis with Boyeson.

At times, Brill also divulged information to Dodge about his patients and their consultations with him, as indicated in his letters to her. He refers to his treatment of Everett Marcy, a young writer romantically involved with Dodge for about two years beginning in November 1925. Brill writes to her on January 8, 1926: "In reference to Everett: He has done much better of late and I feel that a lot can be done for him. He is interested and seems to react well." On March 16, 1927, he reports again on Marcy: "When he wrote to me I asked him to come. When he got here, I gave him regular appointments, but he failed to keep his appointments, often coming late, etc. He was very unsettled, consequently I got tired and told him to wait until he is settled enough to do regular work….I have neither the time nor the patience to give to people who are not seriously bent on working with me." In fact, Dodge had paid Brill for Marcy's therapy with the handwritten manuscript of D.H. Lawrence's *Sons and Lovers*, acquired by her directly from Lawrence's wife Frieda in exchange for a 160-acre ranch near Taos that she had once purchased for her son. In addition to Marcy, Brill wrote to Dodge about his consultations with others, including the writer Carman Barnes and Susy Hare, the daughter-in-law of her friend Elizabeth Sage Hare, a painter and patron of the arts (Everett, 2016, pp. 98, 101, 103–104, 119, 191, 207, 279–280). And in his correspondence with Brill, Freud occasionally mentioned names of patients, such as in a letter from February 20, 1920: "I am now treating a New York dentist, whom you also know, Dr. Bieber. He is making very good progress" (Freud to Brill, February 20, 1920 [translated by Hildegarde and Hunter Hannum], SFA). When Brill's daughter, Gioia Bernheim, was in analysis, Freud revealed that her analyst, Lillian Delger Powers, was a former patient of his whose "interest at the time was devoted entirely to squirrels" (Freud to Brill, November 25, 1934, SFA).

Note:

1   This case has not been located among any of Jelliffe's published articles in the *Psychoanalytic Review* from 1913 to 1918. Years later, Dodge wrote an unpublished account of her emotional struggles, "Notes Upon Awareness" (1939), identifying herself as manic-depressive: "This book is a consecutive summation of the attempts of one manic-depressive character to discover how to free herself of her disability & vacillation" (p. 1). On April 29, 1939, she sent the manuscript to Jelliffe, wondering if he "might like portions to use in yr journal—particularly the piece on manic-depression." He replied on May 20, 1939: "I do not find enough that is tangible for the psychiatrist in the Manic Depressive chapter."

δ

40.
[undated, circa early February 1916]

Dreamed about motoring to Jelliffe[']s—flowers—4 sick men.

δ

41.
[circa February 10, 1916]
[written in red in Jelliffe's notes from February 10, 1916]

Made up mind I would dream last night. Not much: just a fragment.

Looking out of window of mo's house: saw father[']s mo.[1] coming c. a present of a necklace. Gold & dark blue enamel: I and mo[']s. f.[2] 7 ft tall: (Little Less F. Gd [3]) went down walk to meet her:

Jelliffe's notes from February 10, 1916:
Father[']s mo. Very droll character: short round and dark trying not to die—go now, in bed now, said she was going away, ticket: very amusing type.[4]—m[arried]. once, very feminine....Great many childish reminisces. Buffalo Club opp. used to watch men.[5] Small town type:/ All bankers in the family:/ Character:/ lively amusing, never depressed, nor bored nor blue [6]/ used to go to see / liked the freedom of the house. Used to get couple of girls & spend the night. Ghost stories: goodies & ghost stories: she would be kept awake all night. Church every Sunday:# Opposite type was Mo's father:/ They say I look russian or polish. She polish. Mo's side, Engl. & scotch:/ Bath Steuben Co. mo's family Cook....: Stern & high ridge noses, deep set fine cold eyes, absolutely silent man: Friend of <u>very</u> conservative people. Hard as nails/ made units of money.

Personal recollection of him...$1. silver first idea of money—he had the sense of power of money: He had that only thing, I recall. Terribly proud:/ This is a silver dollar:/ I've spent a fearful amount of money for <u>things</u>. "Buy a lot of things on a rainy day"—...Will give away anything I want. "Charge" things. Soda water animal crackers etc ++, Hair ribbons, jewelry:/ At school, charges to his gdmother. "Gold & Blue" Yellowish green & greenish yellow, disturbs me./....

Something sticks in me:/ I wake up comfortable & happy. Idea of contacts:/ conscious contacts.

Blue/ Favorite color....used to like green but as girl. Of later years—blue. Colors awfully important to me. Always kept certain colors away violet, mauve, heliotrope./ Blue & gold chain/ Grandmother wears it: would be natural to her:/ Rather like gdm. on lighter side: feminine rather catty. May be md. to some young clergy man:/ waiting any time/ She is going to leave me her money:/ Attitude just something that can be used:

just let it flow all away: They tied it up for me: monthly# They all feel that I might give it away to the first person I liked./ They think I am unbalanced re money.[7]/ None of them like anything I am:/ She is droll, is droll. Arrogant attitude: they would better pay my bills:/ No affection for mo. & F./ They stopped my charge accts, 16:/ They did it in one way or another:/ always getting something.

Notes:

1 i.e., Grandma Ganson, who, like Dodge, lived on Delaware Avenue in Buffalo, in a brick house with a cupola and an iron fence. As Dodge writes in *Background* (1933a): "I loved her as much as a child ever loves any one [*sic*]. That is, I liked going to her house. It was warm and home-like and nourishing. I liked to go in there and feel secure and loose all over. At home I never could feel so at ease" (p. 109).

2 i.e., mother's father, meaning Grandpa Cook. Dodge reports that he "stood six feet and some inches and was very slender" (1933a, p. 120).

3 i.e., possibly father's grandfather. This reference is unknown, although it may refer to the height of Dodge's paternal great grandfather.

4 As a child, Dodge remembers feeling "full of joy and good spirits" from her visits with Grandma Ganson. Given Dodge's marriage in 1923 to Antonio Luhan, a Pueblo Indian, Dodge's feeling of closeness to her grandmother is made more interesting by the following rumor: "When Grandma was a young girl the Iroquois Indians were all about in that country. I have heard it whispered, when I was quite small, that she had Indian blood, and this was fascinating to me" (1933a, pp. 102, 104).

5 In *Background* (1933a), Dodge remembers that the Buffalo Club, "the club of the middle-aged and elderly gentlemen," was adjacent to Grandma Ganson's house: "As she knitted she peered over her spectacles towards the Buffalo Club....She knew all the men who frequented all these places, and she was openly and earnestly interested in them all....And all the men knew her and always looked towards her bay window, and lifted their hats whether they saw her there or not" (p. 103).

6 Dodge must have welcomed such vitality in her grandmother, since her own mother was often depressed and cried, telling her daughter, "'I feel so blu-u-u-e'" (Luhan, 1933a, p. 37).

7 Although her mother did control the money she received, Dodge eventually felt grateful: "For, after all, whenever I was sick she paid; she continued to give me an allowance no matter what happened; and besides, she helped me out with unexpected expenses like sudden taxes" (1933b, p. 4).

δ

42.
February 14, 1916 (1 of 2)

I am with Maurice in a small plain house, his mother's house, I think. He is going thro' a trunk. He comes across a garment which he looks at. He says it belonged to his little niece [1] who died & he says regretfully that he thinks he would have loved her.[2] I am outraged at the possibility, & angry & discouraged & I get up & go off a long way.[3] I come finally to my mother's house [4] where the dream is forgotten but where I am occupied in trying to forget Maurice since I am not the only one he could have loved.. it is the old revolt at the non-selective male, but finally a letter comes from Maurice telling me he loves me now whether he would have loved his niece if she hadn't died, or not. I feel the reality of his love & its real intrinsic value & I am reassured.[5]

This comes from a desire that love should be the result of the contingency of two especial elements, and not the state of being in love heat & meeting for mutual single satisfaction.

This morning a letter from Maurice [6] gave me this sense of his love for me.. different feeling from my fear that he wants love—from anyone anywhere. This gave me the sense of its being a special brew & contingent upon us two.

Jelliffe's notes from February 14, 1916:
I want M.S. to be analyzed: Possibly ☉ [7] have personal judgment I down or he up:# Everybody has/ If ☉ consider great differences, going to act on this. Resistance to analysis: possibly. Your lacking comprehension of artist type =

Notes:

1 Sterne was one of six children born to his parents. In his memoir, *Shadow and Light* (1952), he writes that his niece Ida, a doctor in Russia, had died in the typhoid epidemic during World War I (p. 76).
2 Sterne recalls his niece as "a lovely young medical student" at the time of his visit to Moscow in 1909 who "begged me to take her with me to Italy, as much, I am afraid, out of schoolgirl infatuation as political considerations" (1952, p. 76).
3 Dodge's violent jealousy of Sterne's unrelenting attractions to other women was a constant presence in their relationship, identified as her primary presenting problem in her initial session with Jelliffe, as recorded in his notes (*"Main trouble: Jealousy"*). In this dream, it is Dodge who leaves Sterne when she is incensed with jealousy, whereas in her non-dream life, she often sent Sterne away, to such

places as New York City, Maine, or New Mexico. In fact, at the time
of this dream, Sterne was in Pennsylvania, where Dodge had sent him
to paint. He had written to her on February 13, 1916: "What hurts me
more than anything is the suspicion that you don't want me to come
back so soon....I long for you all the time. Only you I love" (Sterne,
1952, p. 117).

4   A curious choice of a refuge for Dodge, since her mother's home was
certainly not such a place in real life. However, the appearance of
Dodge's mother in this dream about infidelity may relate to what
Dodge referred to in *Background* (1933a) as "my mother's secret life....
Sometimes little signs would make me feel she knew, intimately, people whom we never saw" (p. 60). Dodge admitted: "She herself had
beaux. Quite early I sensed this and was terrified by it" (p. 25). One
man named Randolph appeared off and on over the years and Dodge
sensed betrayal: "Why had I assumed some secret thing between him
and my mother? Something hateful and terrifying?" (p. 65). On one
occasion, Fred Pratt, one of her father's friends, was so animated and
focused on her mother that her father dramatically left the scene and
wrote Pratt a letter "forbidding him ever to come to the house again"
(p. 66). Dodge certainly knew about one of her mother's affairs, with
John Parmenter, their family doctor, who was sexually involved with
not only Sara Ganson but also with Dodge at the same time. In "Doctors: Fifty Years of Experience" (1954), Dodge describes interrupting a
liaison between her mother and Parmenter: "I went up to my mother's
house and his buggy was at the door....I crept to my mother's door and
it was closed and I heard low voices inside and rashly opened the door
as quietly as I could. Parmenter raised himself from the couch upon
which my mother was lying and she hastily pulled down her skirts"
(pp. 18–19).

5   *Dodge constantly needed this kind of reassurance to fill her up again with
certainty, however temporary, about being loved. She relived, over and
over, her early and "barren experience of being an only and unloved child"
(Luhan, 1933b, p. 1).*

6   Dodge may be referring to either Sterne's letter from February 13, 1916,
quoted in note 3 for this dream, or to one dated February 10, 1916,
written from Pottsville, in which he reassures her: "Mabel, it is perfectly wonderful to me how my love for you has grown from day to
day. Even the 'storms' which every time they came I expected would
uproot it, only made the roots take deeper root in me" (Luhan, 1936,
p. 448).

7   Although not a standard medical symbol, this sign appears frequently in
Jelliffe's notes and seems to indicate when Dodge refers to Jelliffe, i.e.,
"you."

δ

INTERLUDE 5.

In his February 10, 1916 letter from Pottsville, Pennsylvania, Sterne writes to Dodge at Finney Farm with two of his dreams, as she presents in *Movers and Shakers* (1936):

> Last night I dreamt that I went back to Croton to get my things. I was packing, you were reclining on the couch and watching me with an expression of indifference in your eyes, whilst your *husband*, a man with a blond *mustache*, was conversing with you. I was so sad to go, every moment I wanted to go and tell you: it's no *use*, I can't go—but your stony look held me back. She doesn't care, it is better that I break with it all! At last I couldn't control myself longer, I went up to you and said: "it's no use, Mabel, I can't leave you." Then your expression changed, the indifferent look gave place to one full of tenderness and love. "That's right, darling, stay," you said. I awoke with tears in my eyes. Every night lately I dream of you. The other night I was also at Croton. I came unexpectedly and imagine my disappointment when I was told that you had only that morning gone to Pottsville to me....I didn't know what to do, to go back or wait, when suddenly you came in and we greeted each other *cordially*, for we were not alone. Mary Foote was in the same room. You complained that you felt tired and lay down in your bed when we were left alone. I went up to you, we embraced and my head became all *dizzy* in your embrace. My brain felt just like a wave when it has reached its utmost force upward and is about to collapse. I awoke bewildered and with a feeling of dizziness. You must think I am getting interested in psychoanalysis to be writing down my dreams. No, I still have my old apathy for it, but I thank you nevertheless for offering to present me with a Dr. Jelliffe curse (pardon me, I meant course). If I should find out that I need it, I'd be glad to accept, but at present I feel that I don't need it, and never shall need it. (pp. 448–449)

In addition, an undated note written by Dodge on Finney Farm stationery may belong at this place among her dreams:

I think this unknown anxiety has been one reason why I have plunged into love affairs for relief from it. I have always been able to get over it at the beginning & in the middle of love affairs: until they began to make me suffer more than before?

Tell Jelliffe
about expecting a letter
& about having a guilty secret
and about envying other people's interest in the common life while only
    bluffing it myself.
Tho['] feeling it necessary to pretend feeling it!

δ

43.
February 14, 1916 (2 of 2)

Bayard & I & a couple of dogs or monkeys [1] are in Dr. Jelliffe's office. Suddenly Mrs. J.[2] appears in the doorway, or just outside in the hall. She waits & we wait. She seems to be about to put on her hat [3] & either come in or go away. Dr. J. doesn't want to hurry her but he begins to be impatient. He wants to shut the door but not to seem to shut her out. Then to our panic—all three of us—she comes in. We feel guilty but we don't show it because perhaps that would give us away—all three of us—I don't know what we are guilty about. She comes in slowly & looks at us. She sits down in Dr. J.'s chair. She then has Dr. J.'s face. Then we wonder if she is going to have it out with us. But no—she begins to analyse us & we see it['] s all right. She's impersonal, it[']s not about our secret,[4] whatever it is she could accuse us of in a personal way, she doesn't. We all relax & lose interest.

> Jelliffe's notes written at the end of the dream:
> *Your interpretation.* ☉ [5] *think I have some secret resistance* [6]: *Mrs. J. might know something. B[.], I &* ☉ *& Mrs. J. might accuse us. She sat down & began analysis*:

Notes:

1 This may refer to the pair of monkeys that Dodge bought for Finney Farm. As Sterne recalls: "The male was a cruel and ugly brute, who promptly broke the female's neck, sulked in his cage for a few days, and died himself a short time after. Dr. Brill pronounced the beast to have died of suppressed desires, but I preferred to think he died of a broken heart" (1952, p. 116). There is no mention of dogs at the farm.

2 i.e., Mrs. Jelliffe, who died suddenly on March 3, 1916, less than three weeks after this dream.

3 *Freud (1900) believed that "a woman's hat can very often be interpreted with certainty as a genital organ, and, moreover, as a man's" (pp. 355–356). In this dream, Mrs. Jelliffe takes over as Dr. Jelliffe, by sitting in his chair and beginning to analyze them, a substitution that may speak to Dodge's curiosity about Mrs. Jelliffe and what she knows about what goes on in her husband's office.*

4 This is the third time (dreams 36 & 38) in two weeks that Jelliffe, Boyeson, and Dodge appear in a dream together. *The secret she fears being accused of, could this connect with Boyeson's homosexuality, the sexual tension expressed in dream 38 when Dodge longs for Jelliffe to notice her? Or a sexual feeling between Jelliffe and Boyeson?*

5 As before (see note 7 for dream 42), this symbol likely means "you" when Dodge refers to Jelliffe.
6 *What might this secret resistance be? To Jelliffe's interpretation of her erotic transference to him?*

δ

44.
circa February 16, 1916
[written in red in Jelliffe's notes from February 16, 1916]

Night before last./ C. [i.e., with] mother, in her house: I had to go away somewhere & she was helping & I said lend me some of your rings. I reached in a jar. 3 little rings, little finger diam[ond] ruby sapph[ire].[1] on 4th f[inger]. 3 rings, graying pink stones: star rubies, just a little light in them, then went out saw houses all decorated c. red white & blue [2] flags, holiday, celebration.

> Jelliffe's notes from February 16, 1916:
> *Almost a compulsion to tell of rings.*[3]
>   *Rings/ These remind me of ♀ in Buffalo/ Emily Leeming,*[4] *Nina Rumsey Bull,*[5] *staying c. me: interested in psa.*[6]
>   *Rings: articles of decoration: rarely wear.*[7] *Earlier Ideas/ Did once wear. Always felt boy['] s hand.*
>   *Holiday. Patriotism:# Fourth of July.*[8]

Notes:

1 In *Background* (1933a), Dodge describes five of her mother's rings, the first three corresponding exactly to those in this dream: "For rings she had a set of three in rows of rubies, sapphires, and diamonds, her solitaire engagement ring, and a large single pearl" (p. 61).
2 The colors of the American flag are also the colors of rubies, diamonds, and sapphires.
3 *What might this compulsion be about? Was she stealing her mother's "jewels"? Rather than asking her mother to borrow the rings, Dodge demanded, saying "lend me."*
4 Although not mentioned in *Background* (1933a), an Emily Leeming appears twice in the Statue of Liberty-Ellis Island Foundation passenger records (1906 and 1923, listed in 1923 as residing in Buffalo, New York) and would have been 45 years old in 1916, eight years older than Dodge. In *Brooklyn Blue Book and Long Island Society Register* (1912), a Mrs. Joseph (Emily Alvord Howland) Leeming is listed as living at 217 Summer Street in Buffalo. Both references likely point to the same Emily

Howland Leeming who was a Buffalo poet. *Dodge's mention of "Leeming" could also be an association to the previous dream that features Mrs. Helena Leeming Jelliffe.*

5 Nina's middle name "Rumsey" is the maiden name of her deceased biological mother.

6 i.e., psychoanalysis.

7 In *Background* (1933a), Dodge recalls the changing pattern of jewels that her mother preferred: "always exchanging them to follow the fashion. And now she has scarcely anything but pearls. She has accumulated pearls as I have accumulated experience, all these years since she pinned on herself an emerald lizard....I have no pearls or emeralds but I do not mind, for I have had the years" (p. 61).

8 This idea of patriotism may be connected to World War I, although Dodge claims she was "hardly aware" of it: "It seemed unreal to me. I never did really experience the War but I had some observations to write about it" (1936, p. 425). After the sinking of the *Lusitania* on May 7, 1915, Dodge appealed to Arthur Brisbane, editor of the *New York Journal*, to publish her piece, addressed to the United States government: "We women want the war to stop. We want it more than anything else in the world. We are not satisfied with the outlet the Red Cross is giving us....we don't want to go on knitting and nursing and binding. We want to live and help others to live. We want peace" (1936, p. 425). Her article was never printed.

δ

45.

February 21, 1916

[date written in Jelliffe's hand as "Feb. 21," followed by his identification: "Dodge"]

I was at a concert with Bayard & my mother & others, but I was not listening, I was unconscious or sleeping.[1] Soon everybody got up to go, it was over & I woke up. But this sleep had been very benumbing & I couldn't move my legs easily or breathe easily or follow them. I was always behind them as I struggled against the weakness in me. Then they got out of the building before me, & I lost them.[2] I was very troubled because I found it was far to town & I was too tired to walk home & had no money to ride. I saw I was up on Madison Aven[ue] at 72nd St [3]....I felt as tho' the air pressure outside of me was too great to get thro'. I knew the weakness was in me but it felt as tho' it pressed against me from the outside. Then I saw a hotel & knew I could get some change from an aunt of mine [4] who was there, if I would go and ask. Then I would be able to take an omnibus or something. I knew it was the sleep that had had such an effect on me & disabled me. So I went in & found Hannah [5] with some plants. There was one plant that seemed important.

Hannah saw the thing to do was to break off all the leaves so it would grow. That it had ceased growing as it was, but to break off all down to the stalk would make it grow. So she began to do it tho' it seemed risky & dangerous & important, to me.[6]

Notes:

1 *Perhaps Dodge was in such an unaware state because she did not want to take in her surroundings or have to listen to others, particularly her mother.*
2 *This image of Dodge's mother leaving her behind when she was weak and tired resonates with accounts of Sara Ganson's preoccupation with everything in her life except for her daughter and her lack of tolerance for any signs of vulnerability.*
3 This is only blocks away from where Dodge's grandparents, Grandpa and Grandma Cook, used to live on the corner of Fifth Avenue and 78th Street, a neighborhood that gave Dodge her first exposure to the city when she visited from Buffalo as a child (1936, p. 8).
4 This could be any one of Sara Ganson's three sisters, Marianna, Louise or Georgie. There is no record that Dodge's father had any siblings.
5 Dodge's Irish cook who worked for her at 23 Fifth Avenue and had never left New York. As Dodge recalls in *Movers and Shakers* (1936), after Hannah's first and only visit to Finney Farm, she refused to return and "begged to go back to 'civilization,'" complaining, "'I never knew you had to walk on the *dirt* in the country'" (p. 345).
6 This description of radically removing the dead parts of a plant in order to foster new growth is remarkably similar to Dodge's analogy about psychoanalysis in her paper "Psycho-Analysis with Dr. Brill" (1938b): "Does anyone suppose there is no pain involved when a tree drives its roots deeper, and expands its girth? Well, a psychoanalytic experience is as mysterious, as solemn, as organic as such a growth. And then, added to the blind imperious drive of nature consider the scientific, conscious, rational, directive force of a human being who is wise enough to let nature take its course, while at the same time he steers the course upward. He must stimulate growth, *he must prune away dead matter*" (pp. 4–5, italics added).

δ

46.

[circa February 23, 1916]
[written in red in Jelliffe's notes from February 23, 1916]

Last night./ In a rattrap, a piece of cheese:

All I can remember.

Jelliffe's notes from February 23, 1916:
Rat trap—not sure:/ knew it would be a nice touch [1]: *You think I think I am in a situation:/ ⊙ [2] think I am giving myself away* [3]:
 I am not satisfied peaceful, not upset:…..He [i.e., Sterne] says it is stable, he is rooted he said/ I am when he is with me & living to his best./ I realize I am extreme:/

Notes:

1 *Does this suggest Dodge's desire to please Jelliffe with evocative symbols such as a rattrap? Is she communicating a sense that she is trapped in her relationship with Sterne? Or that she is the cheese and thus luring either Sterne or Jelliffe into a trap?*
2 As before (see note 7 for dream 42), this symbol likely means "you" when Dodge refers to Jelliffe.
3 This may indicate Dodge's sense that Jelliffe objected to her relationship with Sterne because she gave him shelter and money.

δ

47.
[circa February 24, 1916]
[written in red in Jelliffe's notes from February 24, 1916]

Parrot,[1] & another animal, blackbird. Then I saw 3 green young parrots at bottom of cage. Later on, outdoors in snow, c. someone, saw some people skating, had to go through bushes or under bushes to get to it.

Jelliffe's notes from February 24, 1916:
Parrots./ I have one [2]:/ *Because mo. had a parrot* [3]:

Notes:

1 After they returned to Finney Farm from Provincetown in the fall of 1915, Sterne had persuaded Dodge "that to have a real farm we needed more animals, and she agreed." She bought two Persian cats and two turtledoves, the latter which were promptly eaten by the former, and then a red and green parrot that she soon gave away to her butcher because she was offended by its vulgar sounds (Sterne, 1952, pp. 115–116).
2 Dodge reports that she kept two green parrots in the Green House, an outbuilding at the farm where Boyeson often stayed, and where Jelliffe saw the birds when he visited one weekend: "He had seen the two large, green macaws…and had observed them with a small, knowing, psychoanalytical smile" (1936, p. 441).

3 Dodge remembers they had many animals in her childhood home, including cats, canaries, dogs, and "forever a parrot....The parrot habit
   seems a queer one" (1933a, pp. 55–56).

δ

48.
Thursday night [circa February 24, 1916]

Driving with Bayard & some other person,[1] two skirted small horses. Bayard is driving on the edge of a precipice, it is a narrow path & curving, a
curve so sharp that he cannot see that as we go round one horse is on the
glassy ivy path & the other walks off into the air...It is the horse on the right
side yet somehow Bayard can't see him & I can tho' I sit on the left. I seize
the reins & call out "He's over" or something like that—& we begin to haul
him up. We get him up all right.[2]
   Later it is I who am over the precipice which is straight up & down &
made of glass. Bayard is leaning over & pulling me up...I get up.

   Jelliffe's notes from February 26, 1916:
   *Third person in the dream/ 3rd person to right:/ B. & I together pulled
   up the horse./ Horses = B:/ 3rd person./ Bayard could not see & I could./
   round to right/ B. like in life/ Impossible:/ Will admit I cannot help him
   over. B. cold self[-]conscious techni[que]....Calculating/ think about himself./ Substitution:/ I...was not satisfied with seeing his minor traits: Really over.[3]/ have a real conception of friendship:/ In the ☿ relation no
   peace I think: no wish for it, apparently.[4]*
      *Then a dream of release: & today "breathe freely" & then another inter-
   esting thing* ͨ *yesterday before: usually c. depression & anxiety, now easily
   and no disturbance.[5]*

Notes:

1 Could this be Jelliffe since he has appeared in three recent dreams with
   Dodge and Boyeson?
2 *Although this dream describes going over a precipice twice and surviving,
   there is little fear here. What are these images about? Dodge goes over
   herself and survives, and Bayard helps her up. Is this related to Jelliffe
   welcoming Boyeson into her dreams and encouraging their connection over
   hers with Sterne? According to Freud (1900), "smooth walls over which
   the dreamer climbs, the façades of houses, down which he lowers himself—
   often in great anxiety—correspond to erect human bodies, and are probably in the dream recollections of a baby's climbing up his parents or nurse.
   The 'smooth' walls are men" (p. 355). Might this dream have to do with
   Dodge's early (and unfulfilled) wishes of reliance on a stable parent?*

3 In July 1916, Dodge summoned Boyeson to the main house in Croton and told him that she "meant to break up our life at Finney Farm because it wasn't doing anyone any good. 'I wanted to make a place where people I liked could come and be free to do work,' I told him. 'But it's a perfect failure. I am injuring you instead of helping you. You must go back to Athol in the fall and make your own life, Bayard'" (1936, p. 478).

4 It is not known if the intercourse Dodge refers to here is an attempt that she and Boyeson made together or a sexual relationship he had with another person, presumably a man.

5 This recalls Dodge's observation of a disturbance she feels when Sterne is away from her (see note 10 for dream 33). Whatever this symbol refers to (perhaps masturbation, see note 4 for dream 33), she clearly had a different experience this time.

δ

49.
Friday night [circa February 25, 1916]

Dreamed I was in some hotel hall with Maurice talking—he talking earnestly to me. When we got up to go out the door I looked back thinking him right behind me. He was asking the man at the door something in a low confidential way. The man was answering in the same secretive way. I saw their eyes were on three women one of whom was looking at Maurice intensely & smiling. I knew he was asking her name & getting any information he could about her. I impatiently called to him to come along.

Afterwards he was sitting talking to her & she was saying as he got up to join me: "An artist—to be an artist must live <u>beautifully</u>." Later we were leaving each other, we were in the midst of some actors or singers, & he was one and I was one. He was leaving. He was packing—I walked thro' a corridor to his room & he was with his italian friend Gigi.[1] He was gentle & sad but it was necessary to go. He was trying to make me think something different from the way it was & was saying "You know it[']s not a sign the ocean will be as low as it was high..." or some words like that.[2] I rather knew he was leaving because of a woman tho' I knew he loved me—tho' not as he had. Gigi was joking & laughing in a strange language. He pointed to something out in the port (we were on the sea) & said something with a laugh, that means "Small guns" tho' not in the naval sense he laughed. I couldn't see what he meant at first then I did.[3] I remember I was feeling no sorrow at Maurice leaving.

Jelliffe's notes from February 26, 1916:
Type of sexual joke annoys me:/ Don't like that type of joke./ hate cleverness & wittiness. Don't like a laughing attitude towards relations....

Felt in dream he was leaving for some reason he was not telling. Ac-
tors & singers. This seemed like Emmanuel Reicher [4]: *whom I have seen*
lately....They were talking professionally; Bobby was talking of legs & his
costume last night [5]: *Going back on a whole plan of life, which I feel sad*
about; Don't feel distressed: Feeling ♀ trying to get him away from me: not
spiritually beautiful: Blonde, greyish green eyes, pink cheeks, 3 ♀[.] *She*
was one with dark circles under her eyes. ♀ can't remind me of anyone:
maybe German, maybe this ♀ Maurice is interested in is German.[6] *Not*
jealous of him! Have dismissed him: I have feeling I have acted like a man
in this thing.[7]/

Notes:

1 In *Shadow and Light* (1952), Sterne recalls his 1908 trip to Italy when he
   met Gigi:

   I found a large studio and with the help of Gigi, a dashing neighbor, I
   was able to heat it fairly well. Gigi was the most exciting local character: handsome, vain, boastful, and always acting a part. He got into
   all sorts of scrapes, and tricked me badly several times, although I always seemed to find him out before too much damage was done. Gigi
   remained my friend through it all because I greatly enjoyed watching
   his playacting and I think he respected me for not being taken in by
   him....My greatest Italian compliment came one afternoon when I
   was having a drink with Gigi and he looked speculatively at me and
   said, "You know, for an American you're pretty smart." (pp. 70–71)

2 *Although the meaning of this statement is elusive—could he be saying that*
   the sadness is not as great as the joy?—common themes in Dodge's dreams
   are low and high, depths and heights.

3 *This double entendre with its erotic suggestion demonstrates Dodge's en-*
   thusiastic embrace of the language and play of dream interpretation. As
   always, she likely was pleased to be dreaming dreams that had elements
   that would capture Jelliffe's interest.

4 See note 1 for dream 32.

5 Jones and Reicher were both involved in Percy MacKaye's *Caliban* that
   was to be staged in May 1916. Reicher played the Ghost of Hamlet's Father and Jones was the set designer (and may already have begun working on his designs). See note 1 for dream 127.

6 Dodge was always jealous of a married German woman, referred to
   as "B." in her memoir, but most likely Mira Sohn, as discussed below,
   whom Sterne knew before he met Dodge. B. loved Sterne but refused to
   betray her husband. As Dodge reports in *Movers and Shakers* (1936):
   "She was the only woman he had ever really loved.... He had loved her
   for years; he had lived near her in Rome....He had tried in every way

to recover himself; but no other woman had reached him so deeply as she....I often accused him of being still attached, spiritually, to B., I felt he was attached *some*where, for he didn't seem free to give himself completely to me and make me feel fulfilled by him; so it seemed to me B. must be the element that held him" (pp. 366, 457). Dodge also talked about B. in her session with Jelliffe on April 27, 1916: "*Has strong hold on him. Basis of my distrust—would leave me & go to her.*" Sterne himself wrote about his unrelenting captivation with a married German woman, Mira Sohn, whom he met in Berlin in 1910 and immediately fell in love with: "From that first moment in her home I felt that a power stronger than I could cope with was robbing me of my will and of my freedom....Mira was my completion; I was a fragment away from her, in tangible physical pain" (Sterne, 1952, p. 82). Sterne could also have written these sentences about his relationship with Dodge, as he could feel diminished and trapped by her, but also miserable when away from her.

7 *Could this relate to Dodge's statement in a circa May 24, 1916 letter to Jelliffe that he told her she had been using "my femaleness malely"? See Interlude 17.*

δ

50.
Sunday, February 27, 1916 (1 of 2)

Large, huge covered place, a great shed even acres big, made of unpainted timber. In one corner I see are very early aztec [1] carvings, huge architectural stuff, something that is being arranged, built. I observe that, while I hear a good deal of indescribable noise in this large clear space, still there is much less than outside of it. I note that much noise is shut out.[2] I know that all this is a preparation that [Stephan] Bourgeois [3] is making for something, for an eastern exhibit perhaps.

Jelliffe's notes from February 28, 1916:
Aztec:/ Big supports: like his work, preparatory work [4]....
   Noise: of winds not hammering: of nature./ hurricane:/ heart intestines./ unassimable [sic]/ I can't digest him.[5]
   Bourgeois/ represents: a mentor, director of Maurice: good fine type for a business man./ He is so plainly out to make money. I am a picture dealer: must study to hang my pictures.[6] Always took medicine for intestine:/ Colitis: later: pills every night:/ none now for a couple of years. this last year more:/ I used to have p.c.[7] habit. Wind/... flatulency at times: related to depression, rarely c. colic. In last 2–3 mos. deep down on left side a sore spot in the groin, intestine tied in a knot, always in same

decided complex or auto intox[ication] & don't get rid.[8] *Always look to
see, colitis days. Vary in color & in size—lately very dark: ordinarily less
so: darker constip. coarse whole wheat bread: bothered since psa. I think
more of intestine.*[9]

Bad breath. Am curious about self: no test./ Cigarette smoking,[10]
possibly:/ Father gave me first when I was 17,[11] *don't call it a habit: Have
stopped, never have had distinct craving: "No compulsion about it."*

Notes:

1 In his memoir, Hutchins Hapgood recalls "a curious thing" that happened after a peyote party at Dodge's 23 Fifth Avenue apartment in 1914:
"Many of us, for days and weeks afterwards, had dreams in which there
were many Aztec symbols, and…Mabel, on a visit to the museum, found
the statue of an ancient Aztec with a peyote button carved on his breast"
(1939, p. 366).

2 *The inside is loud but not as loud as outside of the space, the sound is kept
out. Could this image relate to digestive sounds inside the intestine, with
the world outside being louder? Dodge could be preoccupied with the workings of her bowels, as indicated in a number of Jelliffe's notes, including
those for this dream.*

3 A French dealer specializing in Post-Impressionism who opened a New
York gallery in 1914 at 668 Fifth Avenue and who was Sterne's dealer
at this time. In March 1917, Sterne had an exhibition of drawings and
paintings at the Bourgeois Gallery.

4 This "great shed even acres big" may relate to the preparations for
MacKaye's *Caliban,* a performance staged in a large stadium. See note 1
for dream 127.

5 *Dodge's interpretation that she cannot digest Sterne—she cannot assimilate him into her body or psyche, she cannot process him, he is not nourishing for her— is similar to her assertion that Jelliffe "felt that my subjective
feeling for Maurice made me sick" (1936, p. 456).*

6 This may be a reference to the fact that Dodge had begun to paint watercolors at this time. Leo Stein remarked in a letter to her from March 31,
1916: "I haven't yet received any of your handiwork though I saw some
at Jelliffe's." He wrote again, circa early April 1916: "I got your picture
all right and think it very good indeed for one so young though perhaps
it[']s a trifle casual." Stieglitz mentioned Dodge's watercolors in a March
27, 1916 letter—"So you are water-coloring! That is a surprise"—and
inquired on April 6, 1916: "I wonder what they look like. Am I to see
them?" Her only extant watercolor is in the collection of the Beinecke
Rare Book and Manuscript Library, a painting of tulips inscribed on the
frame "For Dr. Brill," likely from 1916 or 1917.

7 i.e., "after meals," medical shorthand for Latin post cibum.

8 *Dodge's associations to intestines—with mentions of colitis, constipation, and a knotted colon—combine with her linking the noise of the wind with both flatulence and depression to create a feeling of dark turmoil and stuckness. She cannot "get rid" of her "complex" and is suffering in her dependent relationship with Sterne.*

9 Through her psychoanalysis with Jelliffe, Dodge came to understand the connection between excrement and money, and therefore constipation as a symptom with meaning. See note 7 for dream 39 about "fecal erotics."

10 Dodge smoked cigarettes when she was in Europe in 1904, a habit for women that carried immense social stigma, with associations to questionable morals and erotic life, but also signaled emancipation. Dodge recalled her first dinner in Paris with Edwin where "we smoked a great many cigarettes" (1935, p. 64). When her grandmother Ganson arrived in France for their wedding months later, Dodge immediately asked if she had any cigarettes, and her grandmother replied, "'No—but you shall have some, honey,'" and arranged for someone to buy them. Dodge then took a cigarette "under Grandma's pleased and beaming smile" (1933a, pp. 111, 112), a feeling that must have been extremely gratifying for her in her growing quest to challenge traditional views of women.

11 Dodge recalls her father smoking "hard cigars" and admits that since childhood "I have loathed the smell of cigar smoke in the house" (1933a, p. 118). Her memory of her father giving her a first cigarette in 1896 is striking given both the social mores around women smoking at that time and also his forbidding "kissing games" when she was younger.

δ

51.
Sunday February 27, 1916 (2 of 2)

Later I am trying to think of a name & an address to write on an envelope, a letter. I can only remember half of it—Leo Stein—who is the most maddening person if one is impatient [1]—is trying to tell me what I want to know but he can't get it to me fast enough. He says: "Oh yes, Nichols…Why that's old Murry Nichols [2]…Yes, let me see"…"But the address, Leo," I beg. "What's that?" he delays, refusing to give it up tho' he knows I'm in a hurry. "Oh! For God's Sake, Leo, what's the address," I shout to him. I get it, I think, finally. No satisfaction.

Complex met complex [3] in that dream. Leo hung on to his information & refused to understand my immediacy!

Jelliffe's notes from February 28, 1916:

Last night we had L.S. galloping all over the place [4]: *Anxiety:/ Part of science of discussing B[oyeson]. & M[abel].D[odge].:/ teasing him/ his anti-socialism....*

Leo S[.] trying to tell me what I know.

Notes:

1 Dodge described Stein's stubbornness as revealed in "an obstinate look on his face that so resembled an old ram" (1935, p. 321). She was often impatient with others, a theme that appears in a number of her dreams (#s 49, 77, & 90). This impatience could take a violent turn, as in the following event that Dodge reported in *Background* (1933a, pp. 164–167) and to Jelliffe, as recorded in his March 25, 1916 notes (see Figure 5.2): "*Impatience, 9 & 10 [years old], almost criminal....at Newport, nurse stupid & slow—I flew into a rage, tried to throw off cliff, succeeded, very nearly killed her.*"
2 Unidentified.
3 Dodge enthusiastically embraced this language of psychoanalysis.
4 Stein was likely visiting Dodge at Finney Farm.

δ

52.
Monday, February 28, 1916 (1 of 3)

Dreamed I was in the country. I had taken an old[-]fashioned house & meant to do it all over, plant a garden & fix it all up. I was planting a lot of box plants & green borders & also a lot of yellow chrysanthemums. My mother was about, mixed up in it. Perhaps we were going to take the house together.

(Does this mother-hate & golden flowers-money-complex coming back mean I <u>want</u> *to get pleasantly fixed up with my mother?*[1] *I often dream of her vaguely lately.)*

Jelliffe's notes from February 28, 1916:

Last night: Mother hatred: Yellow chrysanthemums: more pleasant c. her. Seen her in Nov. or Dec. in N.Y. Make each other terribly uncomf.[2] *She rubs me wrong way. Very dominating: 63–64. Looks as young as I. Well preserved. m[arried]. last year* [3]*....Yet I must urge her each mo[nth].— Edw[in]. [Dodge] pays taxes & mortgages etc: She gives & gives & gives.*[4] *All intermixes.*

Notes:

1   As Dodge relates in "Family Affairs" (1933b), it was to be years before she would be freed from her antipathy toward her mother—in fact, not until 1933, when the first volume of her autobiography was published: "'Background,' then, delivered me from my hatred for my mother. You can't hate what you are sorry for, you can't hate others when you understand that they can't help what they do and say" (p. 3). Within months after the publication of *Background*, Dodge's mother died. *Dodge's wish to have a more loving relationship with her mother is expressed in this possibility of working on and living in a house together, planting gardens and flowers, an activity strongly associated with her mother (see note 1 for dream 53). The money complex may refer to Dodge's immense financial dependence on her mother.*

2   In "Family Affairs" (1933b), Dodge admits: "We were uncomfortable together, for she criticised [*sic*] everything I did and all my friends; while I, who felt contemptuous of her two husbands, Admiral Reeder and Monty, and all her friends, had generally to keep my mouth shut" (p. 2). However, Dodge did not always hold back, as revealed in an undated letter from her mother, written in all capital letters: "I DON[']T WANT YOU TO SAY SUCH THINGS AS YOU DO ABOUT MONTY FOR HE HAS NEVER SAID A WORD TO ME OF WHAT I SHOULD DO ABOUT YOUR LIVING OR ANYTHING AT ALL. [AFTER] ALL HE HA[S] DONE FOR YOU IT[']S NOT RIGHT FOR YOU TO SAY WHAT YOU DO OF HIM. I NEVER SIAD [*sic*] TO HIM WHAT YOU SAID FOR I WOULD NOT MAKE HIM FEEL YOU WERE SO IN-HUMAN." Dodge (1933b) describes the physical pain she experienced in her mother's company: "those terrible, unexpressed resentments and depressions that I had had to endure whenever I was with her, feelings that were physical and that came, either like serpents coiling or uncoiling in madness in the vagina, or like an iron hand clamped inwardly upon the contents of my belly, so that heart, stomach and liver were squeezed temporarily dead" (p. 3). Unfortunately, Sara Ganson left no written accounts of her experiences of being a mother to her daughter, although she often communicated harsh tones in her existing letters to Dodge, made even more shrill by her writing with all capitals: "I CANNOT STAND ALL THIS WORRY FROM BOTH YOU & JOHN [Evans]. I THINK YOU ARE MAKING A GRAVE MISTAKE...HE SHOULD BE MADE TO LOOK OUT FOR HIMSELF & FAMILY" (June 26, 1925).

3   Dodge's mother had recently remarried a man named Montague, nicknamed "Monty." Mabel's father had died in 1902 and her mother had married Admiral Reeder, who died in 1911. Dodge describes these two men: "I had small opinions of the men she chose to marry—for the pink

and white admiral, so pompous and full of strut; or the small business man, 'Monty', also pompous and round and only a year older than myself" (1933b, p. 4).

4   This reference to taxes and mortgages most likely concerns the Villa Curonia, which Mabel and Edwin Dodge still owned, as a letter among Edwin's correspondence to Mabel indicates that the Villa was not sold until 1935. In a letter dated January 24, 1916, Edwin had reassured her: "You need not fear that I shall go back on my word regarding the payments." In 1924, Edwin writes that he has a possible buyer and reminds Mabel: "You will remember in 1916 you were conferring about handing over to her [Mabel's mother] your share in the villa." Dodge's mother often helped Mabel with expenses, including paying for her psychoanalysis, despite her own intense disapproval of it. In a June 26, 1925 letter, she lashed out at her daughter for relying on analysis to help solve problems: "IT[']S ALL ROT TO HAVE BRILL SEE HIM [i.e., John Evans] & ANOTHER PARTY TO WORK BOTH YOU & ME. YOU MUST WORK THIS YOUR SELF. I DON[']T BELIEVE AT ALL IN BRILL & HE WORKS YOU LIKE EVERYTHIN[G]. WHY SHOULD YOU OR JOHN HAVE A STRANGER TELL YOU OR JOHN HOW TO LIVE YOUR LIVES. WHAT IF MONTY IN HIS YOUNG DAYS HAVE TO HAVE A DR TELL HIM WHAT TO DO TO MAKE HIM SELF A RE[A]L MAN." Dodge describes the effect of her mother's financial support on their relationship: "Because my mother was giving me two thirds of the income I lived on...I had to be as nice as I could to her" (1933b, p. 2). She also speculates: "I think part of my mother's generosity to me came from an instinctive need to balance the budget of our relationship" (1933b, p. 7).

δ

53.
Monday, February 28, 1916 (2 of 3)

Later I am in a flower shop ordering flowers.[1] I want a certain kind but they haven't it & they ask me if they can send me a lilac, a beautiful plant, they say, & they describe it so I <u>smell</u> it & feel it, & I take it.[2]

Notes:

1   Dodge was drawn to flowers from an early age, but rejected her mother's approach to them. In *Background* (1933a), she describes her mother's tulip bed at their Buffalo home and her protest at the rigidity of the precise rows of color: "the whole thing so mathematical and so ordered that all the spontaneity and flowerness of growth couldn't be felt at all. It was

like a slaughter of innocents to plant those hardy bulbs and make them come up in unbroken and undifferentiated rows....So that I, who loved flowers so much and who used to try to assimilate each kind into myself by a passionate sniffling, followed often by a more passionate tasting, could never bear that flower bed" (pp. 18–19). In her memoirs, Dodge's descriptions of both the Villa Curonia and Finney Farm include close attention to flowers and trees.

2 *This dream shows Dodge as uncharacteristically receptive to the suggestions of another when she has already set her mind on something. Perhaps this suggests her openness to the process of analysis and its consideration of alternate meanings?*

δ

INTERLUDE 6.

In her next dream (# 54), Dodge recalls driving in a vehicle with Sterne. Less than two weeks before, he had written to her, circa February 17, 1916, from Pottsville about *his* dream of driving *her* car, reported in *Movers and Shakers* (1936):

I must tell you the dream I had the other night. I was driving your car. I don't remember who else was in it, only Albert, or rather his voice, for I don't remember seeing him. I went along smoothly and at high speed when suddenly I came to a place that looked like this: [drawing]—the street where I intended to go all torn up and excavated. Through the scaffolding one could see deep holes in the earth. I didn't know how to stop the car, in fact there seemed no way of stopping it. I realized that to go straight ahead would destroy me. I then decided to go straight for the protruding wall, but before the car could touch it, I shot out my legs and received the blow with my feet. Then the car bounced back a moment but didn't stop, but went for the wall again. This kept up a long time, I always by shooting out my legs and pulling up my knees saving the car from ruin.

Gradually the driving force of the car seemed to lessen and my strength was leaving me, but Albert's voice always encouraging me on. When I had the car stopped, a very important-looking man, big and fat, with a bundle of tools, came up saying he'd stop it. I remonstrated, feeling that I ought to get the credit, but he didn't mind me, got busy with his tools, and when I looked at the bottom of the car I found that he had made a deep round hole in it.

Strange dream, isn't it? I have interpreted it in my own way. Shall I tell you? Your car: our relationship. I was driving full speed to destruction. The brick wall: Pottsville. I batter away at Pottsville and save our love. Then Dr. Jelliffe with his psychoanalytical technique, comes along and claims the credit for something I did myself.—But I don't like the hole in the bottom of the car. (p. 451)

Earlier in this letter, Sterne explained his interpretation about Jelliffe's proprietary involvement in their relationship, expressing his exasperation about the psychoanalytic process and his feelings of betrayal when he learned that Dodge had revealed to Jelliffe intimate details of their interactions: "I have always thought it crude and vulgar when that which two feel at moments of deepest self-revelation and self-giving is revealed to a third. When I knew that what to me are wonderful mystic rites, you were laying bare on the psychoanalytical operating table, I felt outraged and insulted. I suppose the reasons you did it and the object in view should be considered, but I can't! This is the *true* cause of my jealousy of Dr. Jelliffe" (Luhan, 1936, p. 450). Sterne is wary of returning to Finney Farm until Dodge is finished with her analysis: "Mabel, how long do you think your psychoanalysis will take? It just occurred to me that since most of the trouble between us began when you started the course, it would perhaps be advisable that I stay here until you are through with it" (p. 450). Dodge was discouraged about Sterne's refusal to enter analysis himself, and even disappointed in the quality of his dreams: "I kept on trying my best to lure him to be analyzed, too, by Dr. Jelliffe, but he never would, although he began to watch his dreams and tell them to me, hoping, I think, that I could recount them to the analyst. His psyche dealt with him as though he were a child and presented him with the most kindergarten dreams that he could scarcely fail to understand. They warned him of an imminent catastrophe, when showing Dr. Jelliffe as a mechanic with a bag of tools!" (p. 454).

δ

54.
Monday, February 28, 1916 (3 of 3)

Later in the night I am driving in a carriage or motor with Maurice…

Prefer to tell details of this dream.[1]

An apparent diary entry in Dodge's handwriting appears here after the dream, dated Monday, February 28:

> *After a long time of thinking & associating last night I came to a realization that I don't want to be always the dominator. I want to give in but only to my superior in all ways. I don't want to give in, so long as I am the superior, to another's mind or will. But I could if another's heart were bigger than mine & if another's truth were more honest than mine. I have never known a man whom [sic] I felt was greater than I in both of these—so I always said God was the only possible satisfactory lover.*

But I know I would be glad if someone would say—"Stop & be quiet.
Stop kicking—it's all right"—& I could believe it. Then I would relax.
Tho' not till I was sure he was the greater in heart & truth.[2]

Notes:

1 No more details of this dream are recorded in Jelliffe's case notes.

2 *As much as she seemed determined to lead with her dominating ways, Dodge*
   longed to surrender to another who was wiser and "superior" in "heart &
   truth," someone she could trust so she could stop "kicking" and then be able
   to "relax." This was a lifelong search for her, given her early childhood dep-
   rivation of love and her inability to trust her caregivers with her heart and
   truths. She had trained herself—in spite of her urgent strivings to find a man
   to complete and protect her—to rely on inner resources, as unreliable as
   they could sometimes be. Dodge recalled a moment in Sterne's disappointing
   company: "I felt terribly alone in the world and it was he who made me feel
   it....I tried to retire into my secret self and to commune with the reassuring
   presence there that never failed me in those days" (1936, pp. 365–366). In her
   initial intake session with Jelliffe on January 3, 1916, she talked about her
   strategy for protecting herself: "Now safe, reached security: now grown up. I
   found it in self:/ nothing can hurt me. Then another ♂./ Seriously involved."

δ

INTERLUDE 7.

Tuesday [circa spring 1916]

Dear Dr. Jelliffe,

I have just read over a letter written to Nina Bull in answer to one of
hers about my change of faith—etc[.]—etc. It seems to me to sum up a typical experience—it must be so—in psychoanalysis, so I am sending it to
you to read—if you care to—& then you can post it to her—please. I will
be in Sat. at 3–5 please instead of 4–6.

Faithfully,
M.D.

Nina Bull, a Divine Science practitioner, was treating Dodge at this same
time when Dodge was in analysis with Jelliffe. Although Bull expressed
impatience and scorn for psychoanalysis in her letters to Dodge, she was
also intrigued by it, as excerpts from some of her 1916 letters to Dodge
reveal: "I'm so glad about psychoanalysis—& I want to hear about what
it's doing to you. Jelliffe must be a wonder. I'd like to know him"; "First
are you still going to Jelliffe? If you are, I don't think I can treat you, for
I feel his influence over you to be very strong, & decidedly harmful just

now, & I should be working with a tremendous handicap. You have gotten all you can get from him for the present—of this I'm very sure"; "You have immersed yourself in a psychoan. atmosphere for months now—& have absorbed it thru every pore. Why not give the other thing—the real thing—a chance? It alone can give you what you want. You are only wasting your time without it!" In another letter from 1916, Bull explains to Dodge about what she considers the shortcomings of analysis: "Psychoanalysis focuses all the consciousness on a plane which isn't the highest—& of course that has a bad effect if carried on too steadily....I am doubtful if I shall ever be analyzed....I have yet to hear of the person who has been psychoanalyzed into a state of higher spiritual consciousness." Despite her objections, Nina Bull eventually did enter analysis with Jelliffe, likely in the 1930s.

δ

55.
Tuesday, February 29, 1916

Was walking across the fields with John towards the Duncan School.[1] One of the teachers there showed us a picture of a little place of hers she had lived in. She said it was so beautiful & loved it. It looked common & suburban to us. Soon John had to go into a church for a lesson and asked me to come along. It was a kind of confirmation lesson. I went after him. We climbed up into a kind of chair loft & sat down. Presently a woman came in. I knew it was the teacher who would be influencing John if she could so I looked at her with curiosity & some worry.[2] I saw it was Mrs. Glenny.[3] *Mrs. Glenny always drank in Buffalo. Very handsome & world[ly]. She "reformed" afterwords* [sic]. *But is half witted now.* She was looking like a saint. All in white, her hands clasped over her breast, her eyes down, her hair undone & hanging down each side of her face. I knew she hadn't been a saint because she had always drank, & I wondered if she could teach John just as well if he didn't know it. Her cheeks looked flushed.

Then I knew I was sitting in Nina Bull's lap. I felt her warmth.[4] Then someone was standing by & telling me things against the teacher, Mrs. Glenny. She said: "You see she'd stopped to speak to Harry Bull.[5] Of course that kind of man would be speaking to her." I note to myself that of course a horsy man like Harry Bull would like her. *(He isn't horsy but he's a hypocrite, to my mind. This dream is all about hypocrites.)*

Then the person, whose name & personality I forget now, goes on to say things against Mrs. Glenny and I am more & more thinking she's no one to teach John or persuade him into the church. This person says Mrs. G. is hard up, that she & May Palmer [6] (a homosexualist) are living together, etc., & I see she is disreputable & scheming & bad. She comes in, "makes an entrance," very slowly & effectively. After this is over others begin to make entrances. It is as tho' we watched them from a gallery...& were judging their technique. As tho' they were all pretending or acting.

A little oldish woman is brought in in a chair. She is lame or crippled, in great pain. She wants to be gotten into a certain place & she is dumped in the aisle instead. Her eyes shine with pain & her brows contract but she smiles & gives directions firmly. She also is pretending, a good kind of pretending. One tries to lift or push her chair to where she wants it & fails but she just, with great firmness & character beckons to another. It is a large sensible looking woman, I cannot remember the face.[7] This one lifts the whole thing & she is finally gotten into place, somewhere, I don't know where. Meanwhile the saint got up & walked out in real character, in quite a hurry, bowing sociably to everyone, & disappeared. I am somewhat relieved she won't be there to influence John.

Jelliffe's notes written at the end of the dream:
I can imagine getting into my f[ather]'s desk [8] but I cannot get into my mother's womb and as for nursing at my mother's breast [9] it makes me sick.[10]

Jelliffe's notes from March 2, 1916:
Mrs. John Glenny: (drank, husb[and] drank) all sorts/.... This woman: always worldly: like a saint: I wondered if she could teach John/ Do not lie to each other:/ Not a mother & son attitude:/....

Nina Bull:/ warmth of body buttocks, no sex glow, skin glow./ My back her front# I have been her model in a way/. I suddenly recall how my father was in l. c. her mother [11]: mothers not friends. Play c. Nina, early period: try to shock her: Angle worms: eat them. I could pretend to put in mouth & throw over shoulder.[12] Mabel Ganson:/ N. Bull[']s history interesting, done much same things. Our divorces about one month: later. How funny: Mrs. Wilcox—takes a town Buffalo size: Nina's step mo: This sister had always liked F[ather]. Awfully glad I was strange & ate worms. Made her productive: Something in Buffalo:/ All out of rebellion./

May P:/....Went to ♀/ Paris./

Years of pain/ anxiety/ Smiles. She also is pretending.

Anger...& pink toe: mother took me into her bed & made me cringe: terrible pain [13]:/ Any idea of similar type, feels in clitoris.

Notes:

1   At the time of this dream, John Evans was 14 years old and a student at the Morristown School in New Jersey. In Jelliffe's notes from March 2, 1916, he records Dodge stating that John wants to come home from

school. At some point, she did withdraw him "from the atmosphere of the stuffy boarding school and I gave him" to the Elizabeth Duncan School in Croton, where he was at first the only boy (Luhan, 1936, p. 347). However, Evans was back at Morristown in the fall, as a report card from November 8, 1916 lists him enrolled in the fourth form (MDLC).

2 *Even though Dodge rejected her son in his early years, she made efforts toward providing him with a stable home (by marrying Edwin), seeing to his education by hiring tutors in Italy, and then, when they were returning to the United States, finding him a good school. In this dream, she is concerned with the influence of others on him.*

3 A woman from Dodge's childhood Buffalo. In *Background* (1933a), Dodge makes a pointed contrast between her art teacher at St. Margaret's, Rose Clark, who was a real artist and had a studio, and women in Buffalo who painted, such as Mrs. Glenny, who "were just married women living in their houses" (p. 225).

4 *The warmth of a lap is a powerful image and sensation for Dodge, who described the cold atmosphere of her childhood: "Probably most people have some memories of their earliest years that contain a little warmth and liveliness but in my own I cannot find one happy hour. I have no recollections of my mother's ever giving me a kiss or smile of spontaneous affection" (1933a, p. 23).* See note 3 for dream 1. Even Dodge's father could not extract a kiss from her mother, as she relates to Jelliffe on April 27, 1916: *"Only one kiss....He laughed & he tried to kiss her. She not affectionate at all....Only angry words."* In Background (1933a) she described this scene: "I never saw but one affectionate gesture from my father to her and that was on a Christmas Eve when I was very small indeed." When Dodge's father opened a gift from her mother, he was so pleased that he exclaimed: "'I'm afraid I'll have to give you a kiss for that.' He bent over her....[and] approached her gingerly. She gave him a brusque push backward as his mouth drew near her cold cheek. 'Oh, get out!' she said, and the kiss slid off and dissolved in the darkness" (p. 25).

5 Nina Bull's husband.

6 A 1916 portrait of "Miss May Palmer" by the German-born American photographer Arnold Genthe (who also photographed Isadora Duncan and other dancers in New York at this time) very likely depicts the woman that Dodge mentions (LOC). A May Palmer is also listed as an actress in the films *The Flame of the Yukon* (1917) and *One More American* (1918) (Internet Broadway Database, www.ibdb. com).

7 *Could this represent Dodge later in life, physically compromised but still forceful and demanding?*

8 In *Background* (1933a), Dodge elaborately describes the excitement of exploring her father's childhood desk in the home where Grandma Ganson still lived, and reveals her compassion for his eventual plight:

> I used to sit down on the floor and pull open the little door in the side of the old walnut desk. Behind it was a row of drawers reaching to the floor. And in them lay some gritty turquoise beads—of strange shapes, strung on an old string—some strangely shaped pipes of transparent browns and yellows, queer-looking, giving a feeling of darkness and danger in dusky rooms far away. These pipes had tortured curves and forms—there was nothing matter-of-fact about them, as there was about the pipes one was accustomed to in dull, ruminating hands in Buffalo! Accustomed! Everything was familiar and so safe! That was the trouble. Safe and comfortable as in Grandma Ganson's or safe and sad and dreary at home.... But these queer, almost eery pipes and the strings of rough, oblong beads of turquoise—they carried one away from home. The beads had a delicious, indescribable odor of another land—sweet and acrid and different. And the pipes! Oh, they smelled of a life so far away and so alluring! To a child sitting on a green carpet before a black-walnut desk, the pipes seemed the quintessence of an almost painfully beautiful life. I put the turquoise, shell, and amber between my teeth and drew in the faint, far-away odors of the East...of tobacco grown in Egypt...and smoked by—my father, yes, but my father in another life than ours. In a life free and far away and ennobled by the strange dangers he passed through, my father before he was caught and pinned down in Buffalo by my mother and me and Grandma Ganson. (pp. 113–114)

9 Given Sara Ganson's extreme reserve and lack of affection, it is unlikely she ever nursed her daughter. See notes 3 and 4 for dream 17 for a description of Dodge's childhood fascination with a breast that squirted milk.

10 *Dodge's affinity for her father is apparent here, as she can imagine a closeness with him, due to her understanding of and identification with his mental illness, perhaps an undiagnosed type of manic-depression that she also considered a possible diagnosis for herself (see Interlude 10). In contrast, an imagined closeness with her mother makes her sick and repels her. Dodge's longing for a mother was fueled by her repulsion toward her own.*

11 In *Background* (1933a), Dodge remembers: "Nina Wilcox [later Bull] is one of those whose destiny and mine have been linked together from the earliest days. My connection with her began when, as they told me, my father fell in love with her mother. But he married my mother and she married Ansley Wilcox and Nina and I were the outcome" (p. 68).

12 Dodge recalls: "I made Nina think that I could eat worms—by holding one in thumb and forefinger close to my mouth and then swiftly throwing it over my shoulder" (1933a, p. 80).

13 *This disturbing image of her mother taking her into her bed—an act usually associated with the promise of comfort—and then somehow inflicting pain, symbolizes the distress that Dodge felt even in the close presence of her mother.*

δ

INTERLUDE 8.

The day after Jelliffe wrote these notes for Dodge's analytic session, his wife died suddenly. According to the date of his next note, he and Dodge did not meet again until March 13, 1916. Jelliffe had fallen in love with Helena Leeming 34 years earlier and they had five children together. In his "Notebook of General Observations" (1905–1944), he recorded the facts of his wife's death, in much the same way he noted weather conditions and water levels at Arcady, their Lake George home: "March 3, 1916. Mother (Helena) died suddenly of brain hemorrhage. Had been well and over-busy. Her will leaves ½ Arcady to me: ½ to the children undivided" (SJA). Nowhere does he record his emotions at her sudden death. It is only in reading a series of handwritten notes from William Alanson White to Jelliffe immediately following this unexpected news that some of his deep grief is implied. On March 3, 1916, White wrote from Washington, D.C.:

> My dear Jelliffe[,]
> Have just this minute hung up the phone. I was inexpressibly shocked by what you told me & could not find words to speak my feelings as I felt also that you could not for I caught the tremor in your voice. I know that this will mean a very great readjustment for you in all sorts of ways that just at this moment of course are not clear. If I can help you let me know how. After all perhaps I know you better than anyone else so therefore perhaps I may be able to help better than anyone else. I feel deeply that you thought of me & wanted me to know. Give my love to all the children & don't forget all the wisdom that we have been trying to work out for other people. I have had to take many a dose of it myself & perhaps a good old fashioned tablespoonful may help you now. Then philosophy if only it can be brought to bear as the right time. Try & use all there is in it now. I shall want to see you very soon. You will be constantly in my mind.
>
> With my deepest sympathy & sincere affection[,]
> Wm A White

He sent another letter to Jelliffe the next day, March 4, 1916:

> My first impulse yesterday was to get on the train & go to NY. But after all I wasn't sure that that would be wise....However[,] if you need me in any way let me know.
>
> I hope after the immediate confusion settles down & the necessary adjustments are made...you get right after the work. After all that's our best friend so get at it just as soon as you can....
>
> Be good to yourself these days.

And then again, two days later:

> How are you? I am wondering. I am thinking that soon I shall commence to write business letters to you, not for you to answer but to help you back to work....
>
> I haven't said anything in any letters about Mrs[.] Jelliffe but I've known her as long as I have you & her going was the very last thing in my mind. I feel her loss in a very personal way. She had come to occupy a taken-for-granted position in my life....
>
> However, get to work & may even this sorrow be a stepping stone— an empty phrase to any but a psychoanalyst, but you know what it means in all its reaches.

On March 8, White invited Jelliffe to accompany him to New Orleans on April 1 for medical meetings: "What do you say about going along. It might help if you felt you could." On March 9, he responded to a communication from Jelliffe:

> I have your note of yesterday. What you need is a good sleep. How about a Turkish bath at the club, a good rub down, a dose of veronal & then select 2 or 3 of your patients who are suffering most & try as hard as you can to help them. Then you will find, as I often have, that the good advice you give them is quite as applicable to yourself. The giving of yourself this way I think will help. Don't let it all drive you too much into the unreal. Death has always been the greatest Harvester & then those that are left must go on living just the same. Face the whole thing as simply & directly as you can, get a good sleep & go to work.
>
> Work is the best medicine.

Helena Leeming Jelliffe's death was announced in the *Medical Record* on March 11, 1916, according to Jelliffe's handwritten notation in the margin of the clipping he saved, found loose at the back of his scrapbook from 1935–1943: "the wife of Dr. Smith Ely Jelliffe, who died on Friday of last week of cerebral hemorrhage, was a woman of unusual ability in many lines of human endeavor. Although not a physician herself much of her literary work was in medicine. She was the translator of a number of works in neurology and psychiatry and was also the writer of many editorial contributions" (SJA).

When Jelliffe and White revised their 1915 textbook, *Diseases of the Nervous System*, for a second edition in 1917, the dedication read: "To Helena Leeming Jelliffe, whose lofty purpose, ideal striving, and never-failing coöperation, have been a constant stimulus to progressive endeavor, this book is dedicated as a token of love and esteem."

Jelliffe wrote to Dodge on March 8, 1916, likely in response to a condolence letter from her:

Dear Mrs. Dodge,
    It all came so soon—and was over. She only had twenty minutes of pain— she had a ruptured blood vessel at the base of the brain. She has been a wonderful everything to me since I was a boy of 16, and I cannot yet know the full truth. I cannot believe it. With many thanks for your sympathy.

Very sincerely,
Smith Ely Jelliffe

δ

56.
[circa March 13, 1916]
[written in red in Jelliffe's notes from March 13, 1916] [1]

Recall no dreams. One spot of a dream:

Holy Grail—yellow—green—(these upsetting to me). Also coarse shiny common porcelain: Another feature of it—bands around it of common level, machine made base brass. Soldiers, I held it up—sort of an attack by more soldiers, unchained toys, then one of underbrush or ambush.[2]

> Jelliffe's notes from March 13, 1916:
> *Why so displeasing:/ not right task, not high level: something bad* [3]: *blue green high level, yellow not. Female organ = Holy Grail* [4]: *Lance & Grail = male & ♀/ Whole idea of common metal, lowest order color... Three things I loathe—(1) color (2) common pottery & (3) and machine made—all these used at once.*

Notes:

1 This is the first dream recorded and the first session notes since Jelliffe's wife died on March 3.

2 *Although these soldiers may be an association to World War I, the "ambush" here may refer to the sudden and unexpected death of Jelliffe's wife.*

3 *The appearance in this dream of "upsetting," "displeasing," "not right," and "something bad" may suggest Dodge's response to the death of Mrs. Jelliffe.*

4 *Dodge's association to the vagina as the holy grail, something earnestly pursued, is quite striking given her knowledge that Jelliffe is grieving over his wife.*

δ

57.
[circa March 16, 1916]
[written in red in Jelliffe's notes from March 16, 1916]

Seated in W[alter].L[ippmann].'s lap: Relative size of child & grown up person, recalls nurse[']s lap.[1]

Jelliffe's notes from March 16, 1916:
Canadians [sic] nurse: brown hair, brown eyes, sitting in her lap looking out of windows: horses racing....

I recall another little girl Dorothy [Scatchard] [2]....bathroom c. her, her doing something, urinating some fascination. She was trying to make me see this, to touch her down there. 5–6–7./ I recall some feeling. She had it & through her I had it./ She reminds me [of] Chevy Chase girl. Bdg [i.e., boarding] school, handle & caress her genitals: ♀-♀: made my mo. take me out. I assume ♀ role./ I got vague feeling of pleasure:/ She simply lay there. It made me glow, but never led me to seek self....

Odors/ I recall the fact that fingers smelled—Probably ordinary urinary odor.

Jelliffe's notes from March 23, 1916:
My first idea: Sanatorium idea: nurse's lap: also recalled when year or 2 old: Avon Springs Sanatorium: recall general effect: certain smell. linen. sunshine—certain experiences. Can recall being in verandah c. some nurses. Pale blonde sad lady looking down road. As I now think: acute melancholia. Always expecting him to come back—a propos of that: 5–6: Father aside: remember mo[']s mo & mo tried to take us away from him. Heard later F[ather]. had been in a sanit. [i.e., sanatorium] just after marriage. Probably reason why I was there: Later on someone told me F. crazy & had been locked up, for self-abuse [3]—after was in: Also had learned about Prince letter.[4] F. & m. together:....

After nurse[']s lap recollection—came to Avon Springs. Little tiny springs: In book as good a description page 643 text book.[5] Exact prototype: almost as such as that:/ Something happened 33–34: When I

left Edwin:/ Higher degrees of satisf[action] & lower dep[ression]. after
Reed:/ Dark night of the soul as the mystics would call it./ In a way I felt
saved, save them.#
    So much color:/ Delicious smell of linen & cookies/ Whether any horror/
Screaming & convulsion dream. 13–14: voice: smell: recognition of evil.[6]
/ Might be Avon:/ May be Springs. Swallowing.
    I have strong sense of ablutions, washing before and after.[7]

Notes:

1 This theme of sitting on a lap is repeated from dream 55, where Dodge
   was sitting on Nina Bull's lap and "felt her warmth." ***This carryover of the
   content of a comforting lap may be related to Dodge's response to Jelliffe's
   sudden absence after his wife's death, as she dreams of Lippmann, a trusted
   friend for whom she feels no sexual attraction. He, therefore, is free to be a
   source of non-sexual contact and reassurance. Dodge is the size of a child
   in the dream, another indication of her vulnerability and neediness when
   Jelliffe was away from his practice.***

2 A childhood friend from Buffalo whose aunt Emily Scatchard married
   Seward Cary. Dodge provides more sexual details of this same event in
   her associations to dream 122, as recorded in Jelliffe's May 16 notes.

3 i.e., masturbation. See note 1 for dream 15 and note 9 for dream 77.

4   This may refer to Dodge's 1914 letter to Dr. Morton Prince, see
   Interlude 10.

5 On page 643 in Jelliffe and White's textbook, *Diseases of the Nervous System* (1915), is a photograph entitled "Pseudobulbar palsy from syphilitic
   disease" to illustrate the following passage from the chapter on "Syphilis
   of the Nervous System": "Monoplegias are not infrequent, one arm, one
   leg, one side of the face, possibly the cortical speech areas with, in case
   of double lesion, pseudobulbar palsy. Minor speech disturbances are extremely frequent, tremors of the facial muscles usually accompanying
   the stumbling, stuttering or drawling speech." Page 643 also begins a
   section called, "Parenchymatous Types.—General Paresis." Could this
   be Dodge's remarkable recollection of the page number from Jelliffe's
   textbook or instead Jelliffe's note to himself written during Dodge's session? ***Is this reference a suggestion that Dodge's father, confined to a sanatorium, had syphilis?***

6 See dream 15 for a connection between a "peculiar smell" (of semen?) and
   evil, and note 3 for dream 61 for connections between the smell of semen,
   syphilis, and evil.

7 Presumably this refers to before and after sexual intercourse. In their
   co-written paper, Jelliffe and his patient Zenia X— had published an
   account of her ritual washing, as she admits that in her 20s "the idea
   that sexuality, therefore impurity, had crept in to separate me from

my duties....This idea was present with me probably even in child-hood. I was much given then to washing and cleansing my hands" (1914, p. 369).

δ

58.
[circa March 23, 1916]
[written in red in Jelliffe's notes from March 23, 1916]

Motoring: to r [1]: village: lots of people all sick, looked very attractive at first: only realized that after I got in.[2]

> Jelliffe's notes from March 23, 1916:
> *When I woke up, I laughed: all sick, all need some treatment./ I said to Bayard. I grudge the trip:/ does me good:/ I get tired in & out of motor:/*

Notes:

1 i.e., rural?
2 *This realization that surface attraction can hide illness may relate to Dodge's growing appreciation of the universality of neuroses and complexes, perhaps among her guests at Finney Farm such as Boyeson and Hartley. She says in her associations that she laughed when she woke up from the dream, possibly indicating that she triumphed in noticing the deception. It could also be a reference to people at the sanatorium who may have appeared "very attractive at first" but actually needed "some treatment."*

δ

59.
March 24, 1916 (1 of 6)
[typed]
(see Figure 5.1)

Sometimes I dream of an old hag—torn and demented, who is ushered in by a servant, who can't control her, to me. She has lost control of herself and demands that I give her a place *(as a servant)*. I firmly refuse and tell her to go away. She gets raging and flings her arms up and threatens me—I don't know what—but some kind of exposure. She threatens she has read letters and remembers all she has read. I suppress a momentary fear of something [1] and seize her arms and bend them down and hold her and conquer her and put her out.[2]

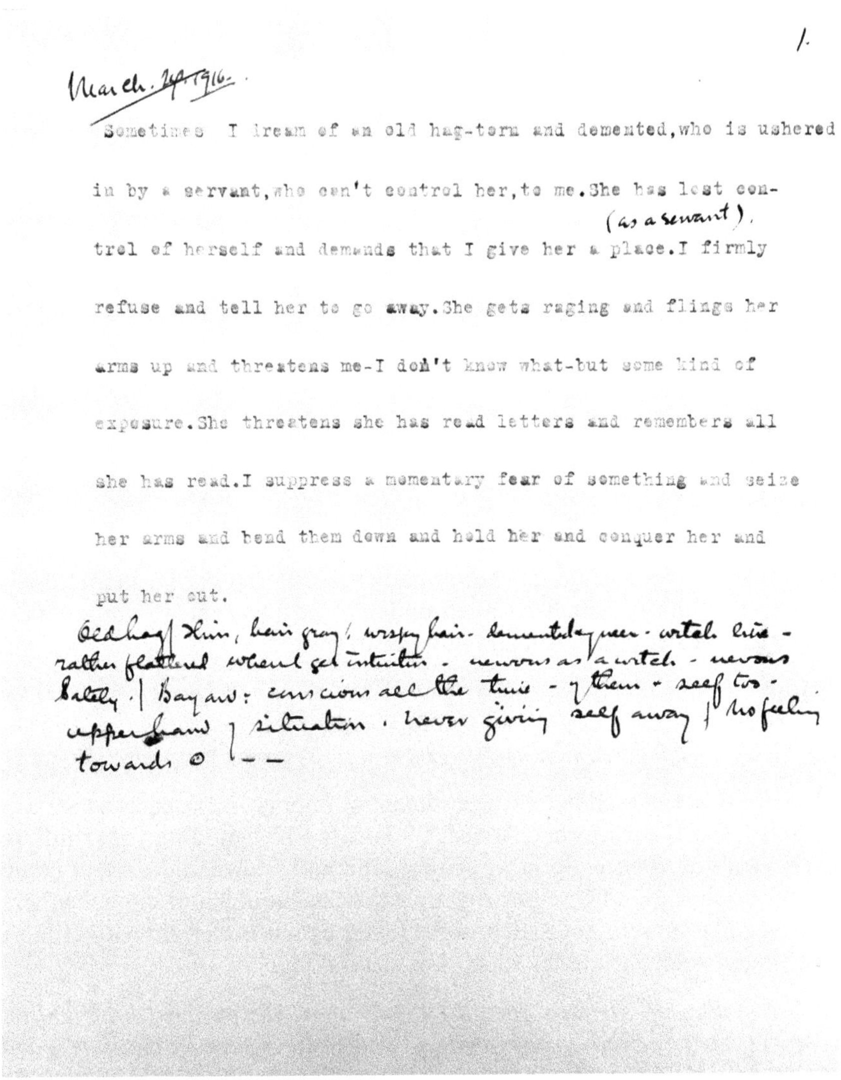

1.

March. 24. 1916.

Sometimes I dream of an old hag-torn and demented, who is ushered in by a servant, who can't control her, to me. She has lost control of herself and demands that I give her a place. (as a servant). I firmly refuse and tell her to go away. She gets raging and flings her arms up and threatens me-I don't know what-but some kind of exposure. She threatens she has read letters and remembers all she has read. I suppress a momentary fear of something and seize her arms and bend them down and hold her and conquer her and put her out.

Old hag/ Thin, hair gray, wispy hair- demented & queer - witch like - rather flattered when I get intuition - nervous as a witch - nervous lately. | Bayard: conscious all the time - of them & self too - upper hand of situation. never giving self away | No feeling towards ⊙ —

Figure 5.1 Mabel Dodge's dream, March 24, 1916, typed, with Jelliffe's handwritten notes. Courtesy of the Beinecke Rare Book and Manuscript Library.

Jelliffe's notes written at the end of the dream:

Old hag/ Thin, hair gray, wispy hair, demented & queer, witch like, rather flattered when I get intuition, nervous as a witch, nervous lately./ Bayard: conscious all the time, of them & self too, upper hand of situation, never giving self away./ No feeling towards ⊙ _ _

Notes:

1 Dodge certainly wrote scores of letters that contained her own secrets
and those of others. As she admitted, "Everybody says I tell everything,
my own and every one's [*sic*] secrets, and it's true! I cannot, to this day,
resist that peculiar urge to tell what is not really mine to tell....I used to
be sorry I did it and ashamed people knew it and said it and called me a
sieve. But I don't know that I feel particularly sorry any more. The less
secrets the better—of my own or anybody else's. Need any one [*sic*] *ever
feel ashamed*? I doubt it" (1933a, p. 10).

2 *Here Dodge displays her characteristic willfulness to "bend" the other and
her need to be in control.*

δ

60.
March 24, 1916 (2 of 6)
[typed]

On a boat going somewhere. Also Florence Bradley [1] and her sister [2] and
others. Some stranger rather fantastically dressed and her husband. She is
assisted upstairs by him, his arm around her. She unexpectedly smiles at me
and offers me her <u>pipe</u> to try.[3] I am nice to her.

*(Assoc.—I remember seeing my neighbor Mrs. Strong and her husband [4] for
the first time the other day as they preceded me up the drive. He had his arm under Mrs. S. helping her. I remember I have never returned her neighborly call.)*

Florence B. seems well but strange somehow. I notice her linen and lace col-
lar and cuffs.[5] We approach a beautiful coast—blue mountains. I think in
the dream it is Greece. Soon we see the land and a town and a street going
steeply up the hill.—There I hear people talking about it and someone there
who <u>won't</u> be subservient to Schroeder,[6] though he is all right with Gilbert
Rae [7] and someone quotes what "Freud says."[8]

*(Assoc.-[Lincoln] Steffans [i.e., Steffens] is in Mexico [9] (the beautiful
country). Steff's friends in Greenwich [Village] are Schroeder and Rae—and
Bursch.[10] Mrs. Bursch disapproved of me. S[teffens]...is in Mexico with
[Pancho] Villa [.] [11] Villa won't be subservient to Carranza,[12] will he be so
to S[teffens]. Beautiful country—My mother is in California.)*

Notes:

1 Bradley and Dodge had first met on a boat from Italy to the United
States.
2 Alixe, mentioned in *European Experiences* (1935) as living with Florence
Bradley in Paris and painting (p. 432).

3 A radical habit at the time for women and a reference to emancipated, perhaps louche, behavior. *This could be a reference to erotic feelings for a woman, perhaps even the "upstairs" while Dodge remains relatively below her.*

4 Most likely neighbors at Finney Farm.

5 Dodge describes Bradley's appearance when she first met her: "She was smart too, in the careful carelessness of her boyish, tailored clothes, her severe, white linen shirts" (1935, p. 429).

6 Probably Theodore Schroeder, identified by Lincoln Steffens as "a well-known New Yorker who was spending his life and his livelihood fighting for liberty" (1931, v. I, p. 327).

7 Unidentified.

8 Likely a common refrain at this time, with Freud's significant influence in the United States and the popularity of psychoanalysis in Dodge's circles.

9 Steffens (1931, v. II) devotes three chapters of his autobiography to his experiences in Mexico. He describes his early understanding of the conflict:

> I learned very quickly that the Mexican revolution was in the civil war stage and that one must be careful which side to go in on. Two new leaders, Venustiano Carranza and Pancho Villa, were rising against Victoriano Huerta, the dictator whom President Wilson was refusing to recognize. He was doomed, but Carranza and Villa, both fighting him, were fighting each other, too. The reds in New York who were watching Mexico were on Villa's side, but the only reason they gave was that he was at least a bandit,…whereas Carranza was a respectable, land-owning bourgeois. (p. 715)

In Vera Cruz, Steffens first met "Carranza the unapproachable, who received me but did not for months open up." When Carranza assumed the presidency of Mexico, he invited Steffens, in his role as journalist, to accompany him on a months-long train journey around the country: "For a while Carranza was cold and mute to all the correspondents, but he gradually warmed to me, on the side" (pp. 717, 728).

10 Unidentified.

11 Pancho Villa, born Doroteo Arango, was a Mexican revolutionary who had raided the border town of Columbus, New Mexico on March 9, 1916, in violent rebellion against the United States for publicly supporting the opposing leader, Carranza, for president of Mexico. At this time, the United States military forces were pursuing Pancho Villa in Mexico, where he had escaped to after his attack. In 1913, John Reed had gone to Mexico to write articles for *Metropolitan Magazine* about Pancho Villa, a mythic figure who captured the imagination of many.

12 Carranza was a Mexican revolutionary leader seeking the presidency of Mexico who had currently joined forces with the United States to capture

Pancho Villa in Mexico. As the headlines in *The New York Times* announced on March 26, 1916, two days after Dodge's dream: "BANDIT NOT SURROUNDED...All Going Well...But End Not in Sight...TWO CARRANZA ATTACKS Villa Got Away Both Times" (p. 1).

δ

61.
March 24, 1916 (3 of 6)
[typed]

Dreamed of an obscure charming house exclusive, hidden, kept by a dear oldish woman. I was living there or wanted to. I noticed she had something the matter with her nose,[1] though a sweet face. I was frightened of syphilis and afraid I would catch it. Then young Raeder [2] was ther[e] and he seemed to have something secret the matter. He had to consult a doctor. The woman said "You know what it is?" I said "Yes," meaning syphilis, but she said "His breath, you know."

(Associations. Edwin's syphilis [3] and my unconscious fear of catching it—the breath connected with this excluded. Apart though charming house-anti-social trend.)

Notes:

1 This likely indicates saddle nose, a collapse of the bridge of the nose that is associated with syphilis.
2 Unidentified.
3 Edwin Dodge had told Mabel before their marriage that he had syphilis. It turned out that Sterne also had syphilis, unknown to him at the time of this dream, but soon uncovered by A.A. Brill, who first suspected the diagnosis from the content of Sterne's dreams presented during his consultations (Luhan, 1954, pp. 33, 34). In addition, Mabel was to contract syphilis from Antonio (Tony) Luhan before their marriage in 1923. This dream, with its mention of the nose and the breath, connects with another of Dodge's dreams she later told to Brill, suddenly recalled when she smelled a blood-streaked sheet that Tony had draped over himself when he returned home one night after sex with another woman, as she recounts in "The Statue of Liberty" (1947b): "The dream was overwhelming, yet it was only about an odor. A strange unknown effluvia that assaulted me with menace and threat and it was accompanied by a voice I had never heard before that uttered meaningly [*sic*]: 'That is the odor of evil.'... For I recognized then for the first time what the nature of the odor was...For me now the primitive, physiological character of the smell of the seminal fluid was evil, deadly and destructive" (pp. 166–167).

δ

Transcription of Jelliffe's March 25, 1916 notes:

Couple of things I wanted to speak of. Impatience, 9 & 10 [years old], almost criminal. Grpts [i.e., grandparents] at Newport, nurse stupid & slow—I flew into a rage, tried to throw off cliff, succeeded, very nearly killed her./ Then told the parents./ My punishment. I was made

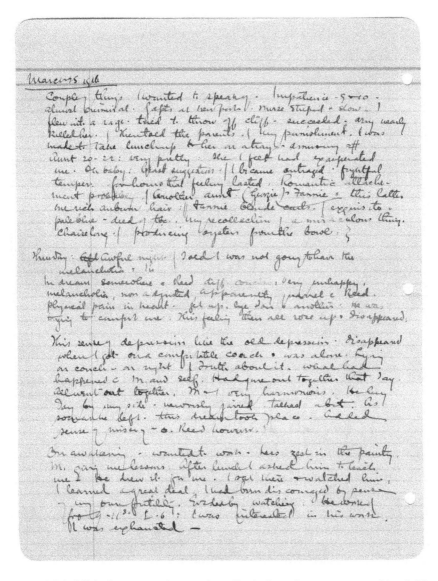

Figure 5.2 Jelliffe's first page of notes from Dodge's analytic session on March 25, 1916. Courtesy of the Beinecke Rare Book and Manuscript Library.

to take lunch up to her on a tray, amusing # Aunt 20–22: very pretty:
She I felt had exasperated me. Oh baby: breast suggestion.| I became
outraged frightful temper. for hours that feeling lasted. Romantic at-
tachment probably.| Another aunt (Georgie) & Fannie: this latter one
rich auburn hair:|| Fannie blonde curls.| exquisite, pale blue—died of
tbc [i.e., tuberculosis]. My recollection| a miraculous thing, chaise
long[ue]:| producing oysters from the bowl.

This first section from Jelliffe's notes corresponds exactly to a passage
in Dodge's memoir of her childhood, *Background* (1933a), when she was
visiting her Cook grandparents at their summer house in Newport. She
admits that she was so incensed by how "stupid" her nurse was that "I
tried to commit murder!" Dodge describes her feelings leading up to the
event: "This poor thing had no ways of her own and didn't understand
anything....She made me want to scream with impatience and to stir her
up in some way." When Dodge saw her standing on a bank above the
ocean, she acted: "I was suddenly engulfed in a wave of anger and disgust
for the anemic girl, so intense and overwhelming that I was lost in it. I
dashed up to her and with all my strength I pushed her over the cliff, hoping passionately to see her fall dead at the bottom of it" (p. 164). The nurse
survived and Dodge reports the aftermath of her crime:

Aunt Georgie came in flushed and damp from playing tennis, her red-
gold curls sticking flat to her forehead. She had on a long full white
flannel dress that had a waist with full puffed sleeves. She wore a
striped belt around her tiny waist and she looked adorable to me—as
she always did.

She stood in the hallway laughing while Grandma Cook told her
what a naughty girl I had been "pushing Annie over the cliff! The
idea!" reiterated Grandma Cook.

"Oh, what a baby!" cried Aunt Georgie. "Doesn't know how to be-
have that's all. Baby! Baby! Baby!" she went on gayly, pointing her
finger at me and making a sort of face. I just stood where I was and
gazed at her, a slow tumult rising in my heart. She could hurt so!

"Baby! Baby! I guess you need dinner now, don't you?" she went
on, and raised her hands to fumble with the buttons of her waist that
followed one another in a long close row down the front. She made as
if to unfasten her dress and lift her breast to me and it broke my heart.
I don't know why. I went to pieces in an instant, touched and broken
up by some magic formula known to her hidden instinct. I opened
my mouth, for a voiceless second of time drew in the great charge of
air to fill my lungs for the blast that followed as I flung myself on the
floor and simply bawled my life out. I cried for an hour and so hard,

so deep, so hurtful it was that I had to remain in my bed for the rest of that day and the next—but why it was, I wonder yet. And that's how I remember Newport. (p. 167)

The second section of this page of Jelliffe's notes is transcribed after dream 62.

δ

62.
March 24, 1916 (4 of 6)
[typed]

Thursday:—Dreamed I was miserable and groaning. Malaise. Changing from couch to couch. Thought it was because I was troubled over Reed— had quarreled.

Jelliffe's notes from March 25, 1916:
Thursday, awful night./ Told I was not going to have the melancholia: In In [sic] dream somewhere c[.] Reed [on] diff. couches, very unhappy, melancholia, non adjusted, apparently quarrel c[.] Reed. Physical pain in heart. Get up, lye [sic] down on another: He was trying to comfort me: This feeling then all rose up & disappeared.

This sense of depression like the old depression, disappeared when I got on a comfortable couch & was alone.[1] Lying on couch, on right/ Truth about it. What had happened c[.] M[aurice]. and self. Had gone out together that day. All went out together. M. & I very harmonious. He lay by my side, nervously jarred, talked a bit. As soon as he left, this dream took place. Added sense of misery—c. Reed however.

On awakening, wanted to work, less zest in the painting. M. giving me lessons. After lunch I asked him to teach me. He drew it for me. I sat there & watched him, I learned a great deal. I had been discouraged by sense of my own futility. Evaded by watching: He worked from 9–11.30, 2–6: I was interested in his work.[2]

Notes:

1 **On a separate couch, Dodge feels better when she is independent from Reed, reinforcing that she can take care of herself when alone, despite her fears to the contrary.** She constantly struggled in love relationships with her overwhelming dependence on the male for her identity, as she threw herself jealously and possessively into these unions. However, Dodge astutely observed in *Movers and Shakers* (1936) that, away from Reed, in the presence of others at places such as her salons, she could achieve "that phenomenon

of power conferred upon one by opinion....But the peculiar thing about it was that when I was living with Reed at home my power seemed to leave me....And he never satisfied me. The substitute for love called power thrilled me more than he, though I always preferred to have him there and to feel uncertain and unsure of him and of myself rather than to triumph, with him away, in what [the poet] Donald Evans so wittily called 'the tragic turnip field'" (p. 264). Dodge repeated similar patterns in her relationship with Sterne.

2 This shows Dodge at her most admiring of Sterne, able to learn from him and receptive to his influence.

δ

INTERLUDE 9.

The previous dream relates to the postscript in the following letter from Dodge to Jelliffe, circa March or April 1916, where she reflects on her crucial contribution to the creation of jealousy in her relationships with Reed and Sterne:

Wednesday

Dear Dr. Jelliffe,
    I have been reading Jung's "Psychology..."[1] for twenty[-]four hours & it has started something in me into movement—I don't know what—but the analysis of Miss Miller [2] awakens in me a recognition of my own complex & its eternal recurrence under manifold forms & symbols;—its past seems unfolded to me now, & in retrospection its history is perceived as my history. I can only today admit the importance of its dominance when I am forced to admit that it appears to me now to be accountable for all that has happened to me & all which I have believed I caused to happen! I understand certain free movements that I have had both as partial sublimations of what would otherwise have been more vigorous assaults of the unknown & unnamed enemy & as avoidances of reality because such reality would have been undoubtedly tainted for me pathologically.
    But altho' I admit all this quite freely & realize it seriously for the first time—still I cannot understand what it is that has been dogging me all this time...I can understand some but not much[....]And I do not altogether see what I was "freed of" in definite terms—, only in symptoms such as heaviness, sorrow[,] disappointment, disillusion[,] malaise, distaste for life & all that. But as for redemption from sin or what sin[,] I have not been able to hit any nail on the head...rather as a highly spiritual & noble soul in an imperfect world have I found comfort or relief or rest in religion or nature-love.

Now <u>do</u> you think we can get on to all this before you go away? I mean back to the incipience of the complex? I feel light <u>could</u> dissolve it.

Sincerely,
M.D.

[P.S.]
Of course I feel now that it is <u>my</u> inconstancy & inevitable spiritual infidelity that I have always resented & which has brought on the neurosis—when I become jealous of others. This jealousy begins as far back as I can remember.

I desire to be omnipotent enough to create Reed—Maurice—or who-not—into stable ideal creatures that I may myself be so. The imperative is not that <u>they</u> shall be so but that I shall be so. It is <u>my</u> inadequacy that makes me finally neurotic thro' jealousy—& no inherent characteristic in the symbol. I will get over being jealous so soon as I become stable myself. It is myself in the symbol—(Reed or Maurice) that I fear & distrust & it is myself who makes me sick.

There <u>is</u> no one but I to myself...This of course is my attitude consciously & unconsciously. It is both right [when regarded curatively—] & wrong—when when [*sic*] persisted in, in a ruthless narcissistic way.

Notes:

1 Jung's *Psychology of the Unconscious: A Study of the Transformations and Symbolisms of the Libido, A Contribution to the History of the Evolution of Thought* (1912) was translated by Beatrice Hinkle and published in 1916.
2 Miss Frank Miller was an American woman whose fantasies were published in 1906 as "Quelque faits d'imagination créatrice subconsciente" in *Archives de Psychologie* (v. 5, pp. 36–51). Jung used this material in his own book to illustrate his theories about the unconscious, explaining that "the absence of any personal relation with Miss Miller permits me free speech" (1916, p. 490). It is likely that Dodge would have identified with, as described by Jung (1916), Miller's "unusual suggestibility, which she herself considers as a symptom of her nervous temperament" (p. 42), and also "her almost magic effect upon another person" (p. 47). She would have resonated with Miller's experience of the "true pleasure to leave the world of inhabited cities—and to enter the world of waves, sky and silence" (p. 49). Even though Dodge had yet to move to Taos, New Mexico, she found refuge in the countryside of Croton and the beaches of Provincetown.

δ

63.
Friday night, March 24, 1916 (5 of 6)
[typed]

Dreamed my mother went out to try a new horse.[1] She said she would drive two little white colts with it. It was a beautiful red roan mare with a fine wavy mane, but I noticed as she went off with it its fault was to bring its head down too much.[2]

Notes:

1 In *Background* (1933a), Dodge remembers an incident that put an end to her mother's horseback riding, something she did often "in the early days of her marriage,…though an accident stopped that. She was riding in the park with Fred Pratt and her horse bolted. She could not kick her foot loose from the stirrup and she was dragged along the ground for quite a distance. And that made her lose her nerve for riding" (p. 48). *Dodge dreams again of her mother, perhaps because the analysis is bringing up childhood memories and wishes.* Here, her mother appears either before she was afraid of riding or while trying to overcome her fear.
2 *No matter what, Dodge would always find fault with her mother's actions.*

δ

64.
Friday night, March 24, 1916 (6 of 6)
[typed]

Then I was I thought in Florence. Lady P[aget].[1] and I put a very stiff old lady [2] in a carriage or motor to send her some place. It slipped away down hill. We knew it was going to be a bad accident. She would be all tangled up inside.

Assoc.—The accident my mother had when the horses ran away with her and my father Xmas night many years ago. How she never lost her nerve over it till next day, Sunday in church. They read a prayer of thanks and she cried and came home.[3] Also her accident riding horseback with Mr. [Fred] Pratt [4] when I was one or two years.

Notes:

1 Lady Violet Paget, an influential member of English society residing in Florence and a writer using the name Vernon Lee. She introduced Dodge to many colorful people who then soon visited the Villa Curonia.
2 Dodge continues to dream about her mother, here in the form of an "old lady."
3 See note 4 for dream 13 for the story of this accident that occurred as Dodge's parents were headed to a dinner party, when Dodge's mother

ended up alone in the overturned horse carriage with "one velvet slipper sticking out of one window and the other out of the opposite window" (Luhan, 1933a, p. 41). Despite this ordeal, Sara Ganson composed herself and went to the dinner. It was not until the following day in church that she began to cry about her misfortune and rushed home:

> "What's the matter, Sara?" asked my father.
> "They pra-a-a-yed for me in church!" she moaned....
> I suppose, her accident having been really a bad one and her escape almost unbelievable, that the minister had offered up thanks to God. Anyway, we all have our limits of endurance and this had proved to be my mother's. She never returned to St.Paul's after that. (Luhan, 1933a, p. 42)

4 The closest friend and college classmate of Dodge's father who had been the best man at her parents' wedding and came regularly to dinner each Sunday when she was a child in Buffalo (Luhan, 1933a, p. 65). This accident is described in note 1 for dream 63.

δ

65.
Wednesday night, March 30, 1916 (1 of 2)

Dreamed for the first time of my father.[1] Dreamed he was driving a pair of horses. He was seated high up over them as on a stagecoach & I was by his side. It was so high up—& there were no sides to the seat—that I felt the danger of losing my balance thro' the movement of the coach.[2] I had to sit quite stiffly. He did not seem to notice any danger but was at his ease.[3] I remember a general feeling of squareness—I don't know how but it came from a feeling that his hat was square & his head was square & the whole configuration of the coach was square.[4]

Later I was trying to convert him to Psychoanalysis.[5] It seemed to me to be just the thing for him.

Notes:

1 In fact, Dodge had already dreamed twice (#s 30 & 35) about her father.
2 *Dodge may fear losing her equilibrium when engaged with her usually volatile father, who in this dream is uncharacteristically in the driver's seat. Even the image of Dodge sitting next to him is highly improbable with its unlikely intimacy and perhaps physical contact.*
3 A rare, if impossible, state of mind for Charles Ganson.
4 This feeling may relate to Dodge's description of her father's childhood home, as "square" with a "square stone front porch" (1933a, pp. 107, 110).
5 See Interlude 10.

δ

INTERLUDE 10.

Dodge's expressed effort in the previous dream to engage her father in psychoanalysis is quite a departure from her characteristically distant approach to him. In *Background* (1933a), she comments about her father's severe moods and often violent behaviors (such as routinely smashing a plate on the floor at a dinner party when he noticed his wife exchanging glances with a man): "His ways were accepted if not understood....I don't believe it ever occurred to any one [*sic*] to try to help him. His peculiarly unsuitable marriage was taken as a matter of course. That he hated my mother was no news to any one [*sic*]." People in Buffalo concluded: "'Charley Ganson is a crank'" (pp. 116–117). However, Dodge sensed even as a child that there were darker, deeper reasons for her father's volatility: "Everyone seemed to know instinctively that he was not really mean and that something tortured him so that he gave vent to it upon any one [*sic*] who happened to be near....His life was so terribly empty of interest or activity....The energy in him turned to poison, stagnating in his veins, and his only outlets were anxiety, jealousy, and querulousness. No child could have taken to him. Of course I didn't like him" (pp. 27–28). Dodge's own work in psychoanalysis with both Jelliffe and Brill likely led to this later understanding of her father's inner torment as described in her memoir.

Two years before she started psychoanalysis in 1916, Dodge had planned to appeal to Morton Prince for help in understanding the similarities between herself and her father, wondering if he could "bring some order out of the apparent disorder." In a 13-page letter to Prince in 1914 (located among Jelliffe's case notes with his handwritten note indicating "Letter never sent"), she described her father "who suffered mental agony all his life because he was not understood—because his case was not rightly diagnosed" and his symptoms:

> What I remember of my father are periods of melancholy—leading up to fearful outbursts of temper, followed by long painful attacks of gout and inflammatory rheumatism. I do not seem to remember his ever being <u>really</u> like other people, for at times when he was well he was much wittier and more amusing than they, cleverer. But these times grew fewer and fewer. His face, as I look back on it now, was mainly tormented, lined, sallow, haunted. What I remember concerning him are such words as "uric acid", [*sic*] "monomania[,]" "depression", [*sic*] and finally a doctor who was merciful enough [in effect] to keep him always under the influence of morphine, then death from an illness that had such symptoms as buzzings in the head, etc., a kind of poisoning, a poison distilled by himself, auto-intoxication. Had he been a biblical character he would have been said to be possessed by devils,—and <u>someone</u> could have cast them out. As it was no one understood,—it is as tho' he lived in the in[-]between time.—I, feeling some strange, analogous suffering, am reaching out to you.

What was true of him is true, with another adaptation, of me. Only I have more vitality. I am terrifically happy in between times....

It is too simple to say that life alternates between two conditions, vitality and depression, yet perhaps all the rest can be confined within the definition of those two terms....And what I want to try to make clear to you is that neither of those conditions are [*sic*] normal. The one is supernormal and the other is subnormal, and both seem to me to be states of emotion [or] being unrelated to objects. My feelings do not seem to depend much on the objects that they think they depend on—the objects do not change, the feelings do. You can suspect in this matter the amount of unhappiness I can bring to others, for on account of my vitality I can almost hypnotically arouse in others the intense emotion I feel in myself,—and which seems to depend upon them,—seeming to blow my spirit into them. And then [all] of a sudden it dies in me with no cause,—the moon was full and then it isn't. A sacrifice is demanded without which I cannot be happy again—all the scheme of things must be altered because I want it so in order to be happy. It is altered and I am not happy. It was not that that was making me unhappy. I can make anyone do anything that I want, but I cannot make myself do what I want.

Sometimes there seems only one reality in the world[—]vitality and its fluctuations. Hegel seemed to think so too. But even so I do not think that it is necessary to suffer the entrance into one of hideous torments because one is empty of vitality. One should learn how to be full of something else, something stable and enduring. For I seem to be only a vacuum. Sometimes the wind that is life is blowing thro' me, sometimes not, and when it is not[,] something else,—painful, tortured—in agony—is in possession. When life is in me I am a part of life and human interests, and of great use, having power to influence people and keen to help and further all that is spirit and going up,—all that will break new roads, let in more light....

But when life is gone out of me, then I am like something banished to the outer darkness, out of touch with all that is human, feeling no recognition of the interests of others, having no sense of relationship with any human being, feeling outside, inhuman, unloving, insentient, an exile from the earth. At such times in a warm lighted room in the evening, with intimate friends, I have felt inside that my spirit was outside, unable to come in, unable to exist there if it should come in—eternally wild and suffering and separate. When these periods come, I get what they call nervous prost[r]ation. I do not know whether these attacks of nerve fatigue are causes or effects. I imagine they are results. Because the mental pain is so great that it breaks down the physical tissue, generates poisons, which in turn react upon the mental condition, and the vicious circle is complete. But because of certain occurrences which I will tell you now, perhaps there is a handle to this situation, which someone like you can grasp and with the aid of my own will, direct.

Dodge writes next about sending her husband Edwin away, believing he was "the <u>cause</u> of my misery," and then feeling "the vitality come back into me"; she also reports on her lover Reed and how he changed in her presence, becoming depressed while she was "better than ever." The letter to Prince ends with her worry that her liveliness is dependent upon the depression of the other:

> And all this is why I am writing to you. Is there a miserable spirit that must exist in me except when I have the force to precipitate it into someone else, when my vitality, drawing their vitality from them leaves a vacuum into which I push this misery? And that has a separate existence that stands <u>outside</u>, alone, sometimes, so that I and one another, with whom I have the right combination, can actually sense it? Hear it? I think that I must be helped to answer to this. I believe that my sanity depend[s] upon it. So I am writing to you and putting it to you as well as I can and if you wish it I will come where you are, if you feel it will do good.

Since this letter was apparently never sent, Prince did not have the chance to address Dodge's questions, but with the letter in Jelliffe's possession, it is likely he and Dodge discussed her concerns.

δ

66.
March 30, 1916 (2 of 2)

Later I dreamed of John. I heard him give a horrible cry—I rushed to where he was.[1] He was small like a baby but mature—he was in moral pain, of some kind. He was stretched out as tho' with physical suffering. I spoke to him, he tried to smile & seemed to make an effort to tell me that what hurt him was small <u>in reality</u> in proportion to the effect on him. He realized the agony he was in was out of scale with the reality of the cause, suddenly carried further out of his reasonable perception, he seized my hand & bit it viciously at first as himself & against his will but turning into a dog as he did it.[2] I felt there was danger in this bite—& horror as well. There was blood in this dream.

Notes:

1 *Dodge's maternal instincts emerge here in a dream about her own son, after just dreaming about her father and her mother in the previous three dreams. John's presence here may symbolize the child who has been overlooked, as Dodge was in her own childhood. To have a mother actually rush to her side would have been Dodge's unmet wish.*

2 It is hardly a stretch to imagine such a scene between mother and son, as they had a highly charged relationship, as revealed in the content of letters and poems Evans sent her over the years. In a letter to his mother from around this time, written from Morristown School, he pleads: "Do you know I don't love you in the same way other boys love their mothers—altho' I love you a lot. You scare me! Can't you make yourself more of a friend than a teacher?" One of his poems from this same time reads: "O my mother!/ My thoughts of you always shall be./ I live—should I love—should I die/ Still my thoughts would be turning to thee!" John Evans's outpouring of love is only one facet of a relationship that could turn stormy and destructive. In another letter from Morristown, John writes in anticipation of their upcoming visit: "I wonder if we can get along pretty well this summer. It is about time we harmonized outwardly as well as inwardly while we are together. I don't doubt that we have ever been 'off' inwardly, but we didn't ever show up very well outwardly." He writes to her in 1919: "Whatever I say and do—I never sacrifice that side of me with which I love you…. My other side fights you in everything that gives it a chance to fight." *This dream scene describes the phrase "biting the hand that feeds you," a dynamic that existed both between John and his mother and between Dodge and her own mother.*

δ

67.
[circa April 1, 1916] (1 of 3)
[written in red in Jelliffe's notes from April 1, 1916]

Something to do c. John & garters. He was trying to adjust something. He said he could do it by cutting off the top part & putting on bottom part.[1]

Note:

1 *This dream follows one where John bit his mother's hand and drew blood. Might Jelliffe and Dodge have considered this a castration dream with "cutting off the top part"?*

δ

68.
[circa April 1, 1916] (2 of 3)
[written in red in Jelliffe's notes from April 1, 1916]

Country church, horse, talk of horse, he said or thought I wonder when Rob is coming?

Jelliffe's notes from April 1, 1916:

Rob: Edw D. brother [1]:/ *rather nice fellow, eyes small, rough skin, nice &
loving c. family, by slow, persevering way. Best law firm. One of his ptnrs
[i.e., partners] my lawyer in getting divorce* [2].... *Been thinking of Edw.
lately. John [Reed] went to Provincetown* [3]: *He told me whole thing
over:/ have been thinking regarding the divorce. Have to go to Salem Mass*
[4]/ *Tired old horse, head hanging down./ My unconscious conscious to
that extent* [5]:/ *Going over relations/*

Notes:

1   Robert Dodge (A.B. Harvard 1893, L.L.B. Harvard 1897) was a lawyer
    in Boston, at this time a partner in a firm that eventually was named
    Palmer, Dodge, Gardner and Bradford, where he was still working at the
    time of his death in 1964.
2   Mabel Dodge's lawyer was Endicott Peabody Saltonstall (A.B. Harvard
    1894, L.L.B. Harvard 1897). In a letter to Mabel dated June 14, circa
    1916, six days after their divorce was official, Edwin wrote: "Saltonstall
    used to be a partner of my brother's. I imagine his honest face and rep-
    utation for general honorable dealings went a long way with the judge."
    Robert Dodge and Saltonstall were partners in Saltonstall, Dodge, and
    Carter, located in Boston, until the firm dissolved in 1910.
3   In the summer of 1914, Reed and Dodge had rented a cottage together in
    Provincetown.
4   The court granting Dodge's divorce was located in Salem, Massachusetts.
5   *Is Dodge referring here to the obvious defeat in a horse's head hanging
    down, as it relates to the divorce?*

δ

69.
[circa April 1, 1916] (3 of 3)
[written in red in Jelliffe's notes from April 1, 1916]

Going after a [illegible], tracking down. There was a table all festive, set,
festive. he [*sic*] [1] was not there. I was looking for him. I must have found
him./ No notion of having seen, nor heard of:/ Agreeable sensation about
it: Human relations new feeling of interest, have other people after an idea,
book or what not.[2]/

Jelliffe's notes from April 1, 1916:

*Perhaps Spring & I want a new interest: When I was young was to add to
my circumference. Now only sense of ascent away. Coupled with warm
flattered sense taking part in the world: "I am responsible" for what is
done.*[3]

Notes:

1 It is uncertain whom Dodge is referring to, although it is likely Sterne.
2 When life came back into Dodge after a period of depression, she could measure her recovery by her renewed interest in ideas and people. She describes one of these periods: "Slowly the inhibited feeling for life began to rise again. That again there seemed to me to be wonderful people in the world and amazing things to tell about them; that color came back into life as the life in me moved once more" (1938b, p. 9).
3 This recalls the way that Dodge felt empowered by the suggestion of Lincoln Steffens that she host salons at 23 Fifth Avenue: "'You have a certain faculty....It's a centralizing, magnetic, social faculty. You attract, stimulate, and soothe people, and men like to sit with you and talk to themselves! You make them think more fluently, and they feel enhanced....Now why don't you see what you can do with this gift of yours? Why not organize all this accidental, unplanned activity around you, this coming and going of visitors, and see these people at certain hours. Have Evenings!'" (Luhan, 1936, pp. 80–81).

δ

INTERLUDE 11.

Around this time, Dodge writes from Finney Farm, a letter that may relate to the chasm in the following dream:

Dear Dr. Jelliffe,

  I hope you will do your best to come out tomorrow night because I notice a little change in Sterne today & you might just be able to "get" him now. Though he made a scene last night against psychoanalysis[,] this afternoon he said: "It is I who should be analysed for jealousy—not you—" and he admitted that he has a sense that his craving for sexual expression all over the place is a morbid exasperation.

Yrs,
M.D.

Please telephone me by 9.30 Sat. a.m.

δ

70.
Monday night [circa April 3, 1916]

An abyss—a chasm between Maurice & me—Suddenly a bridge across yellow very narrow indeed & dangerous. I beckon him to come, & he hesitates. I go across towards him & beckon & encourage him on to it—he comes towards me, to the middle of the bridge, it is to[o] narrow to go side by side. I take his hand & lead him over. I wake up before we reach the other side.[1]

Note:

1 *Dodge dreams here of compromise, of finding a middle space in between what she wants and Sterne wants, although, of course, she is the one to "encourage" and "lead him."*

δ

71.
Tuesday night [circa April 4, 1916]

I have a little new apartment of a few rooms in a house in town. On the right hand side on the ground floor. I live there all alone…/I have much pale cold blue about, once while out with some friends I see a chair covered with this cold grey blue, in a shop. I stop & let them go on, & I try to buy the chair. It is a very tiny pretty chair. The clerk says there are two. I can have the pair for $25.00. I offer $20.00 & I get them.

There is a woman doctor about. She seems to be ingratiating to me because it seems to me she wants to study me. She doesn't really like me for myself as she pretends. I have some symptoms she is interested in.[1] I pretend not to show her I understand her.

Once someone & I are looking out the window at the hard frozen rough streets. It is night. Suddenly a large motor truck rushes thro' the street. It lets of[f] streams of hot water which melt all the hard rough ice & it runs away in muddy rivers.

(assn = my own hardened memory & desire for some mechanical / scientific means to melt or dissolve it, & let my complex run off [2]—)

The woman doctor reminds me of a psycho-analyst someone brought once or twice to my evenings—who seemed most repulsive & on a low level to me. A jewess with hard dark eyes with glasses magnifying them—she tried to get hold of me—& murmured things to me. I had a fierce resistance to her & her personality. I don't remember her name. Was it Dr. [Beatrice] Hinkle?[3] Short, ugly, dark & insensitive?[4]

Notes:

1 *The female doctor suggests Dodge's maternal transference toward Jelliffe. Here she doubts the doctor's motives, considering them as stemming more from self-interest than interest in the patient.*
2 *Dodge offers her own interpretation here: the "someone & I" could be Jelliffe and Dodge as they observe the "hard frozen rough" memories*

of her childhood and, through the work of the analysis, "dissolve" her "complex" so that she is freed from its clutches in order to love and live differently.

3 Dr. Hinkle was a Jungian analyst in New York who had studied with Jung in Zurich and in 1916 translated his *Psychology of the Unconscious* (1912). Max Eastman had met her in 1906 at the New Thought sanatorium in Kingston. In his memoir, he described her in quite different terms than Dodge: "Among those bold enough to believe in mental healing without delusions was Beatrice Hinkle, an attractive, not over-credulous, and intelligent young physician" (1948, p. 248). Eastman returned to her for a consultation in 1914, in which she recommended that he enter psychoanalysis with Jelliffe.

4 Dodge's comments have a strong whiff of anti-Semitism, a curious feeling given that her lover was Jewish.

δ

72.
[circa April 6, 1916] (1 of 4)
[written in red in Jelliffe's notes from April 6, 1916]

Have had a number of dreams, did not put down:

Night before last: Some one [*sic*] going to bottom of sea.[1] I wanted to go along c. him. Found it easy to do. At least twice. Some ground at bottom.[2]

Notes:

1 *The bottom of the sea could mean going down into the unconscious.*

2 *Dodge may be saying here that she is finding it easier to get in touch with her unconscious and, in fact, that she is finding "ground" there, a surer footing or stability. At this point, she has been in analysis with Jelliffe for three months and has associated to dozens of dreams in their attempts to understand the workings of her unconscious. This may be a transference dream intended to show off her accomplishments to Jelliffe.*

δ

73.
[circa April 6, 1916] (2 of 4)
[written in red in Jelliffe's notes from April 6, 1916]

Young ineffectual inefficient person. ♂ had a sister. She quite effectual & ordered cards just day before. They were not kind of cards I liked. They were bright lavender & made of perf. lace paper (Valentines c. French bourg[eois].)

shaped rounded c. edges. Painted or written in color invitation. I raised my voice at last.[1] I wanted white card c. black scrip[t] only.

Note:

1 *In the face of something she does not like (cards with distinctly feminine and decorative elements, even "bourgeois" characteristics that she would likely find "low level"), Dodge has to raise her voice "at last" to protest and assert her preferences. Her desire for plain white paper with black script, with the absence of all color, may speak to some class awareness and feeling of superiority in having simple, unadorned invitations. But could this also mean she is not feeling heard in her analysis?*

δ

74.
[circa April 6, 1916] (3 of 4)
[written in red in Jelliffe's notes from April 6, 1916]

Last night.

One was about Mrs. L.[1] *[a ♀ I have been helping in big Jewish bazaar. Artists['] booth. She also collected book of Exile, Gentiles & Jews. Mr. [Frederick] Howe, Walter [Lippmann], Leo [Stein], John C[ollier]., P[ercy]. M[a]cK[aye]. (7 or 8 of them & J. Reed).]* I dreamed I went to see her in her house. Vulgarly rich house. Big garden, back from road, way back. She in big bed all smothered with lace [2] & things. She finally got up & took all day to do it. Kept husb. & mo. waiting for dinner—husb. vulgar common [3] looking ♂. Going out boy 7–8 plaintive wanted to go & play. She had no time to stop & brushed by him.

> Jelliffe's notes from April 6, 1916:
> *Mrs. L./ Will tell you—I got into this book on the Exile. W.L. & I stopped to see the book—The people I sent were the only people. I was flattered.*
> *In beginning of book she said she had collected them: Hence I made her bad mo[ther] & bad wife & doing something quite unnice—In real life distinctly different.*
> *Child of 7–8./ My painting—I cast around. Color to teacher—pupil./.*
> *Exile./ The Jew:/ To please S.[4] probably:/ Much more apt People of Gift & eminence.—Leo no more an Exile. Men of the hour: Friend./ The different ways—Reed = sublimated ways now./ Percy just a friend you know. Walter likes me to talk to me—just like each other:/ Habit of flattering self as to notable surroundings. Then I fall in love or turn them into friends:*

Jelliffe's notes from April 10, 1916:

The Bazaar & the dream of the other day....Leo takes my work real se-
riously/. I took one of my pictures to him [5]:/ *He wrote me quite a long*
letter [6]:/

Notes:

1 Unidentified.
2 Lace appears in the previous dream as something Dodge does not like.
3 "Common" is a term Dodge has now used several times in her dreams (also in #s 55 & 56), always with negative connotations, and here it is also associated with vulgarity. In dream 56, she degrades something as being of a "common level," and in her subsequent associations, she says: *"I loathe...common pottery."* In associations to dream 71, she describes a Jewish woman as *"on a low level."* Even in the previous dream she seems to dismiss something that is "bourg[eois]." Her distinctions between high and low level betray her judgments based on class and wealth.
4 Very likely Leo Stein, since he appears by first name in this dream and twice in Dodge's associations. Raised in an upper middle class Jewish family in Oakland, California, both Leo and Gertrude had a strong Jewish identity and were acutely aware of their difference from others (Wineapple, 1996, p. 37). (Although less likely, "S." could also refer to Sterne, born into an Orthodox Jewish family in Latvia.)
5 In early April 1916, when Stein was a patient at Mt. Sinai Hospital in New York, Dodge took him one of her paintings. He acknowledged receipt in a letter to her from the hospital and offered his critique of her work (see note 6 for dream 50).
6 See Interlude 12.

δ

INTERLUDE 12.

Here in Jelliffe's case notes file, there is a fragment of a long letter from Leo Stein to Dodge, circa April 1916, referred to in her associations to the previous dream. The continuation of this letter appears as another fragment in Dodge's correspondence from Stein. It is in response to a lost letter from her:

> Your letter is of course most interesting & throws a lot of light on things. It is a central expression that helps a lot to coördinate scattered bit[s] of knowledge and especially the matter that has occupied me so much of your relations to others. You see, this distinction that I made between the common and the rare among men & your tendency in a way toward the common rather than the rare for your contemplated

total attachments, is an interesting fact calling for analysis. Here your letter adds light and confirmation.

You want apparently to be needed on your creative side. You can't create significantly by yourself and such men as Maurice & Reed need your creative urge. Even if they supply form & matter the impulse is rooted in you. It is not merely nourished by you, it is in a sense your will that gets expressed....I can't imagine you really identified with such persons as Bobby or Bayard. They could accept a great deal no doubt but in doing so all they took would become theirs not yours. You would be drained and helpless. With Bayard perhaps, though there I speak from vague impression[,] this might be less because he is less creative. I know I always have that feeling about women in relation to myself & therefore I was so insistent that Nina should have a career of her own. Nobody so far as I have ever seen could play an essential part in my creative life however much they might contribute to it & however ineffective I might be without [end of fragment in Jelliffe file/beginning of fragment in Stein to Dodge file] that contribution. I was trying the other day to think of the kind of person who would faire votre affaire & suddenly it popped into my head that Walter is so far as the balance of qualities is concerned quite typically a case. Of course I am not referring to his "character" but Walter seems to me to mediate between the groups of which I have spoken. He is the public man of genius. He has a genuine productive impulse & still he takes from others. One could it seems to me cooperate with Walter in a sense in which one could not cooperate with Bobby or me or for that matter Bayard.

δ

75.
[circa April 6, 1916] (4 of 4)
[written in red in Jelliffe's notes from April 6, 1916]

Another.

E.A. Robinson[.] I was an emancipated or disembodied person[al] friend of his—so free spiritually, ♂ or ♂, free to come & go on earth. He wanted to see me & have talk c. me (ordinarily reserved type) (never falls in l. c. anybody). He was going to spend night c. me. 2 little rooms in poor location, overhanging Hudson, no embarrassment, nothing equivocal because of my emancipated situation.[1]

Note:

1 Dodge had in fact spent the night at a house with E.A. Robinson, but not in a romantic way. See note 9 for dream 23.

δ

76.
Thursday night [April 6, 1916] (1 of 2)

I dreamed that I was in the Jewish Bazaar.[1] I had had a good deal to do
with it. It was all ready, but instead of a crowd, it was absolutely empty. No
one came. At night I lay down & slept, & one person came, a lady. She had
to step up & down clambering over boxes & obstructions to come in or out
but she was very cheerful about it.

Note:

1 See dream 74 for another mention of the Jewish Bazaar.

δ

77.
Thursday night [April 6, 1916] (2 of 2)

II.
Walter & I were together in my family's house. We staid [*sic*] together all
day & got on very well & had a good time.[1] At dinner time I was glad we
were going to have dinner alone & still have our talk & not be interrupted
but I saw there were three places at the table—& that I had forgotten my
father must be there.[2] He was sick or asleep upstairs. I felt impatient
at this.

Walter & I sat down & were able to remain alone as he didn't come. Walter
said we should go on a trip to—I don't know where. I said "How can we?"
And then I suggested taking someone (some girl I forget who) & he said
"You don't suppose we three could go, do you? No—you should have an
"<u>advocate</u>" (or adjutant I forget which word) a young man to always be with
you, take down your letters, do your errands, attend to your business for
you, make notes for you, etc." He seemed to feel such an appendage would
constitute a chaperone & enable us to go away together without unpleasant
comment. We were getting on better & better. I have a faint remembrance of
washing my hands somewhere in here.[3] Then of Walter coming & bending
over me & putting his cheek quite close so I kissed it. This seemed to us
both in pure friendship & congeniality.—It is much as we really feel, I think,
without the kiss.[4]

Then we went away together. I don't know where. We, or I, was then in
the country with people. Someone pointed out a house in the distance &
commented upon the quaint, interesting people living there. A mother &
daughters, & their intensive family life & ways. I wanted to go see them.
I was told they would be glad to see any one [*sic*] & to show what was
there. I set off with someone in a trap. I don't know who or whether a
man or woman, no help any way as a character. I was sitting on the left

side & driving old Charles.[5] We never seemed to reach the house tho' my companion was always pointing it out just ahead. I kept saying "Which, that one?" & the other "No, that one behind." After a long tiresome time we came near to it. It was a green house on the right hand side of the road, but here the road got so muddy I couldn't go on,[6] or lost my interest or enthusiasm to push on tho' the object was just within reach now. So because there was a little extra room—tho' all mud & water—on the left side of the road, I faced Charles around to the left & there lifted him bodily up by the reins with a good effort, & turned the whole thing around & went back.[7]

> Jelliffe's notes from April 10, 1916:
> *Father upstairs: Always sick or asleep. Always had to keep quiet. Never speak & act naturally. Early parties, 5–6, forbid me c. shaking fingers, no kissing games. F. said I could not play kissing games.[8] He was agst. sex awfully.[9] Just as I am.[10] I carry imagination right through:/....F. always up there: gloomy house. Walter a good time all of the times.*

Notes:

1 Jelliffe's notes from April 10, 1916 for dream 74 indicate that she had recently received a letter from Leo Stein (see Interlude 12) in which he encouraged her to collaborate creatively with Lippmann.
2 *The presence of Dodge's father upstairs—the place where he mostly lived in their Buffalo home, isolated in his misery—would certainly have acted as a deterrent to any desired intimacy between Dodge and Lippmann. Could the third place at the table also have been for Jelliffe?*
3 This recalls Dodge's association of ablutions—"*washing before and after*"—that occurred in response to a dream (# 57) also about Lippmann, where she sits "in W.L.'s lap."
4 Despite the erotic potential in this scene, Lippmann remained for Dodge a rare, trusted friend without romantic complications.
5 An old horse that came with Finney Farm.
6 This recalls the image in dream 2 of a muddy road with "cars stuck in it."
7 *After such enormous effort to reach a place, and many misperceptions about which place was the desired goal, Dodge—who is driving the trap with her horse— abandons her quest and returns to where she started, even though "the object was just within reach now." What could this mean? Given her associations to sex, this dream could suggest a frustrated attempt at sexual pleasure, or the dream could indicate Dodge's ambivalence about pursuing certain goals even after expending great effort.*
8 In *Background* (1933a), Dodge relates this story:

> My father was full of fears about me—....When I was only seven or eight, if I was invited to a birthday party over at Nina's or Madeleine's

he would call me to him just before I left my nurse, all dressed up in my white party dress and white stockings, and he would frown and say: "Now mind! I don't want you playing any kissing games. Remember I forbid it!"

He filled me with the strongest repugnance for himself as he said it—and for kissing games, too. If there was any seduction to be feared in those games of post office, pillow, oats, peas, beans and barley grows, and so on, organized at our parties and supervised by the grown-ups with smiles of amusement and derision at the awkward pecks and bobbings of crimson-faced youngsters when we had to submit to the forfeit—to *kiss* as a punishment—it certainly passed me by. And no boy or girl among us ever knew that kissing was anything but a nuisance. (p. 98)

9   In an unsent 1914 letter to Morton Prince (see Interlude 10), Dodge described her father's relationship to sex: "Soon after he was married [I am told in lowered voice]—he was forbidden sexual intercourse with my mother because it made him insane. It appears he did not heed this—[I am not certain whether he did or not really] but anyway he did become temporarily insane and was for a period in a sanatorium. Then he did come back and lived with my mother. I was a baby then. But I do not think that from that period until he died, when I was twenty-two or three, that he ever had any sexual life." Dodge had also reported to Jelliffe on March 23 (see notes for dream 57) that her father's *"self-abuse,"* or masturbation, was the reason for his institutionalization.

10 It is uncertain what Dodge means here, as she defined "the ultimate sexual act" as "perhaps the cornerstone of any life, and its chief reality" (1936, p. 263). She spent years in relationships seeking sexual intimacy with a corresponding depth of emotional connection. She welcomed sex with Sterne—"we...gripped each other's body and emptied the sadness and venom of the day. Then for that fraction of time we were together, without worry and without thought"—but then concluded: "it is not enough to have the most perfect physical combination unless there is an emotional consolation at the base of it" (1936, p. 428).

δ

78.
Friday night [April 7, 1916] (1 of 2)

Dreamed I was trying to buy some very fine handmade petticoats with embroidery & tucking, but they hadn't what I wanted & tried to make me take a very bad taste kind of knickerbockers of silk & lace, instead,[1] which was to form a combination to take the place of petticoats.

Note:

1 This relates to dream 73 where Dodge feels forced to accept something that is not to her taste, until she speaks up about her preference. High and low fashion figure in both dreams. *Dodge's insistence on her higher class tastes may be her way of reminding Jelliffe (and herself) of her social standing and wealth in the aftermath of sharing intimate and perhaps shameful details of her sexual life (including masturbation and anal sex, topics not widely broached in polite company) in her analysis.*

δ

79.
Friday night [April 7, 1916] (2 of 2)

II.
I was in some big city, & Florence Bradley was coming on a steamer. She was to be met. I sent a boy in with a horse & trap to meet her & bring her to me, but as he drove away I realized I had given him no description of her or her name & he would never find her at the dock. And she didn't know my address so she wouldn't know where to come.

  I was in a panic for a moment & then rearranged it somehow by telephoning somewhere.

δ

80.
Saturday night [April 8, 1916] (1 of 4)

Dreamed I was in our house & we were all crowded together. My father came in very cheerful & good natured for him [1] & said if there was room he'd like to sleep in such & such a room. John was looking for his pajamas but couldn't find any, so I told him to sleep in his underclothes, & gave him a suit.

(*Always dreaming of sleeping arrangements & underclothes.*[2])

Notes:

1 This image of Charley Ganson contrasts dramatically with the tortured, withdrawn man usually described by Dodge. It corresponds to a related image of him as talking "laughingly" in dream 35. However, as revealed in Jelliffe's notes from January 15, Dodge explains that her father was not always troubled: "*My father at first very witty & brilliant, quite a man of world: Waxed moustache very brilliant.*"
2 *Together with dream 78 (from the night before) about undergarments (petticoats), these dreams may reveal how exposed Dodge may be feeling*

in her analysis. Her father had also been sleeping (or sick) upstairs in dream 77, Dodge planned to put him in one of the haunted bedrooms at the Villa Curonia in her associations to dream 35, and she shared a sleeping cabin with him in dream 30.

δ

81.
Saturday night [April 8, 1916] (2 of 4)

II.
Dreamed I was always, in company, with others & someone I loved. So long as there were others we could not show our affection. Finally the others all left & this person I cared for slowly changed into a big black negro & put his arm around me & kissed me & said: "Now I can can't I?" He smelled musty like mice [1] & his lips chattered as dogs [2] do. I felt no aversion but a weariness boredom & disinclination for affection.

> Jelliffe's notes from April 10, 1916:
> *Smelt like/ musty smell: rats & mice: not disgusted: indifferent: I think I like him./ Negro: my own sexuality [3]: That a week ago distrust of self:/*
> *Colors c. me:/ maybe inverted:/ In spite of, want to escape notice/. Hate to have people look at me [4]/: Lips chattering:/ Disgusting: had some at that time…licking other animals: filthiness: licking other animals: that thing about other animals—very trying, licking themselves [5]:*

Notes:

1 **Freud (1900) believed that mice can be symbols of genitals "on account of the pubic hair" (p. 357).**
2 See note 5 for this dream, about licking.
3 In her associations here, Dodge connects her sexuality with the presence of a black man, expressing "indifference," attraction, and disgust. In *Movers and Shakers* (1936), she recalls her aversion to a performance held at one of her salons when Carl Van Vechten brought two black entertainers:

> An appalling Negress danced before us in white stockings and black buttoned boots. The man strummed a banjo and sang an embarrassing song while she cavorted. They both leered and rolled their suggestive eyes and made me feel first hot and then cold, for I never had been so near this kind of thing before, but Carl rocked with laughter and little shrieks escaped him as he clapped his pretty hands. His big teeth became wickedly prominent and his eyes rolled in his darkening

face, until he grew to somewhat resemble the clattering Negroes before him....The unrestrained Negress, whose skirt, now, was drawing
higher and higher in a breakdown jig. (p. 80)

The suggestiveness in their performance unnerved Dodge, both repel-
ling and attracting her.

4   In *Movers and Shakers* (1936), Dodge described a moment of not wanting to be looked at when she visited Sterne on Monhegan Island and he
greeted her at the dock: "[Sterne] embraced me with a loud smack. I felt
the eyes of everyone directed at us: the boatmen, the urchins at the little
dock...—all these seemed to be gazing at us with undisguised interest,
suspicion and disrespect. I tried to become invisible and immediately
retired so deeply into my shell that it took months to get me out again"
(p. 495).

5   *Is Dodge associating here to the commonly observed practice of dogs lick-*
ing the anus of another dog? If so, this may connect to her "repugnant"
experience with anal intercourse as reported in associations to dream
19, and to her acknowledgment of "fecal erotics" in associations to
dream 39.

δ

82.
Saturday night [April 8, 1916] (3 of 4)

III.
I was in my drawing room in town, with others. Elizabeth Duncan was in
the dream. I went out of the room & when I came back I saw something
unfamiliar on the floor which alarmed me. I looked & found it was a piece
of excrement [1] several yards long & very big—& curving like a snake.[2] It
seemed miraculous & magical to me—as well as full of horror, & terror on
account of its coming there of its own accord.

> Jelliffe's notes from April 10, 1916:
> *1st time of excrement/ dreamed & read of power./ "Society of primi-*
> *tive joy:" accomplishment: sensation/ expulsion as quickly as possible:/*
> *To get rid of unused material. Also intellectually:/ When I have the*
> *satisfaction. [3]/*
> *Horror that it came there[.]*

Notes:

1   In *Movers and Shakers* (1936), Dodge presents Jelliffe's ideas about the
symbolic meanings of different parts of the body: "The bowels were the
vehicle of the money power, excrement was gold, hoarded or distributed

in circulation….Jelliffe had taught me the close connection between excrement and gold in the symbolism of the psyche" (pp. 440, 516).

2 *Given the enthusiasm for finding phallic symbols at this time of early psychoanalysis in New York, Dodge notably dreams of excrement shaped "like a snake." As Freud (1900) declared: "above all those most important symbols of the male organ—snakes" (p. 357).* This image also immediately follows a dream from the same night (# 81) where Dodge connects her sexuality with a "Negro" man and associates to animals (likely dogs) licking each other (likely on the anus).

3 *Dodge associates excrement and its expulsion with pleasure and "primitive joy," a linking that Jelliffe would certainly have supported or even encouraged. She may have read Jelliffe's article, "Compulsion Neurosis and Primitive Culture" (Jelliffe & Z. X., 1914), in which he connects the "urinary and fecal phantasies" of the twentieth century's child with the "animistic beliefs of primitive peoples" (p. 362). Jelliffe's co-author and patient, "Zenia X—," admits to her own "compulsion neurosis" and to early "fecal phantasies": "Distinctly fecal are a few outstanding incidents occurring during the period from the age of three or four until nine, ten or eleven years. Earliest is the memory of standing with my brother…in an outhouse playing that we were the Trinity 'creating' a baby of dust and dropping it down to earth, presumably…to the feces below"; "A little older, with my brothers, I climbed a high tree that our defecation might fall over the branches to the ground below" (p. 364). The patient then asks: "Now what light do we obtain upon these early experiences of mine…if we turn to the savage world? I find there first very real fancies full of the sense of the close association of the feces with the mysterious life principle or spiritual essence, that fundamental productive life which finds its concrete expression in the sexual power" (p. 366).*

δ

83.
Saturday night [April 8, 1916] (4 of 4)

IV.
Dreamed that after a baseball game at Van Courtlandt [*sic*] Park,[1] the crowd waited for hours for Jess Willard [2] to appear on the field & show himself. We all waited & waited as for a sacred appearance & a hero. It grew darker & darker & we could hardly see but we waited on patiently. He never came.

Assn = famous Willard continence & sublimation.

Jelliffe's notes from April 10, 1916:
…Jess Willard & no ♂ ….Everybody says he was sexually pure.[3]

Notes:

1 i.e., Van Cortlandt Park, in the Bronx.
2 At this time, Jess Willard was the World Heavyweight Boxing Champion, having knocked out Jack Johnson in 26 rounds in Havana, Cuba on April 5, 1915. An article about him, entitled "CONFIDENCE MADE GREEN GIANT WORLD'S CHAMPION; Jess Willard…Stood Punishment and Studied Tactics, Never Doubting Success," had just appeared in *The New York Times* on March 19, 1916.
3 The meaning of Dodge's comment about apparent abstinence likely refers to intercourse before a boxing match. Jess Willard married Harriet Evans in Kansas in 1908 and they had 5 children, born between 1909 and 1916.

δ

84.
Sunday night [circa April 9, 1916]

I am in Walter's house with him. I think we are breakfasting or something downstairs. His father is sick upstairs.[1] *(This motive [i.e., motif] constantly appears lately.[2] [)]* His mother is in & out & about. He says "Come on up to my room." We go up to the third floor. I am talking in cheerful natural voice, but as we go past other rooms into his, he stops me half laughingly from talking, saying: "My father is not like me." This remark calls suddenly to my notice the fact of anything unusual in my going up to his room—& I regret there is any possibility of its being misunderstood by <u>anyone</u> even if <u>he</u> doesn't himself. We go into his room which has two unmade beds in it, & light wood furniture. This rather surprises me because I have heard his library is very dark & sombre. I see all his books of which I have heard so much—in bookcases. Then we concentrate our attention on the bureau or something which we came up there for.

It is some kind of machine or diagram for particular measurements of some kind.[3] Lots of little balls or hills connected with it. It is very ingenious & interesting, seemingly but soon Walter sweeps me out of the room on account of his father hearing us.

Last night's dreams are all forgotten, yet I feel they were largely concerned with measurements & removing weights from one place to another. (Possibly sublimation ideas.[)] [4]

Jelliffe's notes from April 10, 1916:
Feeling ++ in which dream/. Not strong of any. pleasantest re Walter. good time: pleasantest dream—not in real life, not as in intense relation:/….
Bureau & Instrument/ What it was/ don't know of Mother or Heroes: is this a compensation:

Notes:

1 *The mention of both downstairs and upstairs is suggestive of sexual content, according to Freud (1900): "people 'up above' and 'down below' alluded to phantasies of a sexual nature which occupied the patient's mind and, as suppressed desires, were not without a bearing on his neurosis" (p. 288). In the dream, Dodge is aware of not wanting her motives to be misunderstood as sexual when she goes up to Lippmann's room.*

2 In dream 77 where Lippmann last appears, it is Dodge's father who is "sick or asleep upstairs." *What might be the meaning of this repeated image? Parental figures upstairs or above, watching or monitoring their children's (sexual) behavior?*

3 This image recalls diagrams Jelliffe made during his intake and treatment with patients. These drawings resemble a wheel with spokes, with different points labeled, as in "respiratory libido" and "nutritive" in Dodge's graphic chart from January 5, 1916. In one article, he used such titles for his diagrams as "Schematic representation of fixation of libido in one patient" or "Schematic psychogram of unconscious trends as shown in the dream wish" and measured observations such as "dip in respiratory sector" (1917, pp. 75, 77).

4 *Dodge's sublimation interpretation may relate to the presence in Lippmann's bedroom of "two unmade beds" (with their suggestion of sex) and then "all of his books of which I have heard so much" (intellectual pursuit to channel sexual instincts). When Lippmann hurries her out of his room "on account of his father hearing us," he confirms the concern that they will be discovered together, perhaps with sexual tension between them. Dodge would have been aware of the psychological maturity considered necessary for sublimation and she likely would have been pleased to present her analyst with such material.*

δ

85.
[circa April 13, 1916] (1 of 3)

I.
Dreamed of a young man, a stranger to us all, who came along unexpectedly & unexplained & by his charm & efficiency married one of my girl friends. He looked very bright & clever. His eyes were queer. One was screwed up nearly closed, the other one was wide open & square in shape. The latter was the right eye. He led us along a street & suddenly we came to a barricade of wood & chairs & bricks—he stepped ahead & was apparently horrified at what he found. But I knew that whatever it was, he had done it. It was a woman cut in two. He prevented our looking at it.

Assn = Waite [1]

Jelliffe's notes from April 13, 1916:
Dr. Waite & 2 sides of face: (1)♀ cut in half.

Note:

1 Dr. Arthur Warren Waite was a New York dentist accused of and eventually executed for poisoning his in-laws in 1916: his mother-in-law
Hannah Peck died January 30, 1916 and then her husband John Peck
died March 12, 1916. The newspapers were filled with accounts of this
sensational murder, Waite's trial, and execution. Jelliffe was among the
three state alienists who declared Dr. Waite sane, despite his defense of
"compulsive insanity," stating that a "'little man from Egypt'" told him
to kill his in-laws (*The New York Times*, May 21, 1916, p. 20). He was
arrested on March 23, 1916 for arsenic poisoning of his father-in-law.
Dodge certainly may have known about Jelliffe's involvement in the
case. A week before this dream, Dr. Waite's wife filed for divorce, as reported by newspapers in New York and Boston (Grossman, 2017, p. 213;
see pp. 173–196 for a full account of the story).

δ

86.
[circa April 13, 1916] (2 of 3)

II.
I am out on a rough & stormy sea. It is night. The waves toss the boat, which is
a smallish square one, about. We are blowing horns & the captain is shouting
through a megaphone. I think they are shouting for help but soon I see that
we—& two other ships—are trying to attract the attention of something. I
look out, & make out, in the dark two very small boats tossing in the waves.
The wind is bearing them past us & away. We are trying to get the attention
of a man & woman who are standing up in each of them. They face away
past us looking ahead of them—& we cannot make them hear for the wind
carried the sound away from them. In each boat is a small (sail) mast & each
leans on this, his arm around it. They are being carried on into the storm &
away from help. I feel the tradgedy [*sic*] & their helplessness very much, but I
am <u>occupied</u> in painting it. I am painting the sailor's costume—blue & white.

(Assn = Psy-A.) [1]

Jelliffe's notes from April 13, 1916:
Boats./ If they could hear: They don't know wind, means a lot…

Note:

1 *Dodge's association to psychoanalysis points to one reading of this dream
as representing the "stormy sea" of analysis: Dodge is in the boat with the*

captain (Jelliffe?) witnessing the helplessness of two smaller boats with passengers who cannot hear (who do not want to hear?) and are being swept into the storm, "away from help." Although Dodge feels the despair of their situation, she limits the depth of her response by being "occupied" in painting (sublimation?) the clothes of the sailor. This scene takes place at night, when it is hard to see anyway, and it is also hard to hear on account of the wind from the storm. This dream suggests Dodge's urgent appeal to others, particularly Sterne, to enter treatment. He had resistances to analysis—he did not want to see or hear—and, as in the dream, "we cannot make them hear," i.e., Dodge and Jelliffe could not force Sterne into the consulting room. Dodge was also upset about the mental state of Boyeson, who was then living with her at Finney Farm, and convinced him to see Jelliffe. However, he stopped after only a month, claiming it was too expensive, while Jelliffe reported to Dodge that it was due to "'the resistance'" (Luhan, 1936, p. 464). This dream could also be read as Dodge initially "shouting for help" from others, but then realizing that it is actually the others who need help but are unable to be saved from the storm that is forcing them away from any possibility of aid. Could this be Dodge longing for her parents to care for her but then realizing that they are helpless themselves and unable to offer her the love she needs?

δ

87.
[circa April 13, 1916] (3 of 3)
[written in red in Jelliffe's notes from April 13, 1916]

I had some other dreams but have forgotten them. Felt particularly well & rested when I awakened.

A 3rd I thought of coming in:

III.
On my 5 Ave. 3 Indians go by, looking intense & occupied. I know they are. They & we are at war. Then into room a fourth. Beautiful hands, capable, long time in this dream. He had m[arried]. a young American girl,[1] had taken her away. He had laughingly told me she was going to die. He went into hall, high place, terrace there, he had taken her there, hand & foot & was going to burn her alive.

> Jelliffe's notes from April 13, 1916:
> *Indian:/ My own sexuality [2]: sacrificing high self on top of hill [3]:*
> *Hands/ at this min. H.S. Landor,[4] explorer….*
> *I strove c. none for none are worth my strife Nature/ Love & after n[ature]. art.*
> *I warm my hands before the fires of life[.]*
> *The fire burns low and now I may depart[.] [5]*

Other hands/. Can't think of others[.] God the F[ather]'s in pictures:
Ideal hand/ Fine small bones. like a good machine....long fingers, supple,
quite precise do it in a neat way no fumbling. Some people think with their
bodies:/ M.

My hands/ Writer[']s cramp....

Fifth Av./ Don't know why...3 Indians. down the street/ Always, one
of my favorite ideals, lots of photos about—Indian chiefs 2–3 men I have
known [6]....All fine strong animal integrity. Defy me to find it./ Precision
fineness, imperviousness hardness & abandon in horses etc: Eye true & keen
in measurements: Finer creatures than we are. Finer senses. Secrets of na-
ture, more than we do. One of desires of life—to live in Indian village.[7]

Notes:

1   Dodge was a not-so-young, but an American, girl when she married an Indian man in 1923, see note 7 for this dream.
2   In dream 81, Dodge connected her sexuality with a "Negro" man, who, like the Indian man, was considered perhaps more "primitive" or exotic, thus more associated with libidinal instincts and cravings.
3   *This is a prescient image, as Dodge's eventual marriage to an Indian man demanded self-sacrifice in the midst of rumors and judgment. The headlines in papers across the country revealed the intrigue that her unconventional marriage generated, such as "Why Bohemia's Queen Married An Indian Chief"* (Pittsburgh Post, June 19, 1923). *She admitted: "It had almost crushed John, and John told me it had almost crushed my mother"* (1933b, p. 16).
4   Arnold Henry Savage Landor, English writer and explorer whom Dodge describes in her "Florentine Vignettes" in *European Experiences* (1935), with particular attention to his hands: "It is difficult to describe the effect he made upon one. It was as of one who had been greatly cherished as a child, and he seemed to have been loved and magnetized by love.... His flesh seemed beloved. It had the living glow that comes only from the hands of love, and his hands were small-boned and brown, with long, intelligent fingers, and they too looked satisfied....One sees this fulfilled look, sometimes, in the bodies of children who have warm mothers" (p. 249). *One can only imagine the effect of Landor on Dodge, a woman who was deprived of a warm mother and who was exquisitely attuned to those who did have one.*
5   This is a slightly inaccurate recollection of an 1849 poem, "Dying Speech of an Old Philosopher," by English poet Walter Savage Landor that appears in full at the beginning of Dodge's vignette of his grandson, Arnold Henry Savage Landor: "I strove with none, for none was worth my strife;/ Nature I loved; and next to Nature, Art./ I warm'd both hands against the fire of life,/ It sinks, and I am ready to depart" (1935, p. 248).

6 It is uncertain which Indian chiefs Dodge claims to know, but her experience causes her to praise their "finer senses" and deep connection to the
   "secrets of nature."

7 Her desire would soon approach a reality. In December 1917, Dodge
   traveled to New Mexico to join Sterne, whom she had married on
   August 23, 1917 and shortly thereafter banished to the Southwest to
   paint. They eventually settled in Taos, where she met Antonio "Tony"
   Luhan, a Pueblo Indian from the Tiwa community, who introduced her
   to the wonders of his country and the ways of the Native Americans, and
   was to become her fourth husband in 1923. Dodge was highly aware of
   the monumental leap she had taken in marrying Luhan: "An irrevocable
   step! To pass across from one's race to another is an irrevocable step"
   (Luhan, 1947b, p. 3).

δ

88.
[circa April 15, 1916] (1 of 2)
[written in red in Jelliffe's notes from April 15, 1916]

Going c. B[oyeson]. to see Mrs. McKeever.[1] Apt., large drawing room,
dark red damask, she sang at piano & husb[and]. sang.

Jelliffe's notes from April 15, 1916:
I enjoyed it, others there. Noted furniture—supposed [to] be connoisseur
old Fr[ench]. furniture—he was not.
    McKeever. Friend of B.'s, early experience—I think ♀ in dream a
pt.[2]....
    Dark red damask: all difference in world, modern vulgar. In Italy old
subdued, deep, kind. This the right kind./[3]
    Mrs. McK./ Just imagine—only 2 friends. She is one & the one I don't
like—the wrong influence. The other one I associate c. his drinking. This
one fond of. Nicer person./
    Singing/ I happen to know she sings—little accomplishment./ don't care
much for it./ Don't care for singers themselves. ½ bro of hers. P. Draper
[4] a singer:/ He much like B. always hear from her. B. like him/ This Paul
m[arried]. Muriel,[5] in Florence. He's silly person. Grande Passion c.
most/ Did not go—Just as far as familiarity—few kisses—exciting effect.
Used to make him excited....I think I dreamt that since many times wor-
ried Edwin. He never would know how far I would go.[6]....
    Had a long talk c. B./ Why have you the prejudice ag[ain]st M./ Why
unsuitable. I want./
    I am frightened about giving up the object [7]/ There in country alone c.
B. Massiveness lacking:/ M. massive & weighty.[8] Certain authoritative,

stable qualities:/ Always separated:/ Contempt because mother—not real spiritual values, out of my money:/ I would live in N.Y. or c. M. yes: Not in N.Y. More space:/ I don't like N.Y. Noises +++. Inured to country./[9]
    Mr. McKeever tall & thin & gray, all dim.
    Striking thing. Room. The environment—largeness, ampleness of it. Room like that in Fl[orence]: better: older & darker.
    Red/ All these different kinds. Primitive first color emotional.[10] *& beauty on acct of its unsubtle character:/ Very interesting, lot of interesting psychol[ogy]. Violet always farthest away* [11]—*just this year. Used to like vivid spectral colors. Orange & violet, only like.*

Notes:

1 Unidentified.
2 This is the second time Dodge has dreamed of a patient, likely another patient of Jelliffe's as in dream 39.
3 In her associations to this dream, Dodge again underscores high and low culture—a man was "*supposed*" to be a connoisseur but was not, there is a "*right kind*" of damask, as opposed to "*modern vulgar.*"
4 Paul Draper, acclaimed American tenor whom Dodge had known in Florence.
5 Muriel Draper, an American host of a popular salon in London.
6 In fact, Edwin did have reason to worry, as Mabel deliberately set out to lure Paul Draper to her in Florence, between 1909 and 1911, as she relates in *European Experiences* (1935): "I don't know how it began but Paul thought he fell in love with me. I suppose I must admit I tried to attract his attention for it was a compulsion with me in those days" (p. 257). She believed she briefly succeeded in her goal: "He was well installed in the magical hollow dream I used to create around people, and in which they drew delighted breath for a little while" (pp. 257–258). As Jelliffe recorded in his January 13 notes, Dodge admitted her seduction of Draper that did not end in intercourse: "*Then another ♂ tutor of John's m[arried]. ["Paul Draper" crossed out] P.D.: grande passion, excitement, musician….Had to force him out of bed.*"
7 ***Dodge had come to realize through her analysis that no matter how strong her ambivalence toward a man, she would not easily give him up because of her childhood fear of being left alone and unloved.***
8 In a letter to Jelliffe circa January 1916, Dodge had praised Sterne for "his massive qualities" (see Interlude 2).
9 This relates to an argument later in 1916 that Dodge had with Brill who "was certain from the first that I had no use for the country, that I was wasting my life in Croton" and believed that she should live in the city. Dodge complained: "'I hate the city!....the noise and the smells'" (Luhan, 1936, p. 505).

10 Although her sources (other than popular culture) are not known, Dodge
seems conversant with the psychology of color, an area of scholarly fascination for centuries that looks at the effect of color on mood and behavior. For example, Johann Wolfgang von Goethe's *Theory of Colours*
(1810) posited the psychological effects of different colors on emotion,
such as the color red "conveys an impression of gravity and dignity, and
at the same time of grace and attractiveness" (p. 314). Dodge calls red
the *"primitive first color,"* while Goethe claimed: "this colour…includes
all the other colours" (p. 314).
11 See note 2 for dream 98 about violet and the color spectrum.

δ

89.
[circa April 15, 1916] (2 of 2)
[written in red in Jelliffe's notes from April 15, 1916]

A young ♀ 18–19, just m[arried].? Went c. her to house which her family had
b[ui]lt. White wood wind mill, 2 towers, pergola between, pretty but absurd:
Got there & was to see my baby..then I was she & I had not seen my baby.[1]
Awfully nice, dignity, light green eyes,[2] 3 eyes, one right in center of
forehead.

Notes:

1 Although Dodge was not yet pregnant, she soon will be, conceiving
sometime between May 10 and May 16, see note 3 for dream 117.
2 Dodge described Jelliffe as having "a pair of small, intelligent green
eyes" (1936, p. 439). See note 6 for dream 98 about green eyes and association to jealousy.

δ

90.
Sunday night [circa April 17, 1916]

Dreamed I was going to give a great ball, of the old[-]fashioned kind we used
to have in Buffalo.[1] There was a dinner party before it which seemed composed all of family & also Mary & Conger Goodyear.[2] The members of
the family were mostly in black or dark colors. One was either Mrs. [Helena]
Jelliffe [3] or John's aunt Mary Hollister [4] *(They both look alike anyhow in
real life)*. The dinner party is on an upper floor. The guests are arriving so I
have to hurry to get down to receive them. I rush to the Cabinet, there I have
to hasten urinating with great impatience. The urine is acid & irritating.[5] I
become more impatient to get thro' & down to the ball room…

[I had feelings about this party & all the people coming that most people seem to have in real life but which I have never had. I am eager, excited & pleased, & I <u>hated</u> balls in reality when I was of the age of the dream.[6] []]

Jelliffe's notes from April 17, 1916:

Funny thing last night: urinated in bed last night/ dream….

  One thing/ City vs. country.

  Eager excited pleased feeling, never had it in real life. Hated to go to real balls. All really frightens me to see me get into these tempers. I cry now, impotent rage. Just fighting for my life/ ⊙ [7] are the tyrant:/ Just part of ⊙ temperament./ One great mistake/ You are too apt to forget that other people do not matter in dreams.[8]

  Mary & Conger Goodyear/ Early friend of mine. Thought of her yester-day. Talking to Leo. Constructive c. M.S./ Was changing. (Don't fly into rage c. this.[)] Intense egotism#….

  Congers: just husband, that's all./ I asked her once. She has very nice house & garden [9]: "Just Conger".—Who do you see: More cross/ because/ She does not like Buffalo people.[10]….

  M.S. says I sob & cry in my sleep these nights.# There is so much good will around./ No room in our unconscious:/ All disagreeable [11]….

  Mary Hollister/ Complaining person. Awfully neurotic, always sad…/ John's father's side. She died of cancer.[12]/ Cancer ball/

Notes:

1 As she describes in *Background* (1933a), Dodge officially came out to society at a formal ball in Buffalo at a party for a thousand guests hosted by her parents (p. 288).

2 Mary Forman grew up near Dodge in Buffalo and married Conger Goodyear, called "the Grouch" by Dodge and her friends because he never smiled (Luhan, 1933a, p. 14).

3 Jelliffe's wife had died over a month ago (see Interlude 8). **The family members dressed in "mostly black or dark colors" may indicate Dodge's awareness of Jelliffe's continued mourning.**

4 An aunt related to Karl Evans, John Evans's father who died when John was one year old.

5 Dodge was to develop chronic urinary problems later in her life, as she relates in "Doctors: Fifty Years of Experience" (1954). In the 1940s, she suffered from painful urination, caused by a tumor on her bladder which was then removed. However, after the surgery, she still experienced extreme discomfort and was diagnosed with "Hunner's Ulcers" in her bladder, requiring months of treatment where she was injected with a solution of water and nitrate of silver, finally resulting in the

disappearance of her ulcers (pp. 48–57). This dream may foreshadow these later health problems. ***Dodge also associated jealousy with painful urination (see note 5 for dream 3).***

6 In *Background* (1933a), Dodge's description of her own coming out party reveals this hatred of balls:

> I refused to dance. Four or five hundred polite inviters who had to ask me did ask me and were refused. Hour after hour I "sat out" with Tom, Dick, and Harry....I sat and sat and sat. People began to look more and more disheveled. They ate, they drank, they danced the night through. I was never so bored in my life. I smiled and smiled—and sat....I caught a glimpse of my father's face, growing darker as the hours dragged on. He didn't dance either.
>
> It grew intolerably hot and the ice was melted in the wassail bowl, but the party was going on perfectly, everybody seemed to think. Towards morning, when I felt my face stiffened from smiling, and I could hardly keep my eyes open any more, I saw my father prance out in one of his furious, stamping moods to the middle of the ballroom floor. Raising his calamitous eyes to the musicians' balcony, he began to hiss at them in a burst of anger. Instantly they caught his order and his rage, and in a flash they were playing *Home, Sweet Home....*
>
> My mother and I drove up the street the few yards to our house. We didn't say anything. When we got in, my father was already upstairs....
>
> "Well, that's over with," sighed my mother as she sailed into her room and left me to mount up one more flight. I was "out." (pp. 289–290)

This dream, then, could be a wish fulfillment.

7 i.e., likely "you" when Dodge refers to Jelliffe (see note 7 for dream 42).

8 This sounds like something Jelliffe might say to Dodge to help her dream interpretations by reminding her not to focus on other characters in her dreams, but instead to consider them as representations of herself. ***Could she be appealing to Jelliffe here to acknowledge how difficult this analytic process is for her, calling him a tyrant in his approach to her, and emphasizing her real rage and sadness in her life outside of sessions?***

9 Dodge described their "large, lovely house" in Buffalo as having "white-enameled woodwork and beautifully proportioned rooms" (1933a, p. 14).

10 Dodge explained: "Her life with Conger was restricted, for he was almost always downtown and when he was home he was often grouchy, though not very mean. So Mary and he did not care for 'people.' They hardly saw any one [*sic*] but each other" (1933a, p. 15).

11 ***Is Dodge suggesting here that her unconscious leaves no room for "good will" and only contains "disagreeable" elements, as if all that is unconscious is bad?***

12 According to Dodge, Jelliffe believed that "appearance of a cancer in a person signified hatred. It was the parasite eating away at the vitality of man" (1936, p. 440).

δ

91.
Tuesday, April 18, 1916 (1 of 4)
[typed]

Dreamed of some kind of confinement <u>up</u> high in some building. I had to pull a dumb waiter up from very far down below, as though from down a deep well…in order to get what I was after. I pulled it up but at the end only the rope came out in my hands.[1]

> Jelliffe's notes from April 20, 1916:
> *An unusual dream: Up in high place.*[2]

Notes:

1 *Is Dodge reaching far down into her unconscious to understand something—"to get what I was after"—and then coming up with nothing, just the rope with nothing attached? Is she feeling confined or trapped in her life or in the analysis?*
2 This may relate to another mention of a "high place" in dream 87.

δ

92.
April 18, 1916 (2 of 4)
[typed]

I agreed with M. not to like the "Greenwich village" people.[1] They seemed second rate, affected and shallow to me. There were opera tickets given away by him or me which they got. Blue tickets. The woman said—posing—"I wonder if I can afford six sous to get…to go…..". I saw it was a pose to be so hard up because she had some of my Chinese silk around her neck….

Note:

1 Any of a group of people with whom Dodge was associated in the Village, including Max Eastman, John Reed, Hutchins Hapgood, the anarchists Emma Goldman and Alexander Berkman, and the birth control advocate Margaret Sanger.

δ

93.
April 18, 1916 (3 of 4)
[typed]

I was in love with some one [*sic*] in an idealistic way…a man or a woman. They were away—far off—perhaps abroad. By and by I found out there was no such person. I felt emptied of my love—desolate—insecure—lost.[1]

Note:

1 *At this time in her life, Dodge characterized herself as being incomplete without another, recalling her admission, as recorded in Jelliffe's initial case notes, that she lived through others: "absorbed in or through some ♂." In* **Movers and Shakers** *(1936), when she was ambivalently and tempestuously involved with Sterne, Dodge admits: "Be he ever so unsuitable, a man was what gave me identity, I thought" (p. 482). Her admission in the dream that there "was no such person" could be an interpretation acknowledging the futility of her fantasy that another person could ever complete her.*

δ

94.
April 18, 1916 (4 of 4)
[typed]

A large palace—the windows all blind, covered with some opaque material. I know some one [*sic*] I know is behind one watching me and M. kissing, outside in the empty space, because I see smoke coming from a cigar [1] through the material over the window.

Note:

1 This could certainly be a reference to Jelliffe, in his position of witnessing Dodge in her relationship with Sterne, as she regularly reveals to him intimate details of their sexual life. It also might connect to Dodge's father, Sterne, or even Freud, the father of psychoanalysis, all of whom smoked cigars.

δ

95.
April 20–26, 1916 (1 of 6)

Dreamed I was walking around in the ocean with Acton.[1]

Jelliffe's notes from April 27, 1916:

Acton/. Man in Florence: Big place lot of money:

Note:

1 Arthur Acton, an English art collector and dealer. He and his wife
   Hortense lived and entertained in a 60-room Renaissance villa called
   La Pietra exuberantly decorated with tapestries, paintings, and an-
   tiques and they were among the first expatriates the Dodges met in
   Florence. As she describes in *European Experiences* (1935), Dodge
   and Acton took to each other: "Acton liked to range around all over
   and so did I, and he often took me, or Edwin and me together, to
   visit out-of-the-way villas or to call on queer characters or to hunt up
   antichita....We grew to be good friends....and he would always have
   something new to tell me or to take me to see" (pp. 386–387). He also
   visited Dodge at the Villa Curonia: "Acton used to come often and sit
   there with me for an hour, and once he said: 'You are such a comfort. I
   always feel much better after I have been here with you'" (p. 152). Acton had written to her a month before this dream, on March 22, 1916,
   beginning his letter with "I wish you were here this very minute. Your
   note revived much Mabelness and brought a thrill of joyful surprise,"
   and ending: "Please send me some intimate and personal news about
   Mabelness."

δ

96.
April 20–26, 1916 (2 of 6)

Dreamed I was trying to tear handfuls of loose tenuous phlegm out of my
throat to free my larynx & breathing.[1]

Note:

1 In a letter to Jelliffe from April 28, 1916 (see Interlude 13), Dodge refers to this dream: "I have recalled an episode which will interest you,
   as a result of the dream of removing stuff from the throat." In one of
   his "Technique of Psychoanalysis" papers, Jelliffe (1916) observes: "It
   is a singularly striking fact that the dream material is so rich in these
   transfer phenomena relative to physicians and the beginning analyst
   must be particularly careful in his judgments concerning this transference material which is constantly appearing as directed upon previously trusted general or special practitioners. The analyst finds himself

frequently substituted for formerly employed laryngologists, rhinologists, gastro-enterologists, gynecologists, etc." (p. 395). Dodge had a related dream on May 12, 1916 (# 121) that involved "an obstruction in nose or throat—could not breathe well," inspiring her to write an elaborate letter to Jelliffe suggesting that they "should work together to remove obstacles which impede a free flow of energy" (see Interlude 15). *This is the work of her analysis, both identifying obstacles (resistances) and then removing them.* During the winter of 1912–1913, Dodge's depression had so sapped her energies, by her own account, that she developed severe tonsillitis. The operation to remove her tonsils was conducted in her bed at 23 Fifth Avenue. In *Movers and Shakers* (1936), Dodge reports an insight into her condition that Jelliffe later offered: "Any illness of the respiratory organs, the throat, bronchial tubes, and lungs represented...a failure in aspiration—the breath of God gone wrong....Certainly my throat was testimony either to some lack of aspiration or of failure to achieve" (p. 20).

δ

97.
April 20–26, 1916 (3 of 6)

Dreamed I was very much bundled up, upholstered & walking up stairs with someone. Dr. J.'s office door was at the bottom of the stairs (on the left going up). I decided to fall down stairs [1] backwards as I couldn't go on any more on account of all my upholstering—also I knew this upholstering would prevent my feeling the falling much—I hoped this would attract Dr. J.'s attention—the falling [2] I mean—& its likelihood of hurting me. This was in my grandmother's house.[3]

Jelliffe's notes from April 27, 1916:
Falling downstairs: Gdmother's house: fell down backwards: Father complex. Tried to show off.[4]
Upholst[e]ry. Going to prevent myself from hurting self, prevents me from going up./ Regular spree. I have a hobby, self-indulgence./ Green glass....When in town, to slide into new interest....I'll just stop in importing place. 2 people combing England for old English glass. Extremely rare—rooms full of it. Marvellous [sic] old things. Libido orgy.[5] *Never felt so light & happy. I knew I could not afford it. I never could get to it: $350 worth: I got it all home. Mrs. Sprague & Mrs. Norman* [6]*: (superior attitude). She came out Sat night. Mrs. N. & sat up. told me everything:/ One thing could go out & buy all that glass. how selfish. how many war sufferers: Upholstery....Go through experience—Money between me & life.*

Seemed to make me feel thicker—made me large. It would prevent me from being hurt: Wanted ⊙ to feel I was hurt [7]./ Hard luck story....

Uphoist. Soft things, keep off reality—come between—any "phantasy"—[8]

Notes:

1 *Freud often interpreted movement up and down stairs to symbolize coitus in its rhythmic pattern.*

2 *About falling, Freud (1900) wrote with condescending certainty: "Dreams of falling...are more often characterized by anxiety. Their interpretation offers no difficulty in the case of women, who almost always accept the symbolic use of falling as a way of describing a surrender to an erotic temptation" (pp. 394–395). He also claimed: "If a woman dreams of falling, it almost invariably has a sexual sense: she is imagining herself as a 'fallen woman'" (1900, p. 202).* Years later, in 1938, Dodge, then Luhan, reported three falling dreams in letters to Brill, admitting "I forget what falling means in a dream, specifically" (October 4, 1938, MDLC).

3 Dodge remembers herself going down the stairs at Grandma and Grandpa Ganson's house in Buffalo: "There was a hall in the center with the stairs running straight up to the second floor....They were good smooth banisters for sliding down upon, which was one reason, I suppose, that they became so polished. I slid down them always from the time I stopped going downstairs by the method of sitting down and bumping from step to step—until my skirts became too long" (1933a, p. 107). *Freud's interpretation of such a memory would certainly include sexual and masturbatory elements.* Dodge also records a memory of Grandpa Cook on the stairs at his New York home: "I remember his coming slowly down the grand, gloomy staircase in the house on Fifth Avenue one day when I was about eight years old....When he reached the bottom of the stairs, where I stood looking up at him, he put his hand in his pocket and drew out a shining new silver coin and held it towards me....'Here,' he said to me loudly and impressively, 'here is a silver dollar for you! Look at it! Now take it and never forget it. A silver dollar!'" (1933a, pp. 121–122). See Dodge's associations for dream 41, as recorded in Jelliffe's notes from February 10, for her recollection of this moment with the silver dollar.

4 *Dodge had an extremely complicated relationship with her father, as she both identified with him because of his depression and suffering and found his hidden life fascinating (as when she explored the contents of his desk, see note 8 for dream 55), and yet was repelled by his violent moods and unapproachable state. As a likely consequence, she longed for the attention of men and would "show off" to draw them in.*

5 Dodge had obsessively occupied herself in Florence and New York with furnishing her living spaces. With a kind of "self-indulgence" that here

she labels "Libido orgy," she searched for rare and expensive objects to satisfy her, even if she "could not afford" them.

6 Both unidentified.

7 As a child, Dodge deliberately hurt herself in order to draw the attention of doctors, according to Jelliffe's April 1, 1916 notes: *"Always older men Drs. Drs. Drs.// Used to mutilate self slightly in order to go to Drs. to assuage pain: Would cut warts."* **Does Dodge still believe that she has to present herself in a damaged state in order to capture the attention of her doctor? In this dream, she hopes Jelliffe will notice her and risks hurting herself (although she does protect herself with upholstery) by falling down the stairs.**

8 *Dodge offers her own interpretation here that she surrounds herself with "soft things" to prevent the intrusion of reality, thereby preserving the fantasy.*

δ

98.
April 20–26, 1916 (4 of 6)

Dreamed I thought Florence [1] must call, <u>mustn't</u>, <u>couldn't</u> go on wearing green ribbons. That she must wear another color. So I went to choose some for her & I chose violet ones, which seemed far better.

(Assn: F.W. is jealous of her husband's work = green ribbons & she must give them up for violet ones = the color the farthest evolved, the farthest seen ideal, the most developed.[2] This is my own desire to transform my infantile attitude towards M. into a more evolved & developed one.)[3]

Jelliffe's notes from April 27, 1916:
Fl. Westcott....Not thought of long time. She jealous of husb. work. he brilliant, genius, his chemistry, plays violin, jealous. green ribbons = jealous = Choose violet = farthest evolved in spectrum = ideal = Own desire to evolve own infantile to more developed:/
Violin/ never heard play....don't like violin. like deeper sounds—thin for my taste:/...no partic. consc. assoc:/ I've often thought—clitoris like a chord—like violin. I'll tell you why so sharp, not like cello—. violin has the strained exasperated sharp. right sensation in ♀, c. M. Ø entirely different: Other not on a string—waves of sound also mast[urbation]: outside contact:/ Very intense when I rub his P[enis] agst my ○ [i.e., vagina]/ My own mystic sense more/ Fiddle back & forth:/.[4]
& Color assoc./ Can't connect violin c. violet,[5] nor green c. red, sharp acid:/ I have a strong affect re violet: a strong symbol of aff[ect]: more mature: Eyes last perceived: Eye of artist. or chemist./ History of art:

Green: Having green eyes = jealousy [6] *= something to be overcome. I love green. 1st year I have ever liked violet—now always over house. Always her! Always means jealousy.*

Notes:

1 i.e., Florence Westcott, as identified in Jelliffe's notes. Nothing more is known about her or her husband.

2 As in her associations to dream 88 ("violet always farthest away"), Dodge identifies violet as the most "evolved" color, as it is at the far edge of the visible light spectrum, with its wavelength between blue and ultraviolet. Violet (and purple) are commonly associated with royalty, sophistication, and power.

3 **Dodge desires to move from green (jealousy) to violet (more evolved), as she was tortured by the regressed state that arose from her intense possessiveness toward Sterne and struggled greatly to develop more mature coping.** She writes in *Movers and Shakers* (1936) about Jelliffe's efforts to help her find and trust her own judgments: "That was the way he threw me back upon myself. When I looked within, I saw myself floundering, yet would not—yet—save myself. I continued to believe that somehow, someway, *I* could be fixed, or Maurice could be fixed, so that we would fit together like the covers of a book" (p. 457).

4 If falling down the stairs did not capture Jelliffe's attention, it is likely that Dodge's associations here—the clitoris is *"like a chord"* and *"waves of sound"* suggest masturbation—would appeal to his interest and inquiry.

5 **Although Dodge says she "can't connect" the two words, this sequence of associations from violet to violin, with the final two letters changed, likely indicates an emotionally charged and sexual connection, as she admits to a "strong affect" to violet and a dislike for the violin with its "strained exasperated" sound, relating it to intercourse and masturbation.**

6 The association of green eyes and jealousy goes back to Shakespeare's *Othello* (1604), Iago to Othello: "O beware, my lord, of jealousy!/ It is the green-eyed monster which doth mock/ The meat it feeds on" (3.3.168–168). Also, in *The Merchant of Venice* (1596), Portia uses the phrase "green-eyed jealousy" (3.2.110).

δ

99.
April 20–26, 1916 (5 of 6)

Dreamed I saw John dressed in a fancy costume such as he likes to dress in actually.[1] This time it was a long cape of a patchwork, & I objected because it was too long for him, nearly touching the ground. I altered it for him, shortening it.[2]

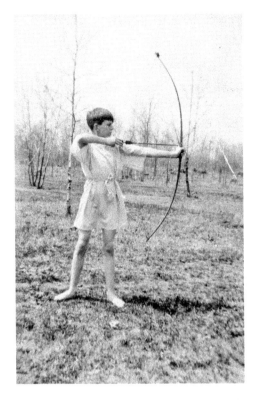

Figure 5.3 John Evans at the Elizabeth Duncan School, Croton-on-Hudson, 1916. "Of course Elizabeth put short, blue drawers and a short, blue-belted tunic on John. Barefooted, with the bow and arrow raised in the archery class, he was beautiful" (Luhan, 1936, p. 347). Courtesy of the Beinecke Rare Book and Manuscript Library.

Notes:

1 A photograph of John at the Elizabeth Duncan School in 1916 (Figure 5.3) shows him dressed in a loose tunic tied at the waist.
2 *Could this be considered castrating or controlling, as Dodge could often be as a mother and romantic partner?*

δ

100.
April 20–26, 1916 (6 of 6)

Dreamed a lot of Jewish women were playing with a small house, with much noise & laughter. They would rush into it together & tilt it forward, then altogether they would move on & tilt it back. This was a game or play. It somehow reminds me of Avon Springs.[1]

Note:

1 The sanatorium in western New York where Dodge's father was insti-
tutionalized when she was one or two years old (see Jelliffe's March 23
notes for dream 57).

δ

101.
April 27, 1916 (1 of 6)

Dreamed I was in a steamer on the ocean. There was one table in the dining room very different from the others—the finest lace and things on it. It belonged to two ladies.[1] Once I told two children who were sitting there that I would sit there with them—but the two ladies appeared & I couldn't stay. I didn't know whether they were dull or fascinating.

> Jelliffe's notes from April 27, 1916:
> *Lace. Very fond of it. Don't recall house, lace all over things, different for summer: Covers & things/ Fine needlework, hand work, vs. mechanical things/ Love….*
> *2 ladies/ Middle aged/ 2 very funny baroness[es]* [2] *in Fl[orence]. funny types. tastes & society in Europe untouched, in house lace. Very funny.*

Notes:

1 This recalls dream 36 where Dodge wanted and then boarded a boat that "belonged" to two ladies from the New Thought Colony.
2 Unidentified. One could be the Baroness de Cassin named in dream 35.

δ

102.
April 27, 1916 (2 of 6)

Dreamed I was standing by someone in a street & across the street at a left angle Mrs. Haweis [1] was speaking to my companion & at the right angle someone else I knew was speaking to her or him. But they ignored me or seemed not to see me. Mrs. H. looked worried.

Jelliffe's notes from April 27, 1916:

N.[2] told me…tumor: fearful tumor—all of insides out. & scientist. Half an hour. 1st source./ Gave birth to an enormous tumor./ She had pulled off this tumor./ She had some knowledge of sex./ Nobody knows.[3]

Notes:

1 Mina Loy Haweis, often referred to by her nickname Ducie Haweis, an English poet, artist, actress, and feminist. While studying art in London, she had met the English painter Stephen Haweis, whom she married in 1903. In Paris, she regularly attended Gertrude Stein's salons and became an early supporter of her work. In Florence, where she and Haweis moved in 1905, she met Mabel Dodge around 1910 and frequently was a guest at the Villa Curonia. Dodge described her as "lovely as a Byzantine Madonna….with dark hair parted and with a great knot on the nape of her white neck" (1935, pp. 338, 340). Dodge became her good friend, a conduit for her poetry, and the godmother of her son Giles. In letters to Dodge (all undated except the first) Mina Loy calls her "My dearest Moose" (March 28, 1913) and "My darling Moose," asking "Do tell me what you are making of Feminism? I heard you were interested…. do write[,] Moose—I haven't a wise companion for the moment," and writes after a failed love affair: "I wonder if hatred is the truth & love the lie….Don't ever live to see the day when the man you want sobs out the other one's name in the ultimate embrace." Mina Loy's poetry was first published in 1914 (by which time Haweis had left her) in both Stieglitz's *Camera Work* and Carl Van Vechten's *Trend*. In late 1916, she moved to New York, soon became a part of the Greenwich Village crowd, and acted with the Provincetown Players.
2 This likely refers to Neith Boyce, or possibly Nina Bull. It is not known whose tumor this association is about, or if it is based in fact.
3 *These associations to the dream—that ends with Mrs. H. looking "worried"—suggest a secrecy around something terrible and "fearful" that is inside, recalling Dodge's associations to dream 90: "No room in our unconscious./ All disagreeable."*

δ

103.
April 27, 1916 (3 of 6)

Dreamed I was in a house hotel or ship—people about—& we were all moving about—and my I [*sic*] heard mother say to my father: "I <u>think</u> we are being persued! [sic] and I think it is by two men." Then they talked about it & one of them suggested these men could get in the window. *[Is this meaning Dr. J. & I after my father & mother complexes?]* [1]

Have recalled definitely episode with D.S.[2]*—revived by E.S.D.*[3]

Notes:

1 *Here Dodge eagerly uses the language of psychoanalysis, likely in the pursuit of Jelliffe's approval and attention.*
2 Unidentified.
3 i.e., Edwin Sherrill Dodge.

δ

104.
April 27, 1916 (4 of 6)

Dream very vague but I think I was very sick—paralyzed or something—& I wanted a man who was a doctor to help me.[1] He was a blind man whom I knew but didn't know as a doctor. He seemed to take charge of me.[2] I was at [Alfred] Steiglitz's [sic] [3] later & we found an inner room unknown to me.[4]

Notes:

1 *Dodge desires a doctor to help with her paralysis, much as she appealed to Jelliffe in a letter circa May 1916 (see Interlude 15) to "remove obstacles which impede a free flow of energy," to help her become unstuck.*
2 *As much as she could assert her independence and control, at her core Dodge craved a man to "take charge."*
3 Dodge visited Stieglitz's 291 gallery often. As she recalls: "It was one of the few places where I went. It was always stimulating to go and listen to him analyzing life and pictures and people....I owe him an enormous debt I can never repay. He was another who helped me to See—both in art and in life. His belief was that he never gave in to anything except what he believed to be the best;...that he cared only for what he called the spirit of life, and that when he found it, he fostered it" (1936, p. 72).
4 *Could this be a hopeful image for Dodge after her wish for a "doctor to help me," finding a hidden internal resource? Or is the "inner room" another place where there are "disagreeable" and "fearful" elements (as in the associations to dreams 90 & 102)?*

δ

105.
April 27, 1916 (5 of 6)

Dreamed I had planted a great rosebush with a trunk ten inches in diameter &
I had transplanted it with a tall very antique stone column that it clim[b]ed on.
I put it in a square garden with an old stone wall around & it seemed to transform this place here & change it into an old italian or english lane very old &
beautiful. I was walking in the twilight & feeling the poetry & beauty of it all.[1]

Note:

1   *The beauty and stability (the rosebush with a substantial tree trunk "ten*
     inches in diameter," the inclusion of an "antique" column) that Dodge cre-
     ates in this dream results in a transformation that pleases her. This more
     hopeful fifth dream in a sequence of six is preceded by dreams with themes
     of fear, intrusion, not being seen, and being sick. Perhaps, then, the "inner
     room" found in the previous dream (# 104) was in fact a positive discovery.

δ

106.
April 27, 1916 (6 of 6)

Dreamed I was dressing my mother—choosing a dress for her & making it
on her. I choose some pale pink & cream striped stuff & then decided to [the
dream ends here, incomplete]

δ

INTERLUDE 13.

Following the session during which she discussed these dreams, Dodge
wrote to Jelliffe on April 28, 1916:

Dear Dr. Jelliffe,
    I liked the way things went yesterday & recalled that we had the same
sense of synthetic consequence the other time I brought in five or six nights'
dreams. I'd like to try it that way for the month of May—coming once a
week with a bundle of dreams, for a two hour séance. I have recalled an
episode which will interest you, as a result of the dream of removing stuff
from the throat, an episode that may be of cardinal importance in having
established a precedent of exasperation which remained—I suppose une-
qualled yet persued [*sic*]. I may be wrong about it, though.
    I will tell you about it Sunday. I won't come in tomorrow—but I have
presented one of my hours to Frances Kavanaugh [1] & written her to let

you know whether she can go & see you at 2 tomorrow. I believe she is a rare specimen & just the one for you & your work—as well as the work for her. Please clinch it with her. She is ignorant of Psycho-Anal. and is raw but sound material—I mean she has real character & insight, & is practical & clear. She, however, needs analysis herself first.

So you do your best to get hold of her. She meant to go to Bryn Mawr & Johns Hopkins, I believe...all unnecessary & takes too long. She has had two years in hospital work.

John will call for Ely [Jelliffe's 17-year-old son] at quarter to five—& I expect you Sunday morning & I will send to the train for you. If you can come out with the boys, do. Don't get any notions in your head that I am having resistances to you or the work. I'm not. I've developed a real sense of friendship & appreciation for you and I have seen that the work works, but I have liked best the way it works when one isn't poking the unconscious every minute!

Faithfully,
Mabel Dodge

Note:

1. Unidentified.

δ

107.
May 5, 1916

Dreamed—

Mrs. Acton.[1] Set of teeth. Surprised her.

Note:

1 Hortense Acton, married to Arthur Acton (see note 1 for dream 95), a wealthy Chicago heiress whose family's banking fortune financed the purchase and furnishing of their villa in Florence. In *European Experiences* (1935), Dodge describes Mrs. Acton as "what they used to call *petite*—pretty, self-conscious, and repressed. She scarcely moved as she sat there, exquisitely dressed in dark velvet, her pink nails gleaming, contenting herself with showing her small white teeth or lifting her lovely, modeled eyelids occasionally in a smile." In one scene around 1905, Dodge notices her husband responding to Mrs. Acton and is devastated: "'Edwin was attracted to that woman,' I sobbed. 'I can't bear it. When I see it, it ruins my life'" (pp. 104, 105).

δ

108.
May 6, 1916 (1 of 4)

Dreamed I was going somewhere—a journey on the water [1]—complained of the food in the basket—& everything. Short journey by boat, then arrived at a little town. The house where we were was nearly empty. Reed sent me to another room to get something & in it I saw a bed with a person in it. I looked & it was a dead person wrapped in a sheet. The face covered. Every room I went into contained a dead person on the bed carelessly wrapped in a sheet.[2] Then we were driving thro' Asolo & we wondered how Mr. Browning [3] was. We saw his house & told Maurice he could stay there if he would like to work there. A river ran rushing in front of it.

Notes:

1   According to Jelliffe's April 27 notes, Sterne was scheduled on May 6 to travel overseas by ship to visit a German woman, Mira Sohn, whom he had loved for years (see note 6 for dream 49 and Interlude 18), in order to make a decision about his relationship with Dodge: *"He must be sure of it....Said he was going to Germany to face the reality:/ Menace to work & to me/ Actually don't know how he would feel—long talk./ Leo [Stein] told him he must settle it. Ryndam = 6th May. Waiting for his passport: I realized he could be trusted."* The steamship Ryndam actually left New York on May 8, 1916 (*The New York Times*, May 8, 1916, p. 15), without Sterne aboard (see note 2 for Interlude 18).

2   ***On the eve of Sterne's intended departure to determine the quality of his attachment to another woman, the appearance of Reed in this dream is striking, as Dodge was ambivalent for years about her love for him. Each room in this house contains a dead body, perhaps a sign of her certainty about the end of her feelings for Reed.***

3   Robert Wiedeman Barrett Browning, called Pen, an artist Dodge had known during her time in Italy, the only child born to English poets Robert Browning and Elizabeth Barrett Browning. In *European Experiences* (1935), she recalls him as "a small, red apple of a man with a plump little figure. He was usually dressed in black and white checks, and he had a round, red, bald head and smooth, red cheeks." She sympathized with his unfortunate appearance: "It must have been hard on Pen to be the son of Elizabeth Barrett and Robert Browning. He told me that he never met people for the first time that he didn't see them start and exclaim to themselves: 'What! Is that the son of those two poets?' For he did look like an apple and that was all there was to it" (pp. 115, 117). Dodge had visited him in Asolo, Italy, where he lived at his family's home and had a sculpture studio. At the time of this dream, Pen Browning had already died, on July 8, 1912.

δ

109.
May 6, 1916 (2 of 4)

I saw Mrs. Norman [1] come towards me. Very angry because I hadn't met her & she hadn't re[a]d my letter. We made it smooth & then she was to go with me to a jeweler[']s. I was to give her or she me something. I was looking at a small watch & they said it was $5000. This seemed to me very much for it.

> Jelliffe's notes from May 23, 1916:
> *Mrs. Norman and letter. Came panting up driveway—Needed you. Bayard took her out to drive. Letter: At lunch, all sex laws to be changed "Woman self sufficient". ["]Woman self reproductive & a higher mind". Much too serious to be discussed. The sex question [2].*

Notes:

1 Unidentified. A Mrs. Norman also appears in Jelliffe's April 27 notes that accompany dream 97.
2 Dodge was very aware of the growing birth control movement, headed by Margaret Sanger (who opened the first birth control clinic in the United States in 1916), and its radical effect on the conversation about sex and women's reproductive rights. As she reported in *Movers and Shakers* (1936), Dodge had met Sanger soon after she moved to 23 Fifth Avenue in 1912: "It was she who introduced to us all the idea of Birth Control, and it, along with other related ideas about Sex, became her passion. It was as if she had been more or less arbitrarily chosen by the powers that be to voice a new gospel of not only sex knowledge in regard to conception, but sex knowledge about copulation and its intrinsic importance" (p. 69). Dodge credited Sanger with teaching her about the immense possibilities of sexual pleasure: "She was the first person I ever knew who was openly an ardent propagandist for the joys of the flesh. This, in those days, was radical indeed when the sense of sin was still so indubitably mixed with the sense of pleasure" (pp. 69–70). Dodge remembers an evening when she and Nina Bull had dinner with Sanger: "she told us all about the possibilities in the body for 'sex expression'; and as she sat there…and unfolded the mysteries and mightiness of physical love, it seemed to us we had never known it before as a sacred and at the same time a scientific reality.…Then she taught us the way to a heightening of pleasure and of prolonging it, and the delimiting of it to the sexual zones, the spreading out and sexualizing of the whole body until it should become sensitive and alive throughout, and complete. She made love into a serious undertaking" (pp. 70–71). When Dodge began analysis with Jelliffe, she had already been deeply affected by Sanger's revolutionary ideas about sex and pleasure. She claimed that

Sanger "helped me…to get rid of some old, old prohibitions, and to raise the curse a bit!" (p. 171).

δ

110.
May 6, 1916 (3 of 4)

Dreamed I was in an appartment [sic] house in bed, & talking out of a window or opening to two or three servants & people, saying to get some work accomplished. Maurice was there. Elena [1] was taking my order but was doing some sex appeal thing to Maurice—sidling up near him, her attention on him.[2] I spoke severely & authoritatively to her, ordered her up to my side, spoke to her like one would to a dog, & threatened her. Soon she left & the others left. M. & I were in bed talking. Suddenly we heard loud noises—shriekings [sic] & crazy crying. Someone came & knocked on the door & said it was Elena. She had gone crazy from grief & wrought herself up to such a pitch. She had crept from her place on the top of the house & was out clinging to a corner of the fire escape & screeching. All the servants in the place were trying to get after her. She was—as in life—like a monkey. The police were summoned, to control her & get her back in. I had to get up & go after her. It annoyed me very much that I had—by my words—brought such a thing about. I was principally annoyed at Elena for cutting up so!

Notes:

1 Unidentified, likely a servant of Dodge's.
2 This is the familiar jealousy triangle that tortured Dodge.

δ

111.
May 6, 1916 (4 of 4)

I have a lot of guests at a long narrow table. I have to discipline them. I try to tell Bobby [Jones], who is at one end of the table, to take a chicken leg away from a dog he had just given it to. I have to repeat the request & finally order him to do it with authority so that the others all see my authority [1] & he is embarrassed. I see he has drunk too much, as he gets up to obey me. He laughs foolishly. This annoys me. I don't like people to drink too much at my table. I feel they are getting out of hand.[2]

Later, part of the same dream.

I am in Provincetown, have a cottage.[3] Someone has died. I am in Mary Vorse's [4] cottage. Jo [5] her husband has died, perhaps I am Mary Vorse.

Someone—a man—perhaps her brother whom I have never seen—is very agreeable & kind. He says he hopes it's all going to be more agre[e]able—that that other meal was just unfortunate. We had just come, & not gotten settled. I try to reply & am pleased but at that moment an upper front tooth on the left side comes out in my hand & embarrasses me very much.[6]

Notes:

1   This recalls the authority that Dodge asserted with Elena in the previous dream.

2   This scene seems to border on debauchery.

3   Dodge rented a cottage in Provincetown for several summers, beginning in 1914 with Reed, then in 1915 and 1916 with Sterne. In 1916, Max Eastman, Hapgood, and Leo Stein, were also vacationing there.

4   Mary Heaton Vorse, a radical feminist, suffragette, and journalist from a wealthy family in Amherst, Massachusetts whose house on Commercial Street in Provincetown was frequented by the movers and shakers of the day. One of the editors of *The Masses*, she also contributed stories about the poor, the working class, workers' movements, and strikes. Her first husband, the writer Albert Vorse, died in 1910.

5   Joseph O'Brien, a radical journalist who married Vorse in 1912 and died in 1915, leaving her a widow for the second time in five years. After O'Brien's death, Vorse became active in helping found the Provincetown Theatre Group with Eugene O'Neill, Susan Glaspell, Reed, and others.

6   *Freud (1900) was insistent about "the interpretation of dreams with a dental stimulus as dreams of masturbation—an interpretation whose correctness seems to me beyond doubt" (p. 387). He particularly believed that teeth falling out symbolize masturbation (pp. 385–388). With the first part of this dream about the dinner party that is verging on being out of control, this reference could refer to sexual urges and expression, particularly when considered with the second dream of this series (# 109) and its associations to "sex laws" and the likely connection to Sanger and her open conversations with Dodge about sexual pleasure.*

δ

112.
May 7, 1916 (1 of 3)

I and another little indian seem away from the tribe. They are up on the hill. We run down thro' the woods to the bottom of the hill. We know they are going to persue [sic] us. At the bottom we meet three old squaws. They smile good naturedly, & tell us to go to the left down a road on the <u>inside</u> of the fence—which hides us from the road. We do—the tribe catch up with us—we are scared—but we run. They run alongside of us on the other side of the fence. Thinking we are ahead of them—then they pass us. We laugh in great amusement.[1]

> Jelliffe's notes from June 7, 1916 [2]:
> *....tribe after us, both run (parallel.) they run & pass us:/ Laughing...: tribe trying to catch up./ Just a kid: no sex, 7–8 [3] ....*

Notes:

1 Running is a frequent activity in Dodge's childhood memories in *Background* (1933a): she and her friends "ran around in the snow" and "ran down Delaware [Avenue]" (p. 87). *Freud (1900) considered that childhood "games of movement, though innocent in themselves, give rise to sexual feelings. Childish 'romping'...is what is being repeated in dreams of flying, falling, giddiness and so on; while the pleasurable feelings attached to these experiences are transformed into anxiety" (p. 272).*

2 Jelliffe's notes date from a month after this dream, June 7 (the last recorded session in her analysis), likely because Dodge often brought in groups of dreams to discuss with him at the same time.

3 This association to *"no sex"* at age *"7–8"* recalls Dodge's description of her father forbidding kissing games (see note 8 for dream 77).

δ

113.
May 7, 1916 (2 of 3)

Dreamed of Florence Bradley.

> Jelliffe's notes from June 7, 1916:
> *Florence Bradley in some relation: before—she crazy—mad & I had driven her mad. Another ♀ in bed. She lying on ground: in spite of all, started to ♀-♀: kiss, mouth full of semen & deposited it in mo[uth]. after having been to ◯: All violent & relentless & horrible [1]:*

Note:

1 Dodge's revulsion for oral sex here is repeated in her associations to dream 122 where she describes her "disgust" for fellatio and her first experience of cunnilingus.

δ

114.
May 7, 1916 (3 of 3)

Dreamed I had to meet my lawyer [1] in Niagara Falls—by a certain train—
overslept & missed the train—tried to get another one—finally I was there
but he wasn't—everything went wrong. A good deal of talk with Seward
Cary over getting two good horses to go with mine to make a four & have
some good driving.[2]

> Jelliffe's notes from June 7, 1916:
> *Seward Cary: He taught me to drive 4 in hand.*[3]/

Notes:

1   Likely Endicott Peabody Saltonstall, her divorce lawyer (see note 2 for
    dream 68).
2   In her adolescence, Dodge and Cary had spent hours riding horses
    together and she loved his company: "He was always happy, and oh,
    it was such *fun* to be with him. Exciting! We accelerated life for each
    other. We, too, were like galloping horses, wild and untamed" (Luhan,
    1935, p. 7).
3   In *European Experiences* (1935), Dodge recalls: "He taught me how to
    drive four-in-hand. How to hold the four confusing reins between my
    short fingers and turn the leaders right or left. Soon after I began to
    drive them leaning against the high seat, for I had to stand because I
    could not reach the floor. I needed to brace myself against the tumbling,
    plunging animals (for Seward *never* had *quiet* horses). He, sitting next to
    me with the long-lashed coach whip in his hand, would begin to laugh
    his gurgling, excited laugh and flick the leaders lightly until they started
    to gallop" (p. 6). Eventually she gained more control over the galloping
    horses: "After I learned to drive four-in-hand, Seward gave me my whip,
    a small, light, long-lashed one, and I've never had more pride in anything
    since" (p. 7).

δ

115.
May 9, 1916 (1 of 3)

Dreamed I was talking to someone about Phoebe [Cary] marrying Arthur
B[risbane] [1]—& how she never suffered over it. I was in my mother's room
in her house & we began to feel water dripping. Soon the ceiling gave way &
a torrent of water crashed down on us.[2]

Notes:

1 A highly productive and influential newspaper editor who at the time was editor of *The New York Journal*, a Hearst publication where Dodge would soon have a syndicated advice column. In 1912, Brisbane had married Phoebe Cary, the daughter of Seward Cary. In Dodge's "Love Letters of a Grandmother" (1947a), she writes: "Arthur Brisbane told me once quite frankly that he believed young men should first love older women and be instructed by them in the arts of the emotional life, and that young women should marry early older men who knew their way around and who could care for them and teach them and give them their first children" (p. 10). At the time of their marriage, Brisbane was 48 years old and Phoebe Cary was 22. In her undated portrait of Brisbane, "A City Father," Dodge writes: "In his family he is a real father....He has a few lifelong prejudices about women that those near him are bound to give in to; he thinks they should keep their ears uncovered and their skirts off the dusty ground....Men are gardeners and women are their flowers, fruit or vegetables" (pp. 1–2). However, Brisbane was quoted at some point in his life as admitting: "There is more in any woman than any man can learn in 50 lifetimes" ("Death of Brisbane," *Time*, January 4, 1937, p. 43).

   Brisbane was a crucial initiator and supporter of Dodge's own news-paper writing, providing encouragement and funding. As she remem-bers in *European Experiences* (1935), around 1900 when she was 21 years old: "Arthur asked me...what I wanted to do in life, what I liked, what I felt....I told him I wouldn't marry and I wouldn't stay in Buffalo like the other girls, but that I would like to live and try to understand more and feel life itself." He then asked: "*Do you want to work?*" and she re-plied: "'I don't know. I don't know what I could work at...I don't know how to do anything. But would you give me something to do on your paper?'" Dodge was later pleased when she heard that he had told some-one: "'Mabel has brains. She has *brains*'" (p. 21). Years later, on January 29, 1917, he wrote to her, after having seen her advertisement for interior decorating services in *The New Republic* on January 13, 1917: "I see you are going to work. Why don't you write? You could really make some money and amuse yourself. Do you want to try it?" He also suggested topics for her column, as in his letter dated September 15, 1917: "Tell why women like to be married—pulling against the stake, like a little goat tied with a string."

2 *Would Freud, and consequently Jelliffe, have considered this a birth dream? Dodge is in her "mother's room" and first there is a slow dripping and then a gush of water. Dodge is about to become pregnant within the next week, so this dream could suggest her preoccupation with birth and foreshadow her desired pregnancy.* Also, Dodge's mother was married

to a man who was only a year older than Dodge herself, a reversal of the age difference between Phoebe Cary and Brisbane.

δ

116.
May 9, 1916 (2 of 3)

I was in some kind of difficult place morally...like one of the mystics' tests. I sent for Mildred Gratwick [1] to make it easier...She read in the margin of a mystic book I had been reading, where I had written in pencil: "My dear, I am growing depressed."[2]

In this dream I had a sense of discouragement & inability to hold out...

Notes:

1 A childhood friend who lived two blocks away from Dodge in Buffalo. In her chapter "Books and Playmates" in *Background* (1933a), Dodge recalls: "Mildred and I made a good combination. She had none of the...somber obedience of Nina [Wilcox], but she was a good play-mate and ready for anything. She was always laughing and opening her eyes wide in fun....Somehow I remember the snow in recalling the things I did with Mildred....We ran around in the snow knee-deep, the unbroken snow of people's lawns." In a poignant closing, Dodge remembers watching from a window as her friend walks away, ac-companied by her nurse, after a day of playing together: "They were out of sight soon and the old silence and desolation would fall on me once more. The house was still, the nursery was still—and again I was left alone in the emptiness that must be fought with and filled with the forms that are drawn from oneself lest misery conquer one" (pp. 85–87, 89).
2 During one of Dodge's chronic periods of despair over her relationship with Sterne, she turned to Evelyn Underhill's *Mysticism: A Study in the Nature and Development of Man's Spiritual Consciousness* (1912): "But empty of my love for Maurice I was empty indeed! Soon an emp-tiness was all I experienced. It was sinking down to the old depressed nothingness, which was all I was without a man....I stayed in bed a great deal of the time and read a thick book called *Mysticism* by Evelyn Underhill. Again I felt that I was passing through 'the dark night of the soul' like the mystics and saints she told of" (Luhan, 1936, p. 482).

δ

117.
May 9, 1916 (3 of 3)

Soon I passed from this to the Duncan School & I was one of the little girls. Maurice was sitting by watching as a visitor. I had only the mind of a little girl—concerned with our dance. I was at the head of the line & Dora [1] behind me & Miss. D. suggested we do a certain dance. I had never done it or heard of it. I had to lead the others & I was much embarrassed. I tried to watch Dora's gestures & copy her. She made some movements that were like a scotch dance & then some very archaic movements with both her hands held up straight in front of her—& then singly held up.[2] I tried to push her in front of me so she could lead & I could copy her. I heard Miss D. explaining to the visitor: "You see this is a very primitive early dance…" etc.[3]

N.B. The gestures with the hands were very singular & beautiful. I have never seen them. Like early Egyptian but earlier.

Notes:

1 Dora is among the girls listed who came to the United States with Elizabeth Duncan in 1915 and assumed the surname Duncan (Luhan, 1936, p. 340).
2 Dodge describes Elizabeth Duncan's passionate instructions to her students about their arm movements as they danced in a room overlooking the hills in Croton: "'Touch the hills!' she would cry. 'Reach out your fingers until you can touch the hills.' The sensitive young flesh quivered and stretched out towards the skyline. The slender arms grew longer, the fingers tapered out beyond their own limited boundaries. When children try to reach the skyline every day, they end by coming really a little nearer to it than if their reach is only so far as the arithmetic book" (1936, p. 347).
3 In a note likely attached to Dodge's letter to Jelliffe circa May 26, 1916 (see Interlude 18), she refers to this dream and links it with her becoming pregnant: "It occurs to me that that dream in which I put someone else before me in that primitive dance, & in which you detected a first appearance of desire to abdicate leadership came the night before the conception. That night was a week ago Tuesday—the date was, I believe, the sixteenth. You can look it up." This suggests that the baby was conceived May 10, but then in her letter circa May 26, she says that the baby is "ten days along," thereby dating its conception to May 16. *Jelliffe's interpretation that Dodge wanted to "abdicate leadership" when she wanted Dora to lead so that she could "copy her" suggests their ongoing dialogue about Dodge's ambivalent desire for control. She seems to credit her successful conception to her (emotional and sexual) receptivity and willingness to have someone else lead.*

In *Movers and Shakers* (1936), while describing a sexual reunion with Sterne, Dodge recalls her profound response to sensuality and her learning the words "archaic" and "primitive" (both of which appear in this dream) from her two psychoanalysts: "He reclaimed me and I sank down, down, beneath that weight of sensual life that poured out of his body and that was rich and somber and real, but heavy, oh, so heavy, weighing one down, pulling one *down*, reaching a kind of bottom, basic, and fundamental. There are levels, true all of them, and Maurice made me, then, truest at the lowest, or perhaps most primitive. Jelliffe had taught me to use that word: primitive. Later, Brill taught me another one: archaic" (p. 455). See note 3 for dream 82 about Jelliffe and Zenia X—'s 1914 article "Compulsion Neurosis and Primitive Culture" where he asserts: "If the child of the twentieth century is a résumé of what has gone before, he too passes through an animistic stage….his notions of the universe at certain stages of his evolution will correspond to those of more primitive races" (p. 362).

δ

INTERLUDE 14.

Although Hutchins Hapgood insists in his memoir that he was never in psychoanalysis—"I have been busily engaged all my life in confessing to my friends, especially my wife, and, as far as I could, the world, so I had no need either of the confessional or the psychoanalyst, nor could I nor any other person of moderate financial circumstances afford that superfluous luxury. Mabel, of course, tried it, as she tried everything" (1939, p. 383)— the following letter from Dodge to Jelliffe from the spring of 1916 suggests he may have consulted with Jelliffe. Dodge enclosed the still unpublished and only privately circulated manuscript of Hapgood's "The Story of a Lover."

[circa winter/spring 1916]

Dear Dr. Jelliffe,

Here is Hapgood's MS. I am really sacrificing my personal sense of integrity to my desire for his good. This MS is to be printed annonymously [sic] and only one or two have seen it. Today he gave it to me to show another mutual friend on condition that no one else should see it! But I believe that it will help you so much to establish a sympathetic relation with him, that I am almost willing in sending it. It is the first deception that has come in a very fine and intimate relationship.

I must have it back by Thursday morning as he has limited my time for having it. So I will send or call for it.

Also I am sending you two books, and two short things he wrote, one about his wife and me and one about me.[1] They will help you understand him.

And soon I want to send you some other documents—some things of mine. I came away exhilarated this morning becasue [*sic*] it seemed to me that there is room to stretch in Freudism (do you <u>call</u> it that?) and I almost saw that in a doctrine I have always been preaching—that perhaps after all there may be in it a scientific validity!....

It is quite settled for Tuesday evening at 6:30. Hapgood will be here.

Sincerely yours,
Mabel Dodge

Another undated letter appears to be from this time, circa winter/spring 1916:

Monday

Dear Dr. Jelliffe,

I have asked John Collier of the People's Institute to come too, tonight, as he is a friend of Mr. Hapgood's & is in the secret & will help the situation. He is a genius in his way[....]and he is interested besides, in other things—including Freud's science—so he'l[l] fit in well.

Sincerely,
Mabel Dodge

Note:

1 The article about Dodge was "A Promoter of Spirit," published in *The New York Globe,* circa 1914. It is included in Luhan's scrapbook "Misc. Vol II" (1936–1939, n.d.). The piece about Dodge and Boyce is unidentified, as are the two books she sent.

δ

118.
May 10, 1916 (1 of 3)

Dreamed I was reading a letter where Hutchins [Hapgood] [1] was explaining how unreliable Neith was, due to her female, congenital, lack of memory i.e. soul [2]—that she could not remember whether she had known Aleister Crowley [3] or not. Yet it had had such a strong influence on her life—& she had so much good will in trying to remember in order to reconstruct their relation (H. & hers) [4] but was obstructed by a purely female characteristic.

Notes:

1 Although one of Dodge's closest friends during this time, this is the first appearance of Hapgood by name in one of her dreams.

2 Dodge had read Hapgood's *The Story of a Lover* (1919) in manuscript form where Hapgood reports, "I often told her she had no soul" and "Our first few meetings showed me that she had no past! All that she could or can remember is that she had worked—worked calmly and quietly, without excitement" (pp. 12, 14).

3 A British writer and occultist who lived in the United States for a period of time between 1914 and 1918. In a letter from April 1915, Crowley writes to Dodge in New York: "I am giving a magic elixir party to a few friends tomorrow, Saturday night, here, at 8 o'clock. Would you like to come? It would give me great pleasure to see you again. And you would find the experience unique" (Luhan, 1913–1917, n.d.).

4 Hapgood (1919) relates the constant efforts he and Neith made to repair and reconnect over many years, through her pregnancies and their respective, mutually-encouraged infidelities. Hapgood recalls his frequent experiences of loneliness and frustration with his wife whose remoteness and "intolerable silence" (p. 92) left him wondering "What place was there for me?" (p. 50). At one point he concludes: "Under the illusion of the senses and the amorous fancy I have felt a real bond....Perhaps it was a real union, a real oneness, but with difficulty maintained, impossible to maintain; continuously, inevitably falling apart, slipping back again into tragic, hopeless separateness" (p. 63).

δ

119.
May 10, 1916 (2 of 3)

Maurice went away for a long journey. I was hopeless of seeing him again tho' he meant to return.[1] So I went abroad with Reed.[2] We were in some foreign place, and he suddenly went back to America to rejoin someone he had left—angry at me—because I had wronged him in some way. I felt awfully sad & left behind & abandoned & conscience stricken because I hadn't waited for Maurice.[3] I got hold of Mary Foote [4] & joined her, but wasn't happy.

Notes:

1 See note 1 for dream 108 about Sterne's planned trip. He intended to see a German woman he still loved, so of course Dodge would have doubts about his return. Reed also appears in dream 108.

2 Dodge had, in fact, traveled to Europe by ship with Reed in June 1913, first to Paris and then to the Villa Curonia. During the voyage, Dodge resisted his advances, arguing: "'Oh, Reed, darling, we are just at the Threshold and nothing is ever so wonderful as the Threshold of things,

don't you *know* that?'" But once they were in Paris, she gave herself over to him and then, in her characteristic way, "nothing else in the world had, any longer, any significance for me" (Luhan, 1936, pp. 213, 215).

3 This is the reverse of what actually happened in 1915, when Dodge did not wait for Reed while he was in Europe from March until the fall. In his absence, she chose Sterne as her lover.

4 Foote often served as a romantic consultant for Dodge in times of crisis.

δ

120.
May 10, 1916 (3 of 3)

Dr. [Bernard] Sachs [1] was talking to me. I was in bed languid, weary & disheartened. He was telling me I had a great future ahead of me. He told me that Mrs. Sachs never ceased talking about my villa. *[n.b. Four years ago when he & his wife went abroad I gave them a permit to visit the villa but never have heard a word of it or thought of it since.]* He went on arguing with me to arouse me but it did no good. I think he was talking of my talent for house decorating.[2]

Notes:

1 American neurologist and psychiatrist who practiced in New York. Dodge had consulted with him in late 1912 when she first returned to New York from Florence, seeking relief from her depressed and nervous state. She was in torment over her love affair with Paul Ayrault, and her subsequent indecision about her relationship with Edwin. As Dodge recalled: "With the most profound unconsciousness of my selfish ingenuity, I persuaded good Dr. Sachs, the psychiatrist who was attending me, that Edwin was the cause of my weakness and depression, so he... explained to Edwin that it would be better for him to stay away until I was stronger" (1936, pp. 23–24). Edwin Dodge moved out of their apartment into a nearby hotel until her mood improved. When Dodge invited Brill to speak about psychoanalysis at her salon a few years later, she invited Sachs: "He repudiated my invitation with the tone of an admiral who has been invited to tea on an enemy submarine. He said he was not at all in sympathy with the subject...and, he added, he considered the subject a dangerous one for me" (1936, p. 142). *Could Dodge's dreaming about her former psychiatrist indicate discouragement in her analysis with Jelliffe? She is "weary & disheartened" here, a state she knew well from the time of her treatment with Sachs, who in this dream is encouraging, admiring, and hopeful. In her next dream (# 121), Dodge expresses some doubt about whether Jelliffe can help her and she decides not to return to him that day.*

2 On January 13, 1917, *The New Republic* ran an advertisement announcing
   Dodge's consulting services as a decorator, a talent she had developed
   creating her visions of the Villa Curonia and 23 Fifth Avenue: "Mrs.
   Mabel Dodge is prepared to assist in the furnishing and decorating of
   rooms, to supply ideas of her own, or to express those of her clients"
   (p. 308). Around this date, Dodge wrote to Jelliffe: "I am 'ready' as they
   say in advertisements—to do home-decorating—furnishing etc[.]—I
   want to help people realize their <u>own</u> taste in their envirnments [*sic*].
   If you remember—will you speak of me—& help me get a job because I
   will do it <u>well</u>."

δ

121.
May 12, 1916

Dreamed I went to Dr. Jelliffe's. Had to wait a little while as he was with a
patient. He had just come back from Washington.[1] I was in some discomfort because of an obstruction in nose or throat—could not breathe well.[2]
In an inner room [3] between the waiting room & office some secretary or
assistant was working on a patient.[4] The patient was in a chair—& worked
over much as a dentist works—Some obstacle being removed or drawn
away. I had some things in my black bag which I took from time to time to
ease myself. A bottle of black powdered stuff like dry sand seemed to help
me—taken in big mouthfuls. I heard the doctor & the patient talking cheerfully & lightheartedly. Soon he opened the door & let the patient out. A
blond. I went in. The doctor commented in some way on his return from his
trip—he spoke in a leisurely way—I was examining some plates of a patient
having much the same trouble as myself. In the first plate the patient was
represented as strapped flat to the ground on the stomach & the mouth &
nose pressed against a square of glass. The following plate represented a
small green mark on the glass produced, from the pressure on the patient,
from his nose or mouth. I felt a doubt that Dr. J. could succeed in my case
as this seemed slow & we had little time that day. He said he could.[5] I soon
found myself outside the office. I was going towards home. I meant to return
to the office later. But I found that I had a long way to go & no money &
was walking. So I turned into a café where I saw Leo & borrowed 5 cents to
telephone to my house or to the doctor. He gave me the money but I found
myself then in my car on the way home or to the doctor's, when I suddenly
saw Mildred [Gratwick]'s house [6] & decided to stop for her & go out &
have some fun as we had done as children when we went out with the pony.
[7] As the car swung up to her door I thought: "The older I grow the less I
mind or feel doing things without my mother knowing." I knew I meant I
had decided to play hookey & not go back to the doctor's.[8]

Jelliffe's notes from May 15, 1916:
Mildred Gratwick...very conventional:/ People talked of me—hard to keep her friends. She m[arried]. & had 7 children. Used to like wild harmless things: Always went to church c. her...very emotional:/ Sex. references in bible vs. uplift asex[ual]. mysticism.

Notes:

1 Jelliffe had attended the annual meeting of the American Neurological Association, of which he was a member, in Washington, D.C., held May 8–10, 1916. *Transactions of the American Neurological Association* (1917) for this meeting records Jelliffe's participation in discussions of seven separate papers, among them: a response to Sidney Schwab's "Intentional Hypertonia" where he argued for more understanding of "psychogenic tonus difficulties, such as are seen in katatonia" as opposed to "physico-chemical" and "vegetative" ones (p. 103); he agreed with James J. Putnam's focus in his "Acroparesthesia" paper on the psychogenic components of this disease and cited a case where "improvement has occurred under psychoanalysis" (p. 327). In addition, at this time in Washington D.C., both the American Psychoanalytic Association and the American Psychopathological Association had their annual meetings. It is certainly possible that Jelliffe went to all three. The notes from his sessions with Dodge indicate a gap between April 27 and May 15.

2 This image is very similar to one in dream 96 where Dodge describes "trying to tear handfuls of loose tenuous phlegm out of my throat to free my larynx & breathing."

3 This recalls the "inner room" that she found with Stieglitz in dream 104.

4 Jelliffe did, in fact, at this time, employ assistants in his practice, as he admits in one of his "Technique" papers, referring to them as "the persons assisting me in psychoanalytic work" (1916, p. 268). He may have borrowed this unorthodox idea from Jung, who had written to him in July 1915 about his own use of assistants: "I trusted the cases entirely to her [his assistant] with the only condition, that in case of difficulties she would consult me or send the patient to me in order to be controled [*sic*] by myself....It is very important, of course, that you keep close analytical contact with an assistant, else you risk constant mistakes. I arranged weekly meetings with my assistant." Jelliffe halted this practice around 1918 (Burnham, 1983, pp. 78, 120–122).

5 *In this dream, Dodge "could not breathe well" due to some obstruction and yet she has to wait while Jelliffe is with another patient and "talking cheerfully & lightheartedly." When he finally sees her, he is "leisurely" and does not seem to grasp the complexity of her situation. Is this Dodge's response to his absence when he was away in Washington, D.C.? Does the "green mark" on the plate indicate jealousy of his time with another patient?*

6 As Dodge describes in *Background* (1933a), "a massive house made of square blocks of granite" that was "very sumptuous inside....In the hall there was a great tiger skin and in the little reception room there was a huge polar bear rug. I adored these animals and we used to sit on them and lie flat on them and dream. I bore them in my mind until the day came when I could have my own tigers and bears—and sure enough, their replicas lay upon the polished floor and the red tiles of the Villa Curonia" (pp. 84, 85).

7 Although Dodge does not mention a pony in recounting her childhood play with Mildred, she recalls "a great game of travel, moving all the tables and furniture about, making trains and railway stations, until...we became more and more noisy," and eating dinner "with gusto and loud shrieks of tomboy laughter" (1933a, p. 88).

8 This dream is very likely the one Dodge refers to in her next letter to Jelliffe (Interlude 15), where she challenges his technique and its effects upon her sense of freedom in therapy, and ends by saying she will not come in the next day. ***By deciding not to return to Jelliffe's office in this dream, and also feeling more liberated from her mother's (and Jelliffe's) judgment, Dodge asserts her independence and feels the freedom to return to childhood pleasures.***

δ

INTERLUDE 15.

Friday [circa May 1916]

Dear Dr. Jelliffe,

A propos of a dream I had last night, I have just formulated in my mind & given shape to what was for some time past a vague feeling. This feeling has been in regard to some elements in your technique of analysis... not at all a resentment towards you "per se" nor towards Psycho-analysis, but rather to your system of procedure. I think your dogmatic trend halts me! I don't feel your right to prescribe a philosophy & that is really what it comes to! It seems to me we should work together to remove obstacles which impede a free flow of energy but I don't believe it comes within the realm of psychoanalysis to impose a formula for thinking, or a set of symbols which you arbitrarily designate in consistency with your particular constitution.

You see in all of us are found to be different tastes & perceptions. In no one of us, except perhaps in the supreme artist, is found the capacity of imagination to realize sympathetically, & to understand, all tastes—& perceptions, so each of us must be left to grow according to the variety we represent—having the color & perfume of our species. Don't you think you rather incline to turn us all into the species of plant [1] of which you are yourself so fine a specimen? I believe in you thoroughly. I wish there were more like you—but I wouldn't like everyone to be like you because

I like different ways of thinking & reacting. "But this" of course you will say—"is symptomatic." Maybe, but not necessarily of illness.

I would like the analysis to go on without the degree of utilitarianism we have split upon—& without the feeling of resistence [*sic*] to dogma & definition that I have felt rising so often…& which results from a clash of personalities in a case where the fact of personality should be practically absent…of course difficult in this case for we are not negative, either of us.

But don't you think you could leave out some of your judgements [*sic*] (mentally as well as spoken—more than spoken in fact) and have a little more leeway for the conceptions of the patient without regarding them as fantasy,—& the present type of letter as regression! This is not at all bad tempered as it seems, but based on a desire for a better understanding.

Sincerely,
Mabel Dodge

I am not coming in tomorrow as promised but Monday if possible for 2 hours—3–5? Tomorrow I have no car—having lent it.

Note:

1   This may be not just a metaphor but a direct reference to Jelliffe's doctoral degree in botany and his lifelong passion for collecting plants. His papers at the Library of Congress include hundreds of pressed flowers and plants.

δ

INTERLUDE 16.

Jelliffe replied fully and without defensiveness, welcoming her letter and eager to engage with her around this topic in their next session. In fact, Dodge liked this letter so much that she included it in *Movers and Shakers* (1936, pp. 445–446), and had written to Jelliffe from Taos circa February 1936 to ask his permission to publish it: "I like it very much & find it intelligent & very fitting in the book, relating to our talks."

[circa May 1916]

My dear Mrs. Dodge,
    I am sorry you feel I dogmatize: I myself am dogmatic that I have no right to do so. As a thorough-going sophist and pragmatist my own philosophy cannot and must not be imposed on another of different experience. With Protagoras, I hold, since we do not any of us act quite alike, so therefore we cannot perceive quite alike and that the only necessity for conformity in thinking is concerned with those things which are "necessary to live"

as I have quoted it so often to you! We vary concerning those things which are not needed for a bare existence and may conduce to a life that is "beautiful and good." I feel sure you cannot find therein a dogmatic philosophy.

I think my dogmatism is concerned with the evidences of your unconscious solely. If your unconscious indubitably says, "This I wish to do—but I, my conscious, knows, it will lead to death, and not to a life that is beautiful and good," then I must confess I am dogmatic. If your unconscious says, "I am a man and I can procreate with my male organ," then I am dogmatic. "You can't and you need not try." This is not forcing a philosophy upon you. This is only telling you you are trying to do the impossible. Perhaps I fail to get this distinction over; if so, then surely I am at fault.

I am not one whit involved in forcing people to do anything. I am only trying to be a mirror in which one may read why one cannot do certain things in certain ways. If my reading and experience and knowledge of evolution has taught it to me from another side, I should not use that overmuch, else it might seem I was putting myself in front of the mirror.

Those things which are most strongly felt as resistances are the direct results of the patient's and analyst's blind spots. One must be very careful regarding the great tendency to displace the affect, born of the resistance, to something quite foreign to the situation.

I hope I can help you to see this on Monday. I am glad you can formulate my dogmatism, as you have; it is one of my difficulties, more born of the desire to hurry people along than to make them conform. I am after all a wretched conformist myself and to be held up as a single pattern, machine maker of souls— although perhaps an [sic] hyperbolic way of taking your phrase—is a shock.

Very cordially,
Smith Ely Jelliffe

How about Bayard? I hope he will write me.

δ

122.
May 13, 1916

Dreamed I had to go away to some small place on the seacoast for a few days to get my divorce—(Salem). I got Mary F[oote]. to go with me.[1] We went to a small sort of boarding house & had to persuade the landlady to give us a room for the place was full. She showed us a horrid irregularly shaped room with a window on an inner court overlooking other windows & people in them.[2] I took it & left M[ary]. while I went out to attend to my business. But I went rather far away—& staid [sic] & suddenly remembered her & thought I must telephone her to come & join me. Then I found myself with the Bramley's [sic] & Dorothy H.[3] somehow. It was Dorothy I had left behind. John [Evans] arrived bringing me mail from somewhere. I tried very hard to telephone to this poor friend who was tied up in this town several villages away—waiting for me. But I couldn't find it in the book—& I couldn't remember the name of the place, or the boarding house. A complete lapse of memory & a sense of my hands being tied. I was expostulating with someone because they wouldn't tell me the name but they didn't seem to understand what it was I wanted to know. At one moment I was back in the place with Mary or Dorothy & trying to leave to go back where I came from—at another I was trying to get into communication with this place. *It was an uncomfortable effortful dream, I was always trying to do something I should do, & being prevented.*[4]

Jelliffe's notes from May 16, 1916:
Been gardening hard—men planted things all wrong.[5] *Yesterday 10 people working./ Feeling very well....*
Re Cunnilingus/ I had forgotten, 7–8–9 or 10. Little Dorothy [Scatchard] & Aunt [Emily]—ran into train of cars./ This little Dorothy. Mrs. Cary. Breasts [6]*/ together in W.C.:/ urinating: I now remember: She kissed my* () *in bath room. She wanted to lean me down to her: My 1st sex exp[erience]. she called it—words came up—"little P[enis]. thing." Why possibly that part of ♂, not interesting—the cl[itoris] inside the* (). *Never any use or service. Dr. [Parmenter]* [7] *always clit[oral] stim[ulation]: at same time: He found out possibly = Edwin. Cunnilingus: So loathesome [sic]:/ Became hateful / Made fellatio c. disgust./ only once #/ Origin/ Dorothy 2–3 times/.*[8]

Notes:

1 Foote would have been a likely choice as someone to accompany Dodge to her divorce hearing, since she had confided in Foote about her marriage during the time of her affair with Ayrault in 1912. At this very moment, from May 1 to 13, 20 of Foote's paintings were in an exhibition at M. Knoedler and Company in New York, including portraits of "Mrs. Mabel Dodge" (see Figure 4.1) and Robert Edmond Jones.
2 *Could this image of a "horrid irregularly shaped room with a window on an inner court" have anything to do with her current or anticipated state of pregnancy?*
3 Unidentified. This could be Dorothy Scatchard (perhaps "H" is the initial of her married surname?), as she appears in Dodge's associations to this dream. The Bramleys are identified in note 7 for dream 35.
4 *Is this a transference comment that also relates to the previous dream (# 121) where Dodge suggested that both Jelliffe and her mother may interfere with what she desires? In this dream, she is "prevented" from communicating with others and keeps trying to reach them. Her son appearing with "mail from somewhere" may also connect to her pregnancy, reminding her of the deep conflict that characterized her pregnancy with him.*

5 This image connects to Dodge's previous dream (# 121) where things are not done to her liking, and to her letter to Jelliffe (see Interlude 15) where she objects to his technique of analysis.

6 As a child, Dodge accompanied Dorothy to watch her aunt Emily nurse her baby, as she recalls in an unpublished passage in "Green Horses": "It was the first time I became conscious of my body and the lovely feelings it held—feelings that rose and spread all through one, delicate and fiery and alive—as we stood and watched the baby suck at the white breast" ("Intimate Memories, Vol. II.," n.d., p. 401).

7 Parmenter's appearance here in her associations may be linked to Dodge's thoughts about pregnancy, as she was uncertain if he or her first husband was the father of her son, John.

8 Likely with Jelliffe's inquiry and interest, Dodge describes her childhood sexual play and her adult sexual relationships with her characteristic openness, while also revealing her revulsion for oral sex.

δ

123.
May 16, 1916

Dreamed Mr. Cook [1] had performed some sort of work—it was a creative undertaking. Everyone was admiring it, tho' only he was able to understand it. He stood as tho' weary from his labors but proud & satisfied. I took his work to look at it. It seemed to me to be a small tablet with some drawing or inscription on it whose meaning escaped one at first but I looked closely & saw that all it amounted to was a number of women in a row, just showing to below the breasts. And I said to myself that all his work amounted to was bothering over a number of women's breasts.

> Jelliffe's notes from May 23, 1916:
> *Geo. C. Cook. Greenwich V. people...Sloppy person, don't care for, not def: loose jointed & great big—haven't you ever seen him, no chin, large dark eyes, lost & pathetic. I know what it means:/ Most of my phantasies = homosex. fantasies* [2]*:*
> *Why ♀ breasts./ I have had many phantasies, one mystical, another dominating: Others persecution & no one understanding/....Look like tablets or frieze to people to waist: Just people to breast:...life to life: pictures which are just breasts....*

Notes:

1 George Cram "Jig" Cook, writer and playwright who, along with his wife, the playwright Susan Glaspell, was among the principal founders of the Provincetown Players in 1915. The members of the Players, who sometimes held performances in their own homes, often incorporated the ideas

of psychoanalysis into their plays, at times satirizing them. Cook and Glaspell's 1915 play, *Suppressed Desires,* is a parody of the unquestioning adoption of basic Freudian ideas and reveals the trap of inflexible application of psychoanalytic mechanisms. In the play, Henrietta, an untiring proselytizer of psychoanalysis, advises her sister, tellingly named Mabel, to discover her suppressed desires so that she can act on them, thereby avoiding possible insanity: "It's like this, Mabel. You want something. You think you can't have it. You think it's wrong. So you try to think you don't want it. Your mind protects you—avoids pain—by refusing to think the forbidden thing. But it's there just the same. It stays there shut up in your unconscious mind, and it festers….It breaks into your consciousness in disguise, masks itself in dreams, makes all sorts of trouble" (in Heller & Rudnick, 1991, p. 283). However, when Mabel begins therapy with Henrietta's own psychoanalyst to uncover the meaning of a dream, the interpretation pronounces that Mabel has suppressed desires for Henrietta's husband. Henrietta then abruptly abandons her previously unbendable belief in the meaning of all utterances and dreams, dismissing the interpretation as rooted in a "ridiculous coincidence," to which Mabel replies: "Coincidence! But it's childish to look at the mere elements of a dream. You have to look *into* it—you have to see what it *means!*" (pp. 289–290).

2 *By acknowledging her recurring fantasies about women, Dodge reveals a preoccupation with the nurturing breast that has haunted her for years, ever since she saw the breast spurting milk across the room as a young child (Luhan, 1933a, as described in her chapter, "The Breast," pp. 29–33), and the taunts from her Aunt Georgie to feed her from her breast when she was acting like a baby (see transcription of Jelliffe's March 25 notes accompanying Figure 5.2). By this date, according to her calculations, Dodge was just pregnant and this dream may also relate to the anticipation of nursing a child as a way of nurturing herself.*

δ

124.
May 18, 1916

I was with C.A.[1] for a while on my way somewhere. To leave I had to jump a great distance—from the window to the street—which I did, with a good deal of confidence tho' some apprehension. I feared the shock of landing but there was none.

Note:

1 Unidentified.

δ

125.
May 19, 1916

Dreamed I was running my fingers over my throat & saying "There is no spot where it can be perforated so that the poison can be drained away."[1] The throat was shaped like a cross.

> Jelliffe's notes from May 23, 1916:
> *Running fingers over throat: throat & cross = Larynx = higher creative channel: Rose bloom in cross: instead of thorn* [2]:

Notes:

1 In her dreams, Dodge's throat is always associated with blockage (as in dreams 96 & 121). *Could this relate to her feeling constrained in expression in her analysis, aware of the workings of resistances that Jelliffe is working so hard to break down, but that she wants to hold onto? She is pregnant now, and so could the "poison" be connected to something bad or dangerous inside her?*

2 As Dodge explains, in Jelliffe's theories of symbols corresponding to parts of the body, the throat is associated with the shape of the cross: "The creative word issued from the throat of man when he reached the true Power of manhood, and this was the birth of the mystic Rose on the Cross of the medieval Rosicrucians" (1936, p. 440).

δ

126.
May 21, 1916 (1 of 2)

Dreamed I had to go very far up town to do my marketing....

δ

127.
May 21, 1916 (2 of 2)

Dreamed I went to the Masque [1] with Bayard & someone else—and left my bag with the the [*sic*] tickets in it in the motor. The performance was going on & we couldn't get in, awfully disappointed...couldn't think what to do.[2] Suddenly the woman in charge said: "Why don't you buy some new seats?" This I hadn't thought of, but I had no money. But then I arranged somehow & got in & found the big place [3] nearly all empty, the seats empty.[4] I saw Percy [MacKaye] directing it all...While waiting outside a grotesquely dressed (in yellow & furs) homosexual man lurched up, quite drunk & annoyed me very much.

Notes:

1 Percy MacKaye is credited with founding the popular movement that revived the Renaissance genre of court masques and pageants in the United States at this time. In this dream, Dodge is referring to MacKaye's masque, *Caliban*, with set design by Bobby Jones, which opened on Wednesday, May 24, 1916 at the Lewisohn Stadium in New York. The headlines in *The New York Times* the following day announced: "MACKAYE MASQUE A RARE SPECTACLE; 'Caliban,' the Biggest Dramatic Entertainment in History of New York. FIFTEEN THOUSAND ATTEND." The article praised MacKaye for creating "a spectacle of memorable beauty" that featured fifteen hundred performers, lasted more than three hours, and was attended by patrons from all parts of society: "People from the shops and factories, many of them, arrived as early as 6:30, bringing their suppers with them. From that time on limousines, taxicabs, trolleys, Fifth Avenue buses and the Subway kept a steady stream of patrons coming." The date of Dodge's dream, Sunday, May 21, corresponds with one of the days mentioned in this article, in a comment about the weather that "cast a chill over the preparations on Sunday, Monday, and Tuesday" (all quotations p. 11). It is quite possible through her friendship with MacKaye that Dodge may have had an opportunity to go to the stadium to observe the preliminary arrangements for the masque but, if not, she would have been keenly aware of the upcoming production.
2 *This theme of trying to do something and being prevented is repeated from dream 122.*
3 Lewisohn Stadium, named after businessman and philanthropist Adolph Lewisohn who contributed substantially to the building project, opened to the public on May 29, 1915 and was designed to hold almost 10,000 people. It was located in the blocks between West 136th and 138th Streets, and between Amsterdam and Convent Avenues.
4 *What could this emptiness signify? Dodge has literally just been filled up with a pregnancy. Does the vastness of the emptiness speak to her fears about ever being fully satisfied?*

δ

128.
May 23, 1916 (1 of 2)

Dreamed I went to Dr. Jelliffe's & we had made a mistake—he had [1]—in the time. There were two men waiting ahead of me.[2] So I rearranged the time & went out.

Notes:

1 *In her circa May 26, 1916 letter to Jelliffe (Interlude 18), Dodge considers him responsible for her becoming pregnant—is this an allusion to "this baby you have brought about" and her fears about its being ill-advised? First "we" and then "he" had made a mistake.*

2 *Who could these two men be? If she is holding Jelliffe responsible for her pregnancy (and not Sterne, who was actually the father), then these two men could be those who have impregnated her before: either Parmenter or Karl Evans (see note 7 for dream 122) and Edwin Dodge (see note 5 for dream 142). Or could they be other patients of Jelliffe's?*

δ

129.
May 23, 1916 (2 of 2)

Dreamed M. & I lost each other in a big many roomed art gallery. I was waiting for him to turn up & an oldish gentleman came up & asked me if I was expecting to meet a friend & said he had seen a man searching in some agitation in the lower rooms. Then I went to meet M. where he said, & he appeared looking scared to death—in a panic at my not having met him.

In a very high room in the same gallery was an old lady who had a kind of sinecure from the gallery. She staid [*sic*] up there all the time. I can't remember what her job was—she took care of something. I think she also made something.

In the lower hall or gallery while I was waiting for M. I was looking at the great paintings on the wall & ceiling. Huge decorations very rich & "baroque" & composed of barbaric groups—dark people—& they all moved back & forth, part of the exhibition was that they could move & they seemed to stretch all their muscles & bodies back & forth in a rhythm.[1]

Note:

1 Dodge sees a large group of "dark people" rhythmically moving their bodies, a dream image connected to her association of "my own sexuality" with the "Negro" (see dream 81). Dodge now suspects that she is pregnant, as she indicates in her next letter to Jelliffe (see Interlude 17). *Could this dream, with its spaciousness, its "big many roomed art gallery" that was a "very high room," relate to what Dodge claims in this letter, that the work of psychoanalysis acted to "open up the walls of the uterus to receive the flow"? Sterne is "agitated" and "scared to death," perhaps his feeling about being a father and of thus linking his life with Dodge.*

δ

INTERLUDE 17.

Finney Farm
Wednesday morning [circa May 24, 1916]

Dear Dr. Jelliffe[,]
Here is a point where I'd like your opinion. I thought of asking you about it & then dreaded a storm—or worse—a gloomy face. But please try & see it as the first case—see it freshly I mean—& not in the light of the conventions. See it as a case in itself— not as a type—& then give me your opinion.

When I started psycho-analysis I told you I did it to get over jealousy which bothered me. Instead of that—so far it has gotten me over a lot of fantasies which I sincerely believed represented the higher & more spiritual part of me...my mystical notions & so on. At the beginning of it I told you I wanted to do some creative work—& we believed I would get my energy freed so that I might. Then one day I asked you to state to me what my problem is, & you said I use my maleness femalely—& my femaleness malely—. At the beginning of the analysis you probed me to find my strongest desires. You will find—in turning back to your notes—that I told you I started life wanting fifteen children.

You have told me repeatedly that no relation between a man & a woman was justified save in that it was productive & I have repeatedly told you that I wanted it to be so. Well—I have never had a relation with a man that I haven't consciously desired a baby; with my whole being I have longed for it. I was meant to have lots of children. But as you said—I was unconsciously using my femaleness malely—& I never conceived for that reason. Now Psychoanalysis has been teaching my unconscious something. Only twice in my life has a certain experience come to pass in me while I was merely passive—noting it. When I was first married & loved that doctor [Parmenter], I tried to keep myself blank to my husband [Karl Evans]. I didn't strain to him & try to seize him as I had. I just tried to preserve my self & my loyalty to the other by a nullified passiveness & one night to my real horror something took me—took place in me—in spite of my not straining to bring it about & in spite of my wil[l]ful non-participation. The event occurred—it was some co-operative understanding between the will-conscious or unconscious of my husband & my unconscious. It left me, I remember, stunned by surprise to find my conscious will overpowered. It was the only time it ever happened to me—& it brought John. [1] I had been on the verge of being unwell & I wasn't. Then for fifteen years—it never happened again. Whatever happened I worked for & tried for—I said I wanted babies & tried to wrest them out of the embrace— but my will was never never strong enough—or it was too strong—& the experience I have just written about hadn't taught me anything. So of course one reason I was neurotic was this struggle between my intense conscious desire to have children which I tried to get in a male dominating way &—according to your theory of opposites—a possible unconscious desire not to receive them. Well—your analysis got under my skin at last… and last week—just on the eve of being unwell[,] the same thing happened again that happened fifteen years ago. It was not only that the orgasm took place in the vagina because that has occurred more or less since the analysis directed it there, but, while my own will—on that night seemed to me torpid, slow, indifferent some other will in me seemed to act, seemed to open up the walls of the uterus to receive the flow. I was amazed at it—recalling another time long ago. I was even at the moment certain it meant a baby—my body and an unconscious will in me had operated to-gether—while I—my own strong self had lain there—hardly doing more than observe. That was a week ago Tuesday & I'm not unwell yet. I have had all the unwell symptoms of pain but that[']s all. I have even begun to feel that marvellous [sic] content & self-sufficiency which I have already described to you—& which I felt only once in my life when John was com-ing—a sense of functioning, creating, & fulfilling. I have tried other things as you know—I have overflowed into all sorts of other channels because this one was closed to me thro' my own perversity, but no other activity compares with this one in pure satisfaction & the sense of rightness. Now I want your opinion of it. When what I have wanted so long has come to pass—thro' psychoanalysis—(which proves indubitably that therefore it is what should come to pass—) when I have such nice children—when the world can use my kind of children—when I am economically able to do it—do you feel I ought to give up having it? In my heart it seems to me only a beginning—perhaps I will have fifteen even yet!

I want you to look at it from the standpoint of the natural laws & tell me if you believe I am in the wrong…and I want you to understand that you must answer me—not as answering to a type but as to an individual. I don't see why I haven't the right to it—if I can carry it off. I am not go-ing to marry on its account—I don't feel sure enough of Maurice nor he of himself—to hurry into marriage. I am congenial with him—& after he goes to Germany to find out if he is released from that other woman & finds he is, I might marry him. But I am not thinking of rushing into it in a panic. If I have the baby I shall face having it by myself—so to speak. And I don't see why women haven't a right to babies this way if they are strong enough to do so without having to lean back on the protecting male. I know that you—as you told me—have chosen to address your-self to the great middle in[-]between class of mind—& you have done an enormous amount of educating in doing so, but I wish that you wouldn't feel you are answering a class when you answer me, because were I in your place addressing them I would reply as you would. They can't do it—they have to work in droves and in the drove, the couple must work together. But I'm not in a drove—and it isn't only money that has set me apart from it, nor have I been excluded. I have the conviction that without money I would still be strong & intelligent—& have power over the drove—because I <u>see more</u> than most of them do. This, of course, is a gift—& a developpable [*sic*] one—& one I have always worked over. Please try & not answer me as you would feel obliged to answer me in a court of law—I want your private opinion.

Call me up & make an appointment—& we'l[l] talk it over.

Faithfully—
Mabel Dodge

Note:

1 Although Dodge attributed paternity of John Evans to her husband Karl in this letter, at other moments she questioned who was the father of her son, Karl or Dr. Parmenter. See note 7 for dream 18 and note 7 for dream 122.

δ

130.
May 24, 1916 (1 of 2) [1]

Dreamed one side of the bed was lacking [2] & I had to get it there. *[I was sleeping at Mary's [3] & one side has the wall, the other was empty.]*

Notes:

1 This dream and the next date from the same day as Dodge's Wednesday letter to Jelliffe (see Interlude 17) in which she announces she is pregnant with a child fathered by Sterne, and in conflict over getting what she has desired.
2 ***This image may represent Dodge's uterus, with a missing ovary (removed years before in surgery, see note 5 for dream 8): "left side where that ovary is gone" (see Interlude 18).***
3 Almost certainly Mary Foote.

δ

131.
May 24, 1916 (2 of 2)

Dreamed I was driving Bayard's Sol [1]—he was walking behind. He had gotten out of the cart to urinate.[2] I was driving Sol down a steep curving stone or brick road. It led to the waterfront like one in Buffalo that it reminded me of. It was very difficult to drive Sol & not have any accident, & not have him get more nervous & run away. When I got to the bottom there was a kind of big place. Lots of people there that I knew, mostly men. It had to do with work & a business like atmosphere—or else it was preparation for the Masque.[3] Walter was there. We were all to have dinner together in a big room, but I perceived that the others, among them Sam Lewisohn,[4] are not at our table while Walter put himself & me at a table alone. He sat opposite me eating & said: "This was Becker's [5] haunt, you know." I hadn't known it. It hadn't any particular atmosphere of things. Soon I saw there was a fat old woman sitting at our table. She wore a bonnet & mantle & had a large bland face with a closed expression. She ate enormously & steadily. I was eating prunes & apricots & some lumps of sugar with it that I crunched.[6] Suddenly she reached behind Walter's head & lifted out a bottle of champagne which she lifted to her lips & drank from.[7]

Jelliffe's notes from May 29, 1916:
W.L.:/ Spoke to him: What about m[arriage]. M.S.:/ Why m. What about ch[ildren]./ Don't think about it:/ I think for J[elliffe]. as conventional:/ He is conventional [8]: revolt: Otherwise:/ Much commotion: Bayard really going to be ♂-♂: Brown [9] & Bobby:/ Bayard stole him from Bobby: distraught....

Notes:

1 Boyeson's horse, identified by him in a letter to Dodge dated October 1916.
2 According to Jelliffe and Zenia X— in "Compulsion Neurosis and Primitive Culture" (1914), urinating outside is associated with forbidden pleasure. Zenia recounts at great length these relished experiences of hers :

> There was always a strange feeling of exhilaration and mysterious un-ion with mother earth if in our play or on some picnic or excursion far from home we resorted to the soil for defecation or urination. Even in adult life on one occasion about twelve years ago, just before the final, conscious outbreak of my neurosis, I was alone in a wild and beautiful region away from human habitation and was compelled to resort to urination upon the earth. The same secret, pleasurable sensation was so marked, so vivid, that I feared to repeat the act, to put myself again in the way of this experience, and when only a year and a half ago it was once more necessary in a lonely spot, there at once arose the struggle with sexual thoughts and feelings to which for many years my illness has driven me....I could not define the feeling accompanying these experiences; it was a mystery, a pleasure secreted in my own body, strange, exhilarating, seeming to draw on the secret springs of my being, and even as in adult life the recalling of these sensations as well as the adult experiences described associate themselves with the

feelings which my knowledge and experience have taught me are sexual, I think that I can interpret the childish sensations as part of the great underlying, sexual power in every life. (pp. 364–365)

Given these assertions, and the connections between the "gushing of water" in urination and "the idea of procreation" (1914, p. 365), this dream could be considered an erotic one, filled with two men who were possible romantic partners for Dodge (Boyeson and Lippmann), and then "mostly men" in a large room where she was to have dinner alone with Lippmann.

3 MacKaye's masque, *Caliban*, opened in New York on this date, May 24, 1916, see note 1 for dream 127.

4 Investment banker, art collector, and philanthropist who lived in New York. He was the son of Adolph Lewisohn. According to Dodge, he donated $500 toward the founding of the Elizabeth Duncan School (1936, p. 342).

5 Unidentified.

6 *Could this be a reference to Dodge's longstanding problems with constipation and preoccupation with things fecal?*

7 *This bottle of champagne could relate to the gluttony of the "fat old woman" (Dodge's insatiable appetites) or could suggest something celebratory, perhaps Dodge's achieved pregnancy.*

8 This recalls Jelliffe's admission in his circa May 1916 letter to Dodge (Interlude 16) that he is "after all a wretched conformist myself."

9 Unidentified.

δ

INTERLUDE 18.

Finney Farm
Friday [circa May 26, 1916]

Dear Dr. Jelliffe,
   The enclosed note was written on Wednesday & not sent. Whenever I have tried to give it to you—as on Wed[.] eve—or mail it since then—my limbs seem to turn to water & my hand seems incapable of the act, because it would mean bringing the matter into <u>actual conflict</u> and allowing a greater menace to the baby—Of course if you read this first you don't know there is a question of a baby but that's what it is & what the other letter is about. It[']s ten days along at present—& just in that time the right side of my body feels like something come alive & in activity, while the left side where that ovary is gone feels so different, dead like a blasted tree. Now the conflict going on in me is awfully strong. I want that baby more than anything else one could offer me. I'd rather have it than paint the best picture or write the best book—& Maurice clings to it & yearns over

it & we both feel we would hate each other if I got rid of it. It[']s so utterly against my instinct to get rid of it…I shudder all over at the thought & my blood seems to curdle in me & refuse…and that is so different from the time I told you of when I first married Edwin & had to have my unwellness brought on because he was sick. Then I had a horror of keeping the baby & I rushed from Florence to Paris in a hurry to get rid of it. This time because it is right-in-nature to have it—I can hardly bring myself to even discuss it, my body is so unwilling to consider giving it up—& the baby might suffer too much & Maurice too. I want to hear from you what practical means there are by which to satisfy all the desires for good in the situation…& not have a conflict. If ever was a psychoanalytic baby—this is one. It has brought about what would have happened naturally but for infantile perversion. It has brought about the submission of the female organs. What a lot of time has been wasted!

The situation would be simple but for two things. Maurice is held by a fantasy built of the hope & desire for that german woman. It[']s his dream. I am his reality. There is no doubt about his real honest love for me & intense desire to have a baby—& make his life here. But he has in him a years-old ungratified desire for that other woman. He hates it—& curses it—& says it is ruining his life & preventing him from living really—and his only hope is in seeing her again after this year we've had together & putting this reality side by side with that dream—in the hope the other will fade[.…]I know he wants to be rid of it. It is a complex, a fixation & the cause of his neurotic tendencies. I know he wants to settle down & make his life here. What does psycho-analysis say of such a case?

Well—so if he goes—who knows whether that meeting will free him as he wishes? The other woman is symbolised [*sic*] now in music, in moonlight, in all the fantasy parts of life & it holds him in an awful grip tho' he longs to be free of it. It has gained a hold on his imagination, & thro' the habit of thinking, his thought channels have been formed for her image to run in! He tried to perpetuate her, & possess her in thought for so long, & now when he would be rid of it, she possesses him so[.…]In other words, she is his religion—he falls back upon it. When we quarrel, he becomes closed to me, absented in a world that he has invented when he is with her. Of course this is bad to live with—as bad for him as for me. He suffers from the possession as much as I. He says it cheats him of all reality—& stands between him & real life.…I think he wants [to] be a father. He has a strong family sense as have most jews. He is absolutely honest & honorable about it all. He begs & begs not to lose the baby & yet when I ask him—can he be a father to it he always replies: "I don't know what I am till I see Mira [1] again after this year with you."

Now in any case he means to go in June as soon as he has finished a portrait, & see Mira to find out where he is at.[2] I have told him I don't want him back unless he is free of this thing[.…]He is willing we should be married before he goes so that I could call the baby something—w[h]ether he is free or not but he doesn't know & I haven't told him yet—that my divorce comes up in June but I don't get an absolute decree until six months after[.…]

I suppose you read my conflict in here, don't you? It is a conflict that turns me into stone & water, alternately!

I know I must decide something soon—to let it go on or stop it[—] for there is no life the first two weeks & also I believe it is not an illegal act to bring on menstruation within that time.

Do you see a <u>practical</u> way for me to have this baby you have brought about? I want it <u>so</u>! Could I go away or something? Or just <u>have</u> it? You ought to see how Maurice is melted by it. He wants children <u>so</u> much. There is nothing he won't do that is in his <u>power</u> to do. He <u>wants</u> the freedom to live, & for 8 or 9 years this other thing has prevented him & driven him into all sorts of strange channels. It is the cause of all his queer neuroses.

Please call me up & see me tomorrow.

M.D.

May 26

P.S. Last night Maurice had the following dream which has some bearing, I suppose.

We were motoring—Hutch Hapgood & his wife [Neith Boyce] & I were along. It went smoothly for a while then we came to an archway thro' which we had to go into a big room or garage—which Albert the chauffeur did— but inside, in order to continue forward we had to take two or three steps down. Albert said he could take them, with care. He put on the brakes & Maurice braced himself to meet the shock. That was done safely—but then we came to a vegetable bed all laid out neatly with young vegetables & flowers coming up. It was directly in our path. We stopped to decide what to do because there was no way ahead but thro' it. M. asked if we <u>could</u> get thro' it & Albert said—"Oh yes—but it will destroy it."—We had to go on so M. told him to do it. But then some tall thin men appeared & protected it & wouldn't allow us to go over it. So M. asked Albert if we couldn't go back & go round another way. Albert replied "No—we could come down the steps but I can't drive the car up them." Then M. asked what we <u>could</u> do. Albert thought & then said: "If you will all get out & rest somewhere—I can get someone to help me—& take the car all to pieces & carry the parts back to where we were—& then put it together again & it will be ready in a day or two.["] And M. told him <u>to do it</u>.

A note on a separate piece of paper appears here in Jelliffe's case notes:

It occurs to me that that dream in which I put someone else before me in that primitive dance, & in which you detected a <u>first</u> appearance of desire to abdicate leadership came the night before the conception. That night was a week ago Tuesday—the date was, I believe, the sixteenth. You can look it up.

Notes:

1 See note 1 for dream 108.
2 This statement establishes that Sterne did not make his planned trip to Germany in May.

δ

132.
May 26, 1916

Dreamed the back of my sofa was clawed up & the woolly material scratched.

δ

133.
May 27, 1916

Dreamed I was going thro' my house where I had not been in some time—with Avery Hopwood.[1] I wanted to see if everything was in its place—someone had been renting it & living there.[2] I saw my glass bottles & things. Avery Hopwood dragged out from somewhere a beefsteak five or six feet large, broiled. I asked if it was alright. I meant to ask if it wasn't decayed from being put away & left there. He said it was all right.[3]

> Jelliffe's notes from May 29, 1916:
> *Avery Hopwood: Lived at Finney F[arm]. before I came there. ♂-♂: nice: intelligent, successful play, regular B'dway type—not interest me.*

Notes:

1 A well-known and successful playwright whom Dodge had introduced by letter to Gertrude Stein in 1915. Around the time of this dream, in the spring of 1916, Hopwood had returned to the United States from Nice, where he had been staying for months. Dodge had possibly seen his farce *Sadie Love*, which ran on Broadway for 80 performances, opening on November 29, 1915 and closing in February 1916 (Internet Broadway Database, www.ibdb.com).
2 *Here Dodge is returning to herself, as she has been away from her home, and determining if everything is "in its place," perhaps an allusion to returning to herself before analysis with Jelliffe.*
3 *At the risk of overly attributing sexual symbolism to dream images, this picture of the broiled five or six foot "large" (long?) beefsteak begs for a phallic interpretation.*

δ

134.
May 28, 1916

Someone was in a small space. I decided to blow it up—there was dynamite in it. I set a match to it & it began to blaze. Someone & I got in a panic & rushed into the hall. Someone else said not to get excited & took the hotel fire extinguisher & began slowly to open a box to get something out. I was in an agony of impatience [be]cause I thought the whole place would be on fire soon inside. But the thing got open & they began to extinguish but this meant a blanket of thick oil over me—over my head, eyes nose & mouth. I was suffocated by it—I tried to save myself & struggled to breathe [1] & awoke.

Jelliffe's notes from May 29, 1916:
Much emotion, woke up screaming. In room, someone in very small space suspended in wall. Dynamite, decided to blow up. Watch blaze: run into hall....began to extinguish. Blanket of thick oil out of me: drowning me./

Someone/ Live human being in small space, wanted to dynamite it. As soon as I start fire, I want to extinguish fire [2]—Aid or helper: More like a woman in hotel....Opened—then the oil blanket seemed to suffocate me.

My first idea:/ if extinguish baby exting[uish] me [3]:/ Oil / not expecting: oil on fire—don't help any a contradiction./ Half time not going to— then reversel no matter which way:/ Have cried so much: So idiotically unfair & then so complicated: M. same terrible doubts: Mother remarried Montague.[4] Electrical dynamo man.

M./ thinks I hate him now. the ☿ wish abated: feeling of hatred when ab[ortion]. thought of. He must go too. Someone else/ a dark vague person: a man possibly./ both rushed to look for something to stop./ Not clear: there was life:/ Have tried to get assoc. one not alone: No one of any help. both felt the same:/ both scared & panicky./ right side of me./. When first woke up. thought M.S.

Does this dream mean destroy/ General conflagration[.] Feeling at first of right—then a sense of great mistake. Set match to it: only then realized what I had done: M.S. not m[arried].

In Hall. ♀ said don't get excited. Small square box: only 2 ♀ now. My feeling of impatience at her slowness in opening the box: lapse—feeling down over face & head. Very very thick, closing: nose & mouth & eyes: as though suffocating. Everything being shut out: Experience/ Drowning like that possibly—afraid of being drowned.

Box:/ square. 8–10 in: flat wood: closed nicely. very well made box, cigar box.[5] not one as neat as a book—pine wood—white:/ does not recall anything/ Always interested in boxes. collected small boxes, mother a mania—This the most important thing in world. Oil came as a surprise. Had thought of a chemical, instead of an acid, oil / Oil & vinegar—salad dressing: expected to be vinegar—: oil. They tell me I put in too much vinegar—Too much vinegar/ I like vinegar—more than B[.] or Maurice./

Mo. & boxes/ Awfully good housekeeper. never throws away [6]*: Mo./ Was going to say—if go into Plaza establish relation: disinherited— establish if go & see mother./ D[.][7] a great transfer agent:/*

Notes:

1 Trouble breathing is connected to three of Dodge's dream images of obstructions or phlegm in her throat (dreams 96, 121, & 125).
2 *This suggests Dodge's urgent ambivalence about satisfying her desires or fulfilling her wishes. As soon as she gets what she wants (fire, pregnancy), she wants to get rid of it (extinguish, abortion).*
3 Dodge was considering terminating her pregnancy at this early stage. See Interludes 17 and 18.
4 i.e., Monty, see note 3 for dream 52.
5 *Again, Freud (1900) considered boxes to be symbols of the uterus (p. 354) and here the box is combined with a phallic symbol of a cigar.*
6 *Does this mean her mother would not get rid of a baby? Dodge associates to her mother at a moment when she is contemplating ending her pregnancy and thus will not be a mother to another baby.*
7 Unidentified, possibly Edwin Dodge.

δ

135.
Wednes. Morn. [circa May 31, 1916] (1 of 3)

Dreamed there was a bush which we decided I need not cut back.[1]

Note:

1 *Does this "we" refer to her and Jelliffe and a momentary decision to not terminate the pregnancy? Is the bush an obvious reference to female anatomy?*

δ

136.
Wed. morn. [circa May 31, 1916] (2 of 3)

Dreamed I was working in a vegetable garden.[1]

Note:

1 *This vegetable garden—with its associations to seeds, growth, and fertility—very likely relates to Dodge's current state of pregnancy.*

δ

137.
Wed. morn. [circa May 31, 1916] (3 of 3)

Dreamed my mother started to drive to the little dressmaker near by [*sic*] in a country village. She had a trap & 2 horses. She clim[b]ed in & put a cigarette in her mouth as she took the reins, & asked me if I minded. I said it was all right but I didn't like it because I was afraid it would hurt people's feelings.[1]

Jelliffe's notes from June 7, 1916:
did not like mo. c. cigarette in her mouth….

Note:

1 Dodge herself had smoked cigarettes for a time (see note 10 for dream 50), a behavior that went against social convention and was considered a sign of loose morals. *Is Dodge threatened by this image of her mother, with its suggestions of erotic life and liberation? Or is her mother a representation of herself as she is considering becoming a mother again to a new baby just conceived?*

δ

138.
June 2, 1916 (1 of 5)

Dreamed I stood on the seashore & watched some sheep from the farm gallop down to the water's edge….I was surprised and delighted at their act because they were black & heavy with manure from lying in confined stalls all winter but they dashed vigorously into the water & the water lifted their wool, & lifted the cloggy manure from it. They came out showing their white skins & white fleece—only the outer edge remained still dark. They were big as horses—& there were 4—& with them a very small woman on a small grey horse. She looked french. She cantered by us back to the stalls, very serious. B. & M. were there. I wondered if they knew her or had her at their place.

Immediate assns with this very vigorous happy & beautiful dream were = sacrificial lamb, only grown large—baptism—immersion—"washed & you shall be whiter than snow."[1]

Jelliffe's notes from June 7, 1916:
Assoc:…Wash & sins: immersion in water [2]*: sacrificial sheep.*

Notes:

1   This passage recalls Isaiah 1:18 from the Bible (ESV): "Though your sins
    are like scarlet,/ they shall be as white as snow;/ though they are red
    like crimson,/ they shall become like wool." *Dodge's association to a sac-*
    rificial lamb—something given up in order to prevent others from being
    harmed—may certainly relate to her fraught pregnancy and her conviction
    that she must sacrifice her baby for the common good, for the survival of
    her relationship with Sterne, or for social conventions, as emancipated as
    she purported to be. The sheep emerge completely cleansed—freed from
    sin?—and white "as snow." As noted before, for Freud (1900), water often
    symbolized birth or life inside the womb (p. 399).
2   This image recalls Dodge's reporting to Jelliffe on March 23 (dream 57):
    "*I have strong sense of ablutions, washing before and after.*"

δ

139.
June 2, 1916 (2 of 5)

Isadora [Duncan] [1] had a new baby.[2] I went to see her & it. It was a day old
but very intelligent. Sitting up. It had gray eyes like her but most remarkable
of all were its hands. Such intelligent hands & very long slender fingers and
in the palm queer lines. I remember something like this .[3] Isadora said
something about D. I knew it was the father & wondered who he was.[4] Then
I went away & passed the room where P.A.[5] was sick in bed, convalescing.
He was huddled in the foot of his bed, watching the door. I asked him if he
were lonely & he nodded & motioned to his eyes to tell me he'd been crying.

Jelliffe's notes from June 7, 1916:
Isadora—new baby [6]*: 1 day old. Intellig. hands….*

Notes:

1   Duncan was currently in MacKaye's masque, *Caliban,* as reported in *The*
    New York Times on May 25, 1916: "Now the entire floor was marked with
    a straight path of light with Isadora Duncan dancing along it" (p. 11).
2   In fact, Duncan had quickly become pregnant after her two children
    drowned in the Seine on April 19, 1913, but her baby died hours after
    birth in 1914. In her autobiography, *My Life* (1927), Duncan reported
    that after the tragedy of her two children dying, she rented a villa in

Italy and persuaded an Italian stranger to have sex with her so she could have another child. While walking on the beach one day, she collapsed in despair after seeing an image of her children running ahead of her:

> I don't know how long I had lain there when I felt a pitying hand on my head. I looked up and saw what I thought to be one of the beautiful contemplation figures of the Sistine Chapel. He stood there, just come from the sea, and said:
> "Why are you always weeping? Is there nothing I can do for you—to help you?"
> I looked up.
> "Yes," I replied. "Save me—save more than my life—my reason. Give me a child."
> That night we stood together on the roof of my villa....When I felt his strong youthful arms about me and his lips on mine, when all his Italian passion descended on me, I felt that I was rescued from grief and death, brought back to light—to love again. (pp. 296–297)

3 Given the resemblance of this drawing to a family tree, the "x" symbol likely indicates a dead offspring.
4 The father of Duncan's new baby is unnamed in her memoir.
5 i.e., Paul Ayrault, who had become physically ill at the time of their affair in 1912, as Dodge wrote to Gertrude Stein on January 27, 1913: "His health is even worse than mine as he has a steady unceasing cough & losing weight all the time" (GLSC).
6 *And, of course, Dodge was pregnant with a new baby at this very moment.*

δ

140.
June 2, 1916 (3 of 5)

Dreamed I was sitting high up on a kind of ledge on a house. It was plenty wide enough not to be dangerous & I was comfortable with cushions but after a while began to get dizzy because I began to think about it.

> Jelliffe's notes from June 7, 1916:
> *High up on ledge. Dizzy: began to think of it:*
> *Precarious:—Then thing happened* [1]*: outraged. Hg2Cl2.*[2] *Then immediately thought of another [dream]:*

Notes:

1 Dodge is almost certainly referring here to an abortion that she induced. See following note.

2 This is the chemical formula for calomel, or mercurous chloride, a substance that was commonly used at this time in medicine, most often as a laxative or to destroy intestinal worms, as well as in the treatment for syphilis. It was also employed to stimulate evacuation from the body of such substances as urine and sweat, and there are infrequent but significant indications in the history of pharmacology that calomel was employed to evacuate the uterus. In *The Columbus Medical Journal* (1908), a "Mrs. W.E.M." from Texas inquired if calomel could cause an abortion and the journal answered: "Any drastic cathartic, in overdoses, is likely to produce abortion....Calomel is a drastic in large doses" (p. 580). A hundred years earlier, Samuel Jennings' *The Married Lady's Companion: Or Poor Man's Friend* (1808), had prescribed a regimen of calomel and aloes for bringing about an abortion (pp. 43–45). In *A Systematic Treatise on Abortion* (1866), Edwin Hale wrote that "older physicians observed that large doses of calomel administered to pregnant women, were frequently followed by abortion" and "more recent writers mention the fact that *calomel* frequently causes abortion" (pp. 101, 102). He then reported that one physician "whose practice lay in a rather disreputable direction...knew of no surer producer of abortion than a massive dose of *calomel*—its hydro-cathartic effect was generally followed by expulsion of the foetus [*sic*]. A woman once informed me that she usually arrested her pregnancies by a large dose of calomel at a menstrual period" (p. 102). These passages point to the strong likelihood that calomel was responsible for Dodge's induced abortion. She had taken calomel before, probably to prevent pregnancy, after conflict-fueled intercourse with Sterne, as reported in Jelliffe's notes from January 29, 1916: "*left me absolutely cold...no satisfaction: then Hg2Cl2:/ Persuaded to come to luncheon I would not come, I could not: Dizzy, nauseated, waves of seasickness, lots of movements: dark brown taste.*" Dodge is dizzy in this dream while sitting on a high ledge. Calomel is no longer used because of the toxicity of mercury.

δ

141.
June 2, 1916 (4 of 5)

I was in my appartment [*sic*] with Mrs. Hapgood [1] & I saw her daughter Ruth [2] & her talking, & as Ruth left the room I saw how she hated her mother.[3]

Jelliffe's notes from June 7, 1916:
Apt. Hapgood: Norm[an]....

Notes:

1 Emilie Hapgood (née Bigelow), married in 1896 (although she divorced him in 1915) to Hutchins Hapgood's older brother Norman, journalist and editor, who at the time of this dream was the editor of *Harper's Weekly*.

2 Emilie and Norman Hapgood's daughter Ruth was at her mother's bedside when she died of a stroke in Rome in 1930 (*The New York Times*, February 17, 1930, p. 17).

3 *Even though Dodge experienced hatred for her own mother, she eventually developed compassion for her parents and their inability to give her what she needed. As she explains in Background (1933a), "I know now they must both of them have been cheated of happier times than they found under their own roof, and that they had no happiness to radiate to a solitary child. We all needed to love each other and to express it, but we did not know how" (p. 23). This mother hatred in the dream could suggest Dodge's self-hatred as a mother, particularly as she considers plans to terminate her current pregnancy.*

δ

142.
June 2, 1916 (5 of 5)

I dreamed I was somewhere where we could see the customs of the natives. I was walking into a large building with stairs up one side & a narrow balcony running around it where I was going to see some strange or cruel practice—all the people—brown natives—come there. They were filling the place—sitting huddled together. They had come to have something performed on themselves—I don't know what—perhaps circumcision—but women came also.[1]

Later, sitting outside with someone, Maurice brought a tiny little dress or two of brown linen I had made for the baby,[2] & he spread them out & we all laughed—as people do at small baby clothes.

Jelliffe's notes from June 7, 1916:
Customs of natives: Strange or cruel practice. possibly circumcise./ Maurice. linen. baby clothes:/
 Had had much corkscrew pain in r. side of uterus. left ovary gone:—Lots of pains next day: no records next day.
 Thursday. Night [3] 2 grs. Hg2Cl2 [4]: Bottle of citrate. Middle of night terrible pain: several dreams. Nothing happened: after writing was unwell [5]:....
 Yesterday: sizing up a girl just as a ♂ would: the male side[.]
 Funny thing that happened today:/ having baby: all physical...no ♀
wish:/ What is this concentration[.]

Notes:

1 In dream 87, Dodge associated *"Indian"* with *"my own sexuality."* Here the natives gather to perform a "cruel practice…perhaps circumcision," *a cutting ritual—"something performed on themselves"—that may suggest the cutting out of her baby from her body.*

2 Dodge was either pregnant or had just lost her baby at the time of this dream. *The joyousness and tenderness in this scene, with Dodge's maternal instincts expressed in her making baby clothes, contrasts starkly with Dodge's "terrible" physical pain and the ending of a pregnancy that she attributed to psychoanalysis making her more receptive—"If ever was a psychoanalytic baby—this is one"— and that she had urged Jelliffe to support.*

3 The Thursday night just previous to June 7 would have been June 1, therefore placing this dream either the morning after June 1, that is, June 2, or the night of June 2, and therefore recorded on June 3. It is not known how Dodge dated her dream records, such as whether she indicated the date as the day preceding the night of the dream or whether the date identifies the day on which she recorded her dream.

4 Dodge indicates here that on Thursday night she took 2 grains of calomel, an amount considered a small dose, unlikely to cause a toxic reaction. (I am grateful to Dr. J. Worth Estes of Boston University Medical Center for this information.) It is unlikely, therefore, that this particular dose of calomel would have induced an abortion, but she certainly may have ingested more either before or after this dose.

5 Dodge's way of referring to menstruation, as in her letter to Jelliffe, circa May 26, 1916, (see Interlude 18) where she refers to a previous pregnancy that was terminated because of Edwin Dodge's syphilis, when she "had to have my unwellness brought on because <u>he</u> was sick." This induced abortion in 1916 is thus the second pregnancy loss that Dodge reveals in her correspondence and dream records.

δ

Appendices

Appendix A

Mabel Dodge, "Mabel Dodge Writes About the Unconscious"
The New York Journal, 1917
(Excerpted)

The Unconscious is so little explored and understood that modern psychologists can only call it by a name which signifies what it is not.

It is not the conscious part of us.

It is not the body, performing its different tasks.

It is not the brain, with its thought-producing mind.

It is not the five senses, telling us what we perceive.

These all lie on the surface of us.

The Unconscious is the vast submerged part of us.

It is, to our conscious selves, as the depth of the lake is to its own surface.

We are eternally fishing in this depth.

All that we know we have brought up from the Unconscious to the surface of us.

All that we will ever know we will likewise find buried deep within ourselves, below the surface of the conscious.

Man's duty to be more conscious of things.

If the whole duty of man were written in one law, it would be to add to the consciousness of life that we have already conquered.

To become conscious of things, more understanding of human nature, more on to ourselves, is the only way to overcome sin, disease, and war.

Besides all the wonderful powers and faculties that lie hidden below your surface, which as yet you know nothing of, are some that you have left vaguely working in you.

Here lie the instincts—the instinct of reproduction, the instinct of self-preservation, the instinct to develop and grow.

Psychologists are developing methods.

Here lies your buried memory—your memory of every smallest act and observation since earliest childhood—nothing lost or forgotten.

Here lies the buried race-memory, right in you, holding all the history of the ages, from amoeba to man.

It lies quiescent or quietly sleeping in the Unconscious; sometimes it stirs, and you recall something from the past.

Psychologists all over the world are developing methods to tap this unconscious memory—both the personal and the racial one; and they are succeeding in wonderful ways.

From the depths of buried memory emerges that "still small voice" that has been called conscience.

This is the guide....

The unconscious is the true fairyland.

I have only mentioned a tithe of what is really all our riches.

All the secrets yet unknown lie in this hidden realm of ours.

Here lies the secret of how we answer our own prayers.

Here lie the secret causes of all the mysterious and devastating diseases.

Here lie the obscure laws of our being which, if we could but read them, would save us from madness and death.

Here in our past lies our future—waiting, waiting the magical awakening touch of the scientist, that patient deep sea diver who in our day is bringing so much to our eyes.

The Unconscious is the true fairyland. The place of marvels and wonders.

Watch yourself; you will see glimpses of it from time to time.

Mabel Dodge, "A Game of Cards—Hearts" *Psychoanalytic Review*, 1918 (vol. 5, pp. 442–444)

Reprinted with the permission of Guilford Press

A Game of Cards—Hearts,—The corners of the big brown room fade in shadow—but the north side of it is brimful of light from a lively fire of cedar logs, which throws up the colors of the striped Indian rugs and the bright Indian blankets that are thrown over two great armchairs drawn up at each side of the fire place [*sic*].

The lamp that hangs from the center of the ceiling falls over a group of three men and three women seated around a polished table.

The six of them are silent and intent upon what they are doing. Their expressions change and shift—their color comes and goes. They frown, or they laugh exultantly, as they make their moves. They are playing cards.

What is "playing cards"?

What is there so fundamental about it—that this custom, coming down to us from most ancient days, continues to charm and engross people of all ages and all tastes?

It must be because, underlying it, there is some satisfaction as common to all people as eating or making love.

What instincts does the game of cards call into activity?

There is the opportunity for prowess—for excelling over the others with its gain of the sense of power.

There is the chance—the accident—that betrays the play of invisible powers through one, which is part of all religion.

There is the uncovering of the "unknown"—which gratifies the desire in everyone for exploring and for discovery.

Then the cards themselves have different meanings. They are symbols of characters who are eternally ourselves.

There is the hero-card.

In "Hearts" the Jack of Diamonds is the hero. The Jack of Diamonds counts thirteen to the good for whoever secures him.

There is the Malevolent "dark-lady,"—the "Queen of Spades" who counts thirteen to the bad for whoever is unlucky enough or unskillful enough to have her foisted upon him!

And the King and Queen of Diamonds would seem to be the father and mother of the Hero, Jack. They "protect" him. Whoever has them has him—so to speak. As for the Ace—"Highest" Card of All— he is the god of the game—protector of them all! Who holds the Ace holds the game—nearly always.

Of course the King of Spades protects the wicked queen, his consort, and takes her wicked part; no godly ace has any power to further her destructive purpose.

Then the Hearts! To hold them in the end counts against us! To give them away as fast as we have them frees our hand for winning!

Isn't this the very game of life, locked up in this handful of pasteboard things?

As we sit together around this table, perhaps we are releasing our pent-up loves and hates—our secret ambitions and some of our unsatisfied instincts which the censor of man within each of us, guarding all our acts, has told us we cannot bring into full play every day.

In a game of cards we may find a substitute for the game of life—a substitutes [sic] that gives us, biologically, a free hand, and which, sociologically, does not offend civilization. For in that fairy land it is not unbecoming for a lady to play quite openly for the Hero, and to grab him if she can, from her rivals—and for the man who secures him—well it is easy to read from his delighted swagger, that he has identified himself with "Jack"—and in fact become him!

The game of cards is the game of love, and in it every repression may seek its outlet, every thwarted instinct may have its release.

Every fresh hand is an opportunity for discovery, and curiosity, unbridled now, may go as far as it can.

This holds true for cards played for the love of the game, or rather let us call it, played as the Game of Love; when it is played for money the standpoint shifts to another set of instincts—and the nutritive self-preserving centers are stirred and animated and unbound.

The game in the brown fire-lit room goes on—and all at once there is an interruption. Some one [sic] knocks at the door—and then opens it. It is a servant announcing two visitors:

"Mr. and Mrs. Average."

They advance into the room and the players suspend the game for a moment. It is amusing to see the various reactions from this interruption.

The players are slightly, very slightly discomfited.

They divide their feelings partly into resentment at being interrupted, and partly into a slight, very slight embarrassment.

This ancient traditional embarrassment at being caught playing cards is as fundamental as the act for which it is the substitute.

The two visitors react also—but differently from the players—even differently from each other.

Mrs. Average feels a slight—very slight anger at the sight before her. She feels herself hardening and resisting the pleasant social scene. She feels a sort of rigidity all along her spinal column.

But almost at the same instant she suppresses these unworthy feelings. She forces a smile and comes forward with an artificial geniality, exclaiming:

"Oh! Cards?"

Mr. Average has had quite another sensation upon seeing the players. He comes forward with real geniality and a ready smile. But in the smile there lurks the satisfaction of finding out fellow sinners. His greeting is the same but his intonation!

"Oho! CARDS!"

Take any six or eight people who know how to play and care for it, and watch them play cards. Watch the courage and the daring, the secrecy, the plotting and the snaring!

Watch the unbridled expression of masculine triumph in overcoming, and, above all, watch the relentless, unmerciful, calculating, unmaidenly play of the female!

One of the great moments to study and understand mankind is while he is playing at cards in the biological Happy Hunting Ground!

References

Blanton, S. (1971). *Diary of My Analysis with Sigmund Freud.* New York: Hawthorn Books.

Brill, A.A. (1939). "Jelliffe, the Psychiatrist and Psychoanalyst," *Journal of Nervous and Mental Disease, 89:* 529–536.

Brill, A.A. (1947). "Psychotherapies I Encountered," *Psychiatric Quarterly, 21:* 575–591.

Brooklyn Blue Book and Long Island Society Register (1912). Brooklyn, NY: Brooklyn Life Publishing.

Burnham, J.C. (1983). *Jelliffe: American Psychoanalyst and Physician & His Correspondence with Sigmund Freud and C.G. Jung.* W. McGuire (Ed.). Chicago, IL: The University of Chicago Press.

Dodge, M. (1917). "Mabel Dodge Writes About the Unconscious," *The New York Journal.*

Dodge, M. (1918). "A Game of Cards—Hearts," *Psychoanalytic Review, 5:* 442–444.

De Stacpoole, D. (1922). *Irish and Other Memories.* London: A.M. Philpot, Ltd.

Dresser, H.W. (1919). *A History of the New Thought Movement.* New York: Thomas Y. Crowell Company.

Duncan, I. (1927). *My Life.* New York: Horace Liveright.

Eastman, M. (June 1915). "Exploring the Soul and Healing the Body," *Everybody's Magazine,* 741–750.

Eastman, M. (1948). *Enjoyment of Living.* New York: Harper & Brothers.

Edelstein, L. (1943). *The Hippocratic Oath: Text, Translation and Interpretation.* Baltimore, MD: Johns Hopkins Press.

Everett, P.R. (1999). "Letters in Psychoanalysis and Posttermination Contact: Mabel Dodge's Correspondence with Smith Ely Jelliffe and A.A. Brill," *The Annual of Psychoanalysis, 26–27:* 333–360.

Everett, P.R. (2015). "The Dreams of Mabel Dodge," *The Annual of Psychoanalysis, 38:* 52–70.

Everett, P.R. (2016). *Corresponding Lives: Mabel Dodge Luhan, A.A. Brill, and the Psychoanalytic Adventure in America.* London: Karnac Books.

Freud, S. (1900). *The Interpretation of Dreams. S.E., 4 & 5:* 339–627. London: Hogarth.

Freud, S. (1905a). *Fragment of an Analysis of a Case of Hysteria. S.E., 7:* 7–122. London: Hogarth.

Freud, S. (1905b). *Three Essays on the Theory of Sexuality. S.E., 7*: 125–243. London: Hogarth.

Freud, S. (1908a). "Character and Anal Erotism," *S.E., 9*: 167–176. London: Hogarth.

Freud, S. (1908b). "On the Sexual Theories of Children," *S.E., 9*: 209–226. London: Hogarth.

Freud, S. (1909). *Analysis of a Phobia in a Five-Year-Old Boy. S.E., 10*: 5–149. London: Hogarth.

Goethe, J.W.v. (1810). *Theory of Colours.* C.L. Eastlake (Trans.) (1840). Cambridge, MA: MIT Press (1970).

Green, M. (1988). *New York 1913: The Armory Show and the Paterson Strike Pageant.* New York: Charles Scribner's Sons.

Grossman, M. (2017). *The Trunk Dripped Blood: Five Sensational Murder Cases of the Early 20th Century.* Jefferson, NC: Exposit Books.

Hale, E.M. (1866). *A Systematic Treatise on Abortion.* Chicago, IL: C. S. Halsey.

Hale, N. (1971). *Freud and the Americans: The Beginnings of Psychoanalysis in the United States, 1876–1917.* New York: Oxford University Press.

Hapgood, H. (1919). *The Story of a Lover.* New York: Boni & Liveright.

Hapgood, H. (1939). *A Victorian in the Modern World.* New York: Harcourt, Brace, & World.

Hartley, M. (1997). *Somehow a Past: The Autobiography of Marsden Hartley.* S.E. Ryan (Ed.). Cambridge, MA: MIT Press.

Heller, A., & L.P. Rudnick, (1991). *1915: The Cultural Moment: The New Politics, the New Woman, the New Psychology, the New Art, and the New Theatre in America.* New Brunswick, NJ: Rutgers University Press.

Jelliffe, S.E. (1894a). "Some Dangers Resulting from the Use of Cows' Milk," *Babyhood, 10*: 293–297.

Jelliffe, S.E. (1894b). "A Report of Two Cases of Perforating Ulcer of the Foot, with Notes and Bibliography," *New York Medical Journal, 60*: 458–464.

Jelliffe, S.E. (1913). "Some Notes on 'Transference,'" *Journal of Abnormal Psychology, 8*: 302–309.

Jelliffe, S.E. (1913–1914). "Technique of Psychoanalysis," *Psychoanalytic Review, 1*: 63–75, 178–186, 301–307, 439–444.

Jelliffe, S.E. (1915). "Technique of Psychoanalysis," *Psychoanalytic Review, 2*: 73–80, 191–199, 286–296, 409–421.

Jelliffe, S.E. (1916). "Technique of Psychoanalysis," *Psychoanalytic Review, 3*: 26–42, 161–175, 254–271, 394–405.

Jelliffe, S.E. (1917). "Technique of Psychoanalysis," *Psychoanalytic Review, 4*: 70–83, 180–197.

Jelliffe, S.E. (1930). "Psychotherapy in Modern Medicine," *Long Island Medical Journal, 24*: 152–161.

Jelliffe, S.E. (1933). "Glimpses of a Freudian Odyssey," *Psychoanalytic Quarterly, 2*: 318–329.

Jelliffe, S.E. (1939). "The Editor Himself and His Adopted Child," *Journal of Nervous and Mental Disease, 89*: 545–589.

Jelliffe, S.E., & Z.X. (1914). "Compulsion Neurosis and Primitive Culture: An Analysis, A Book Review and an Autobiography," *Psychoanalytic Review, 1*: 361–387.

Jelliffe, S.E., & W.A. White (1915). *Diseases of the Nervous System: A Text-Book of Neurology and Psychiatry.* Philadelphia, PA & New York: Lea & Febiger.

Jelliffe, S.E., & E. Evans (1916). "Psoriasis as an Hysterical Conversion Symboliza-
tion," *New York Medical Journal, 104*: 1077–1084 (reprint at LOC, 1–23).
Jelliffe, S.E., & W.A. White (1917). *Diseases of the Nervous System: A Text-Book
of Neurology and Psychiatry.* 2nd ed. Philadelphia, PA & New York: Lea &
Febiger.
Jelliffe, S.E., & W.A. White (1923). *Diseases of the Nervous System: A Text-Book
of Neurology and Psychiatry.* 4th ed. Philadelphia, PA & New York: Lea &
Febiger.
Jennings, S.K. (1808). *The Married Lady's Companion: Or Poor Man's Friend.*
New York: L. Dow.
Kurth, P. (2001). *Isadora: A Sensational Life.* Boston, MA: Little, Brown & Company.
Lewis, N.D.C. (1966). "Smith Ely Jelliffe, 1866–1945: Psychosomatic Medicine in
America." In: F. Alexander, S. Eisenstein, & M. Grotjahn (Eds.), *Psychoanalytic
Pioneers* (pp. 224–234). New York: Basic Books.

Luhan, M.D., Published Works

Luhan, M.D. (1933a). *Intimate Memories: Background.* New York: Harcourt, Brace.
Luhan, M.D. (1935). *European Experiences: Volume Two of Intimate Memories.*
New York: Harcourt, Brace.
Luhan, M.D. (1936). *Movers and Shakers: Volume Three of Intimate Memories.*
New York: Harcourt, Brace.

Luhan, M.D., Unpublished Manuscripts and Scrapbooks, MDLC

Luhan, M.D. (1913–1917, n.d.). "Intimate Memories, Vol. VII."
Luhan, M.D. (1927). "Intimate Memories, Vol. IV: Making a Life, Part II."
Luhan, M.D. (1933b). "Family Affairs."
Luhan, M.D. (1936–1939, n.d.). "Misc. Vol. II."
Luhan, M.D. (1938a). "On Human Relations: A Personal Interpretation."
Luhan, M.D. (1938b). "Psycho-Analysis with Dr. Brill." (Reprinted in full in Everett,
Corresponding Lives, pp. 307–312.)
Luhan, M.D. (1939). "Notes Upon Awareness: Addressed to Krishnamurti."
Luhan, M.D. (1947a). "Love Letters of a Grandmother."
Luhan, M.D. (1947b). "The Statue of Liberty: An Old[-]Fashioned Story of Taboos."
Luhan, M.D. (1954). "Doctors: Fifty Years of Experience."
Luhan, M.D. (n.d.). "A City Father."
Luhan, M.D. (n.d.). "Intimate Memories, Vol. II."

Makari, G. (2008). *Revolution in Mind: The Creation of Psychoanalysis.* New York:
Harper Perennial.
"Public School No. 45" (February 1898). *The Brooklyn Teacher, II (6)*: 1–2.
"Query" (1908). *The Columbus Medical Journal* (1908), *32*: 580.
Rudnick, L.P. (1984). *Mabel Dodge Luhan: New Woman, New Worlds.* Albuquerque:
University of New Mexico Press.
Rudnick, L.P. (2012). *The Suppressed Memoirs of Mabel Dodge Luhan: Sex, Syphi-
lis, and Psychoanalysis in the Making of Modern American Culture.* Albuquerque:
University of New Mexico Press.

Rudnytsky, P.L. (forthcoming). *Mutual Analysis: Ferenczi, Severn, and the Origins of Trauma Theory*. New York: Routledge, Relational Perspectives Series.

Severn, E. (1917). *The Psychology of Behavior: A Practical Study of Human Personality and Conduct, with a Special Reference to Methods of Development*. New York: Dodd, Mead & Co.

Severn, E. ([1933] 2017). *The Discovery of the Self: A Study in Psychological Cure*. P.L. Rudnytsky (Ed.). London and New York: Routledge.

Severn, E. (1952). Interview with Kurt Eissler, Sigmund Freud Papers, Library of Congress.

Steffens, L. (1931). *The Autobiography of Lincoln Steffens*. 2 vols. New York: Harcourt, Brace.

Stein, L. (1950). *Journey into the Self: Being the Letters, Papers, and Journals of Leo Stein*. E. Fuller (Ed.). New York: Crown Publishers.

Sterne, M. (1952). *Shadow and Light: The Life, Friends and Opinions of Maurice Sterne*. C.L. Mayerson (Ed.). New York: Harcourt, Brace & World.

Terry, W. (1963). *Isadora Duncan: Her Life, Her Art, Her Legacy*. New York: Dodd, Mead & Company.

Toklas, A.B. (1963). *What is Remembered*. New York: Holt, Rinehart & Winston.

Underhill, E. (1912). *Mysticism: A Study in the Nature and Development of Man's Spiritual Consciousness*. New York: E.P. Dutton Co.

Van Vechten, C. (1922). *Peter Whiffle: His Life and Works*. New York: Alfred A. Knopf.

Watson, S. (1991). *Strange Bedfellows: The First American Avant-Garde*. New York: Abbeville Press.

Wineapple, B. (1996). *Sister Brother: Gertrude and Leo Stein*. New York: G.P. Putnam's Sons.

Index

Please note: In all entries, Dodge refers to Mabel Dodge, and Jelliffe refers to Smith Ely Jelliffe. When a person appears in one of Mabel Dodge's dreams, the page number for that dream is **in bold**. When there are two or more dreams on one page, or when there are two notes with the same number on one page, for clarification the page number is followed by the number of the dream: 192n1 (dr. 95).

Acton, Arthur **191 (dr. 95)**, 192n1 (dr. 95), 202n1 (dr. 107)
Acton, Hortense 192n1 (dr. 95), **202**, 202n1 (dr. 107)
Albert (Dodge's chauffeur) **109**, 111n11, 139, 233
Auzius, Nina 88n3, 172
Ayrault, Paul 50, 57, 71n3 (dr. 5), 77n1, **238**, 239n5; *see also* Dodge, Mabel: affair with Ayrault

Bernard, Dr. (first name unknown) 117n7
Bernheim, Gioia 118
Birnbaum Gallery 64, 90n3
Blood, Florence **103**, 105n3
Bourgeois, Stephan 95, 96n2, **132**, 133n3
Boyce, Neith 3, 50–51, 59, **89**, 89n1, 101n1, 199n2, **213**, 214n2 (dr. 118), 214n4, 233; *Constancy*, a play by 50; letters to Dodge 50, 89n1
Boyeson, Bayard 46, 51, **79**, 79n1, **89**, 98, **112**, 113n5, **114**, 115n3, 116n2, **124**, 124n4, **126**, **129**, 129n1, 129n2, 130n4, 135, 150, 172, **185**, 204, **224 (dr. 127)**, **229–230**, 230n1, 230–231n2, 236, **237 (dr. 138)**; living with Dodge at Finney Farm 16, 51, 128n2 (dr. 47), 130n3, 150n2; in psychoanalysis with Jelliffe 15–16, 19, 79n3, 113, 115n3, 118, 182–183n1, 220

Bradley, Florence 51–52, **152**, 152n1 (dr. 60), 152n2 (dr. 60), 153n5, **176 (dr. 79)**, **207**
Bramleys **109**, 110n7, **220**
Brill, A.A. xiv, 13, 35, 73, 95–96, 124n1; consultation with Max Eastman 26n1; consultation with Leo Stein 16, 63; determines syphilis in Maurice Sterne 154n3; and Mabel Dodge: first accepts as his patient xiv, 42–44, letters to 118, psychoanalyst of 137n4, speaks at "Psychoanalytic Evening" held at salon of xiii, 3, 61–62, 74n2, talks with about his patients 117–118; and Freud: letter to xvi, letter from 118, loyalty to xix, 22, translations of: *The Interpretation of Dreams* 74n2, *Selected Papers on Hysteria and Other Psychoneuroses* xvi, 12, *Three Contributions to the Theory of Sex* xvii, 12; and Jelliffe: converts to psychoanalysis 13–14, first meets 13, letter to 23, opinion of his "Technique of Psychoanalysis" papers 23; and Jung: translation of *Psychology of Dementia Praecox* 12
Brisbane, Arthur 126n8, **208 (dr. 115)**, 209n1
Browning, Robert Wiedeman Barrett "Pen" **203**, 203n3
Bryant, Louise 62, 94–95n3

Bull, Harry 52, **141**, 143n5
Bull, Nina (née Wilcox) 52, 71n3 (dr. 6), 87n1, 125, 126n5, 140–141, **141**, 144n11, 145n12, 149n1, 199n2, 204n2, 210n1; impression of A.A. Brill 17; in psychoanalysis with Jelliffe 17, 141
Burnham, John, *Jelliffe: American Psychoanalyst and Physician* xiv, 23

Caliban, a masque by Percy MacKaye 131n5, 133n4, 225n1, 231n3, 238n1 (dr. 139)
Camera Work 65, 95–96, 199n1
Carranza, Venustiano 152, 153n9, 153n11, 153n12
Cary, Julia (née Love) 96; rumored to have Indian blood 53
Cary, Phoebe **208 (dr. 115)**, 209n1
Cary, Seward 52–53, 77–78n3, 97, 149n2, **208 (dr. 114)**, 208n2, 208n3, 209n1
Cassin, Baroness de **109**, 110n5, 198n2
Chevy Chase School 37, 78n5, 106n9, 148
Colette **107**, 107–108n3
Collier, John 50, 53, 54, 97, 97–98n3, 170, 213
Collier, Lucy 50–51, 54, **76**, 77n1; *see also* Hapgood, Hutchins: affair with Lucy Collier
Condamine, Robert de la **90**, 91n2; on Dodge 74n3
Cook, George Cram "Jig" **222**, 222n1
Cook, Grandma 59, 69n3 (dr. 2), 73n3, 108n6, 127n3, 148, 156
Cook, Grandpa 59, 69n3 (dr. 2), 73n3, **119**, 120n2, 127n3, 156, 194n3
Crowley, Aleister **213**, 214n3
Cruttwell, Maud 104n2

Dasburg, Andrew 3, 42, 46, 65
Davidge, Clarissa 92n9, 92n10, 92n11
Diseases of the Nervous System, Jelliffe and White textbook 23–26, 147, 148, 149n5; approach to psychoanalysis and dream interpretation 30–31; Freud's and Jung's influences on 24–25; role of unconscious in functioning of body 24–26
Divine Science 17, 31, 52, 140
Dodge, Edwin (Dodge's second husband) 31, 50, 54, 57, 115n2, 149, 202n1 (dr. 107); and Mabel Dodge:

divorce from 42, 109, first meets 56, letters to 111–112n14, 137n4, 166n2, marriage to 2, 56; pays expenses for Villa Curonia 135, 137n4; syphilis of 35, 37, 47, 154n3, 232, 242n5; *see also* Dodge, Mabel: and Edwin Dodge
Dodge, Mabel: abortion/pregnancy loss of xxiii, 42, 232, 235, 236n2, 236n3, 236n4, 236n1 (dr. 135), 239n1, 240n2, 241n3, 242n2, 242n5: use of calomel (Hg2Cl2) to induce 239, 240n2, 241, 242n4; affair with Paul Ayrault 50, 77n1, 215n1, 221n1; affair with Dr. John Parmenter xx, 31, 56, 73n2, 73–74n1, 221, 222n7, 227, *see also* Parmenter, Dr. John; attempt to adopt a baby 84–85n7; attraction to teachers 104, 106n9; baby/children, desire for 73n5, 89n5, 80–81n4, 227–229; boredom of 2, 68n3; breasts, interest in 106n9, 144n9, 221, 222n6, 223n2; and A.A. Brill 3, 186n9: first clinical contact with xiv, 35, 42–44, letters from 118, letter to 194n2, paints a watercolor for 133n6, in psychoanalysis with 3, 43–44, speaks at her salon xiii, 3, 61–62, 74n2; childhood home, feelings about 1, 68n3, 77, 78n8, 110n4; cigarette smoking of 133, 134n10, 134n11, 237n1 (dr. 137); coming out ball of 188, 188n1, 189n6; complexes of 168: father 193, 200, jealousy 27, 33, mother 200; death of 3; depression in 31, 56, 99, 157, 157n1, 162–164, 167n2, 192–193n1, 210, 210n2; disturbance in 104, 106n10, 129, 130n5; and doctors, wanting attention from 195n7; and Edwin Dodge 134n10, 185, 186n6: banished from 23 Fifth Avenue 164, 215n1, divorce from 42, 109, 111–112n14, 166, 166n2, 166n4, 220, 221n1, first meets 56, marriage to 2, 56, sexual relationship/lack of intercourse with 73, 73–74n1, 75n1 (dr. 10), 114, 114n1 (dr. 37), 221; dream interpretation, writings on 45–46; and John Evans xx, 1: ambivalence about birth of 56, early relationship with as a baby 56, 84–85n7, relationship with 143n2, 165n2, *see also* Evans, John; and

Karl Evans xx, 2, 34: marriage to 52, 227, *see also* Evans, Karl; and father *see* Ganson, Charles; fear of being adopted 84, 84–85n7; fear of being alone 1–2, 186n7; as Mabel Ganson 1; Hearst newspaper, columnist for 3, 209n1; and horses 77–78n3, 208n3; interior decorating, advertisement and talent for 209n1, 215, 216n2; jealousy of 35, 38, 68n4, 157n1, 158–159, 227

Dodge, Mabel: and Smith Ely Jelliffe: criticism of for his "dogmatic" approach 20, 218n8, 218-219; dreams about/transference dreams about/in dream associations 29, 46, 69n1 (dr. 2), 69n2 (dr. 2), 69n3 (dr. 2), 70n1, 79, **90**, 91n1, 91n6, **112**, 113n5, **114**, 114n1 (dr. 138), 115n3, **115**, 116n2, 116n3, **119**, **124**, 124n3, 124n4, 168n1 (dr. 71), 168n2, 169n2, **193**, **216**, **225**, 230, 231n8; end of analysis with 41–45; first letter to 33; first meets xiii, 3; first psychoanalytic session with 28, 34–35, 140n2; interested in psychosomatic teachings of 25–26, 178n1, 190n12, 192–193n1, 224n2; in psychoanalysis with xiii, 3, 14, 27–49; and "psychoanalytic baby" with xx–xxi, 226n1 (dr. 128), 226n2 (dr. 128), 226n1 (dr. 129), 232, 242n2; letters from *see* Jelliffe, Smith Ely: and Dodge: letters to; letters and notes to xiii, xxv, 16, 20, 42, 43–44, 58, 95, 98–100, 113, 118n1, 123, 140, 158–159, 167, 201–202, 212–213, 216n2, 218–219, 227–229, 231–233; letters to about end of analysis with 43–44; letters to about her pregnancy by Sterne (Interludes 17 & 18) 42, 73n5; photograph of first letter to (Figure 3.2) 33; writes chapter about in *Movers and Shakers* 35, 39–42, 92n9, 187n2

Dodge, Mabel: lesbian fantasies and affairs of 104–105n2, 222, 223n2; loneliness of 68n3, 70n2, 114n1 (dr. 38), 210n1; and Antonio Luhan, marriage to xxviii, 3, 120n4, 184n1, 184n3, 185n7; as Mabel in Cook and Glaspell play, *Suppressed Desires* 222–223n1; manic-depression, considered as diagnosis of 35, 117–118, 118n1, 144n10; marriages of

2, *see also* Dodge, Edwin; Evans, Karl; Luhan, Antonio; Sterne, Maurice; menstrual period/unwellness of 35, 80, 80n2, 98, 99, 100n1, 227–228, 241; money, relationship with 119–120, 120n7, 228–229; and mother 1: dependence on 136n1, 137n4, hatred of 136n1, 241n3, relationship with 135, 136n2, 142, 144n9, 144n10, 145n13, 160n2 (dr. 63), 160n2 (dr. 64), 218n8; only child, feelings about being 1, 35, 38, 68n3, 122n5; ovary removed 73n5, 229n2, 231, 241; painting watercolors 132, 133n6, 171n5; and parents, feelings toward 120, 241n3; photograph of (Figure 1.1) 2; pregnant, childhood fantasy of believing she was 80, 80–81n4; pregnant by Edwin Dodge 232, 242n5; pregnant (most likely) by Karl Evans 226n2, 227; pregnant by Maurice Sterne xx, 187n1, 209n2, 211n3, 221n2, 221n4, 223n2, 224n1, 226n2, 227–229, 229n1 (dr. 130), 231–233, 235–236, 238n1 (dr. 138), 239n6; pushes nurse off cliff 155–157; and John Reed: first meets 62, relationship with 31, 35, 50, 62, 84–85n7, 157n1, 158–159, 172, 203n2, 206n3, *see also* Reed, John; and salons at 23 Fifth Avenue: xiii, 2–3, 59–60, 61–62, 74n3, 75n6, 87n6, 97n2, 167n3, 168, negro entertainers at 86n5, 177n3, psychoanalysis discussed at 3, 61–62, 74n2, 93n16, 215n1; secrets of 152n1 (dr. 59); sexual life of xx, 174, 174n7, 175n10: early sex play 148, 221, oral sex, feelings about 207n1 (dr. 113), 221, 222n8, orgasms of xx, 87n8, 227–228, sexuality of 177, 177n3, 179n2, 183, 184n2, 226n1 (dr. 129), 242n1; and Gertrude Stein: first meets 63, letters to 63, 239n5, subject of word portrait by 63, 66, 105n3; and Leo Stein *see* Stein, Leo: and Dodge; and Maurice Sterne: banishes from Finney Farm 40, 51, first meets 31–32, 64, 90n2, jealousy toward 76n2, 100, 101–102n2, 121n3, 158–159, 196n3, 205n2, marriage to 44, 65, 76n1, 185n7, relationship with 32–33, 35, 39–42, 64–65, 98–100, 128, 128n3,

133n5, 134n8, 139–140, 140n2, 157, 157n1, 158n2, 168n1 (dr. 70), 178n4, 185, 186n8, 191n1 (dr. 93), 210n2, 215n3, 230, sexual relationship with 99–100, 109, 110n1, 175n10, 191n1 (dr. 94), 195, 211–212n3, 240n2, *see also* Sterne, Maurice; suicide attempts of xiii, 31; syphilis of, contracted from Antonio Luhan 154n3; urinary problems of 188n5

Dodge, Mabel: writings by: "Doctors: Fifty Years of Experience" 56; *European Experiences* 50, 56, 63, 91, 104n2, 208n3; "Family Affairs" 136n1, 136n2; "A Game of Cards— Hearts"xxviii, 44–45, 246–248 (Appendix B); *Intimate Memories: Background* 1, 69n3, 77n3, 136n1, 144n8; "Mabel Dodge Writes About the Unconscious" xxviii, 3, 244–245 (Appendix A), photograph of (Figure A.1) 243; "Making a Life, Part II" 104–105n2; "The Mirror" 65; *Movers and Shakers* xx, xxviii, 3, 14–15, 35, 39–42, 45, 51, 60, 79n1, 219; "Notes Upon Awareness: Addressed to Krishnamurti" 118n1; "On Human Relations: A Personal Interpretation" 45; "Psycho-Analysis with Dr. Brill" 46, 127n6; "The Statue of Liberty" 154n3

Dodge, Mabel: images recurring in her dreams and associations: baby 72, 72–73n1, 85, 86n4, 88, 89n5, 164, 187, 238, 241; bed/couch 72, 100, 157, 203, 207, 215, 229 (dr. 130), 234 (dr. 132); boat/ship 102, 108–109, 110n3, 112, 152, 182, 182–183n1, 198 (dr. 101), 199, 203; box/boxes 87, 88n2, 173 (dr. 76), 235, 236n5; breast/breast squirting milk 82, 82n3, 82–83n4, 87, 87n2, 222; breath/breathing problems 154, 192, 192–193n1, 216, 217n2, 235, 236n1 (dr. 134); car/motor/carriage/ train 68, 71, 75, 85, 103, 139, 160, 208 (dr. 114), 216; cigar/cigarette/pipe/ smoking 112, 152, 153n3, 191 (dr. 194), 237 (dr. 137); clitoris 142, 195, 196n4, 221; colors (red, violet, etc.) 185–186, 187n10, 187n11, 195–196, 196n2, 196n3, 196n5; death: crepe, symbol of death/funeral/death-like feeling/dead person 83, 84n3, 96,

96n1, 109, 203; excrement /bowel movement/manure 72, 72–73n1, 178, 178n1, 179n3, 237 (dr. 138); fat 68, 69n3 (dr. 2), 69, 70, 70n4, 229–230; fire 70, 71n2 (dr. 5), 183, 235; flowers/ plants/garden/bushes/vegetable bed 94, 115, 119, 126–127, 127n6, 128, 135, 137, 138n1, 201 (dr. 105), 221, 222n5, 236 (dr. 135), 236 (dr. 136); food and drink/eating and drinking 70, 70n2, 85, 86n3, 94, 97, 97n2, 102, 107, 112, 114, 127, 128n1 (dr. 46), 203, 205 (dr. 111), 224 (dr. 127), 229–230, 234 (dr. 133); green eyes 187, 187n2, 196, 196n6; hand/hands 81, 164, 183, 184n4, 211, 238; horse/ horses/pony 77, 77–78n3, 84, 84n6, 129, 160, 161, 165, 173–174, 174n5, 176 (dr. 79), 208 (dr. 114), 216, 229–230, 237 (dr. 137), 237 (dr. 138); impotence 73, 73–74n1, 75n1 (dr. 10), 103; Indian people or natives/ Indian vicinity or village 76, 76n1, 89, 90n3, 183, 184, 185n7, 206–207, 241; Jelliffe's office 119, 124, 124n3, 193, 225; Jelliffe's patients 115, 116n1, 185, 186n2, 216; Jew/Jews/ Jewish bazaar 91, 92–93n13, 168, 169n4, 170, 171n4, 173 (dr. 76), 197; lace 169 (dr. 73), 170, 171n2, 175, 198 (dr. 101); lap 141–142, 143n4, 148, 149n1; letter/letters 90, 134, 150, 204, 229–230; money 71, 71n1 (dr. 6), 126, 193, 216, 224 (dr. 127); mother's house/room 119, 121, 122n4, 125, 208 (dr. 115);negro/negroes/black face/dark people 84, 84n5, 85, 86n2, 90, 92n8, 93n15, 93n16, 177, 177n3, 226; negro literature 85, 86n5, 93n16; obstruction/phlegm 192, 192–193n1, 216; old woman/old lady 141–142, 150, 154, 160, 226, 229–230; precipice/high ledge/abyss 109, 129, 129n2, 167, 239; pregnancy 72, 73n5, 80, 80–81n4; sea/ocean/seaside/ water 89, 108–109, 112, 130, 169, 182, 182–183n1, 191 (dr. 95), 198 (dr. 101), 203, 208 (dr. 115), 237 (dr. 138); stairs/staircase/downstairs/upstairs/ ladder 85, 86n1, 90, 91n5, 100, 103, 104n1, 115, 152, 153n3, 173–174, 180, 181n1, 193, 241; throat 192, 192–193n1, 216, 217n2, 224 (dr. 125)

Dodge, Mabel: themes recurrring in her dreams and associations: constipation/intestines/colitis/hemorrhoids /"fecal erotics" 86, 87n9, 116, 117n7, 133, 133n2, 134n8, 134n9, 231n6; evil 80, 91, 93n16, 149, 149n6; incest 102, 102n1, 102n2; intercourse, 73, 86, 87n8, 87n9; jealousy/jealous breath 69, 70n5, 79, 196, 196n3, 196n6; masturbation 103, 104–105n2, 105n4, 105–106n6, 106n7, 109, 110n2, 114, 114n2, 129, 130n5, 195, 196n4, 196n5; primitive: concept of 89, 178, 184n2, 211, Brill teaches Dodge the word "archaic" 211–212n3, Jelliffe teaches Dodge the word "primitive" 90n4, 179n3, 211–212n3; psychoanalysis 161, 161n5, 182, 182–183n1; syphilis 154, 154n1, 154n3; unconscious 90, 91n4, 166, 169n1, 169n2, 188, 191n1; urination/urine 69, 69–70n3, 71n2, 148, 221, 229–230; washing/ablutions 149, 149–150n7, 173, 174n3, 238, 238n2 (dr. 138)

Dodge, Robert **165**, 166n1
Draper, Muriel 185, 186n5
Draper, Paul 185, 186n4, 186n6
Duncan, Dora **211**, 211n1
Duncan, Elizabeth 54, 55, 97–98n3, **178**, **211**, 211n1, 211n2
Duncan, Isadora 46, 47, 54, 55, **107**, 107n2, 107–108n3, 108n5, 143n6, **238**, 238n1 (dr. 139), 238–239n2, 239n3, 239n4

Eastman, Max xxvii, 3, 35, 46, **112**, 113n3, 113n4, 116, 116n6, 169n3, 190n1 (dr. 92), 206n3; consultation with A.A. Brill 26n1, 55; on Dodge's salons 74n3; *Enjoyment of Living*, memoir by 116n6; in psychoanalysis with Jelliffe 17–18, 55
Elizabeth Duncan School 32, 54, 55, 84–85n7, 97, 97–98n3, 141, 142–143n1, 197n1, 211, 231n4
Enemies, play by Boyce and Hapgood 60
Evans, John (Dodge's son) 31, 34, 44, 46, 50, 55–56, **109**, 136n2, 137n4, **141–142**, 142–143n1, **164**, **165**, **176** **(dr. 80)**, **196**, 197n1, 202, **220**, 227; and Dodge: letters to 165n2, relationship with 143n2, 165n2; fear of being adopted 84, 84–85n7; photograph

of (Figure 5.3) 197; questions about paternity of 56, 84–85n7, 222n7, 229n1 (Interlude 17); *see also* Dodge, Mabel: and John Evans
Evans, Karl (Dodge's first husband): killed in hunting accident 2, 31, 35, 55, 188n4; marriage to Mabel Ganson 31, 34, 52

Ferenczi, Sandor xix, 13, 18–19
Finney Farm 15, 31–32, 51, 128n1 (dr. 47), 128n2 (dr. 47), 234; Jelliffe visits 15, 41, 128n2 (dr. 47), 202
Fletcher, Julia Constance 56–57, **82**, 82n1, 82n2, 111n10
Foote, Mary 57–58, 123, **214**, 215n4, **220**, 221n1, **229 (dr. 130)**, 229n3; letters to Dodge 16–17, 57–58; portrait paintings: of Mabel Dodge 57, 221n1, photograph of portrait (Figure 4.1) 58, 221n1, of Jelliffe 16, 57–58, of Robert Edmond Jones 221n1; in psychoanalysis with Jelliffe 58
Freud, Sigmund xx, xxii, 12–13, 152, 153n8, 213, 222–223n1; and A.A. Brill, letter to 118; cigar smoking of 191n1 (dr. 94); on dreams 29, 45, 47–48; interpretation of dream symbols: baby and feces 72–73n1, boxes 88n2, 236n5, childhood games 207n1 (dr. 112), falling 194n2, going up and down stairs 86n1, 194n1, hat 124n3, left and right 72n4, mice as genitalia 177n1, money and feces 117n7, "smooth walls" 129n2, snake as phallic symbol 179n2, staircases, steps, and ladders 91n5, teeth falling out 206n6, upstairs and downstairs 181n1, urination and fire 71n2 (dr. 5), urination and sex 69–70n3, water images and birth 110n1, 209n2, 238n1 (dr. 138); and Jelliffe: correspondence with xiv, first meets xvii, 12, influence on xvii–xix, offers analysis to xvii, *see also* Jelliffe, Smith Ely and Freud; and Jung, rupture with 20–21; on orgasms, vaginal vs. clitoral 87n8; and *Psychoanalytic Review* 20–22; and William Alanson White, letter to 21; writings by: "Character and Anal Erotism" 117n7; *The Interpretation of Dreams* xxiii,

xxvii, 35, 48, 74n2; *Selected Papers on Hysteria and Other Psychoneuroses* xvii; *Three Contributions to the Theory of Sex* (also referred to in other translations as *Three Contributions to Sexual Theory* or *Three Essays on the Theory of Sexuality*) xvii

Ganson, Charles (Dodge's father) 1, 46, 58–59, 79, 79n2, **102**, 103, **107**, 108n4, **109**, 110n8, **161**, 161n3, 161n4, **173–174**, 174n2, **176 (dr. 80)**, 176n1 (dr. 80), 189n6, **199**; cigar smoking of 134n11, 191n1 (dr. 94); death of 136n3; depression/moodiness of 59, 161n3, 162–163, 194n4; desk of 142, 144n8; and Dodge: forbidding kissing games for 174, 174–175n8, 207n3, gave first cigarette to 133, 134n11, relationship with 102n1, 144n10, 161n2 (dr. 65), 162–163, 194n4; funeral of 84n3; jealousy of 35, 59; masturbation/"self-abuse" of 80n1, 148, 149n3, 175n9; in sanatorium 34, 37, 80n1, 148–149, 149n5, 175n9, 198n1 (dr. 100); and Sara Ganson, relationship with 143n4, 162
Ganson, Grandma **119**, 120n1, 120n5, 120n6, 134n10, 144n8, 194n3; rumored to have Indian blood 53, 76n1, 120n4
Ganson, Grandpa 58, 194n3
Ganson, Mabel *see* Dodge, Mabel
Ganson, Sara (Dodge's mother) 1, 46, 59, 69n3 (dr. 2), 80, 80–81n4, 84–85n7, 103, **107**, 108n4, 108n6, 115n2, **125**, **126**, 127n1, 127n2, 128, **135**, 137–138n1, 148, 152, **160**, 189n6, **199**, **201 (dr. 106)**, **216**, **237 (dr. 137)**; accidents with horses 78n4, 160n1 (dr. 63), 160n3; affairs with men 80n3, 106–107n6, 122n4; affair with Dr. John Parmenter xx, 56, 122n4; death of 136n1; and Dodge: control over finances of 120n7, 136n1, letters to 136n2, 137n4, objection to Brill's analysis with 137n4, relationship with 136n2, 137n4, 144n9, 145n13; *see also* Dodge, Mabel: and mother; and Charles Ganson, relationship with 143n4; marriages: to Montague ("Monty") 136n2, 136n3, 235, 236n4, to Admiral Reeder 136n2, 136n3

Georgie, Aunt (of Mabel Dodge) 69n3 (dr. 2), 127n4, 156, 223n2
Ghika, Princess 103, 106n8
Glaspell, Susan 206n5, 222–223n1
Glenny, Mrs. John (first name unknown) **141–142**, 143n3
Goodyear, Conger **187**, 188n2, 189n9
Goodyear, Mary **187**, 188n2, 189n10
Gratwick, Mildred **210**, 210n1, **216**, 218n6, 218n7
Greenwich Village xiii, 46, 60, 190, 190n1, 199n1, 222

Hackett, Francis **107**, 107n1, 107n2
Hannah (Dodge's cook) **126–127**, 127n5
Hapgood, Emilie (née Bigelow) **240**, 241n1, 241n2
Hapgood, Hutchins xxvii, 3, 35, 50–51, 59–61, 65, 101n1, 111–112n14, 133n1, 190n1 (dr. 92), 206n3, 212–213, **213**, 213n1, 214n4, 233, 241n1; affair with Lucy Collier 50–51, 54, 60–61, 77n1; and Dodge: description of upbringing of 60, letters to xxvii, 54, 77n1, 89n1; writings by: *The Story of a Lover* 51, 60–61, 212, 214n2 (dr. 118); *A Victorian in the Modern World* 60
Hapgood, Ruth **240**, 241n2, 241n3
Hartley, Marsden 46, 61, 65, 90–91, 92n13, 93n14, **114**, 150n2
Hausner, Dr. Eric xxv–xxvi
Haweis, Ducie *see* Loy, Mina
Haweis, Stephen 199n1
Hinkle, Beatrice 17, 168, 169n3; translator of Jung's *Psychology of the Unconscious* 159n1
Hollister, Mary **187**, 188n4
Hopwood, Avery 234 (dr. 133), 234n1
Howe, Frederick 116, 116n5, 170

Ida (niece of Maurice Sterne) 102n2, **121**, 121n1, 121n2
Interludes: 1: 95–96; 2: 98–100; 3: 113; 4: 117–118; 5: 123; 6: 138–139; 7: 140–141; 8: 145–147; 9: 158–159; 10: 162–164; 11: 167; 12: 171–172; 13: 201–202; 14: 212–213; 15: 218–219; 16: 219–220; 17: 227–229; 18: 231–234

Jelliffe, Belinda (Jelliffe's second wife) xxv
Jelliffe, Helena Leeming (Jelliffe's first wife) 78n5, 78n6, **124**, 124n2, 124n3,

125–126n4, **187**; death of xiii, 42,
145–147, 147n1, 148n3, 149n1, 188n3;
and Smith Ely Jelliffe: first meets
8, letters from 9–10, letters to 9,
marriage to 8; photograph of
(Figure 2.2) 8
Jelliffe, Smith Ely 3, 182n1 (dr. 85);
assistants, use of in his practice 217n4;
botany, lifelong interest in 8, 219n1;
and A.A. Brill: feelings towards for
taking Dodge as patient 44, first meets
13, letter from 23; childhood of 5–7;
conversion to psychoanalysis xv,
13–14
Jelliffe, Smith Ely: and Mabel Dodge:
appears in dreams of *see* Dodge,
Mabel: and Jelliffe: dreams about;
first meets xiii, 3; intake notes from
first session with 34–38, 80n2; letters
from *see* Dodge, Mabel: and Jelliffe:
letters to; letters to xiii, xxv, xxviii,
3–4, 42, 58, 147, 219–220; notes from
last analytic meeting with xiv, 44;
photograph of intake notes of (Figure
3.4) 36; talks with about his patients
117–118; and "Technique" papers
informing analysis of 27–30; visits at
Finney Farm 15, 41
Jelliffe, Smith Ely: dreams of 6–7, 9;
education of 8–9; and Freud: first
meeting with xvii, 12, influenced
by xvi–xix, 22–23, 48, letters from
xvii–xviii, 12, letters to xviii–xix,
12; and Ernest Jones, letter from
xvi; and Jung: correspondence
with xiv, first meeting with xv, 12,
influenced by xv–xvi, 23, 39; and
Helena Leeming, grief over death
of 42, 145–147, 148n4, 188n3,
see also Jelliffe, Helena Leeming;
loneliness of 7, 10; medical practice
of 11–13; patients of 14–20: Bayard
Boyeson 15–16, Nina Bull 17, Max
Eastman 17–18, Mary Foote 16–17,
Robert "Bobby" Edmond Jones 15,
Elizabeth Severn 18–20, Leo Stein
15, 16; photograph of (Figure 2.1) 5;
photograph of office of (Figure 3.3)
34; psychosomatic medicine xiv, 9,
22, 25–26, 39, 190n12; and William
Alanson White: analyzes dreams with
6, 11, friendship and collaboration
with xv, xvii–xviii, 11–12, 13, writes

textbook with 9, *see also Diseases of
the Nervous System*
Jelliffe, Smith Ely: writings by:
"Autobiographical Sketch" 6–7;
"Compulsion Neurosis and Primitive
Culture" (with Zenia X—) 149–150n7,
179n3, 211–212n3, 230–231n2; "The
Editor Himself and His Adopted
Child" 6; "Glimpses of a Freudian
Odyssey" xiv, xix, 9, 13; "Psoriasis
as an Hysterical Conversion
Symbolization (with Elida Evans) 25;
"Some General Reflections on the
Psychology of Dementia Praecox" 12;
"Some Notes on 'Transference'" 14;
The Technique of Psychoanalysis 23;
"The Technique of Psychoanalysis"
papers xvi, 22–23, 26, 27–30, 47–48
Jelliffe, Smith Ely and William Alanson
White, writings by/editors of: *Diseases
of the Nervous System* 23–26, 147;
Psychoanalytic Review 20–22
Jelliffe, William Munson (Jelliffe's father)
5–6
Jones, Robert "Bobby" Edmond 3,
44, 47, 61, **100**, 101n1, 101n2, 131,
131n5, 172, **205 (dr. 111)**, 225n1, 230;
in psychoanalysis with Jelliffe 15; in
psychoanalysis with Jung 15
Journal of Nervous and Mental Disease
xv, 6, 11
Jung, Carl xx, 12–13, 158, 159n1;
assistants, use of in his practice 217n4;
contribution to *Psychoanalytic Review*
20–21; and Freud, rupture with 20–21;
and Jelliffe xv–xvi, 12, 217n4, *see
also* Jelliffe, Smith Ely: and Jung; and
William Alanson White, visit with 20;
writings by: *Psychology of Dementia
Praecox* 12; *Psychology of the
Unconscious* 158, 159n1; *The Theory
of Psychoanalysis* xvi

Kitchell, Susan Emma (Jelliffe's
mother) 5

Landor, Arnold Henry Savage 183–184,
184n4, 184n5
Lawrence, D.H. 118
Leeming, Emily 125, 125n4
Leeming, Helena *see* Jelliffe, Helena
Leeming
Lewisohn, Adolph 225n3, 231n4

Lewisohn, Sam **229–230**, 231n4
Lippmann, Walter 46, 61–62, **70**, 71n1
  (dr. 5), **75**, 75n2, **94**, 94n2, 94n3, **107**,
  107n1, 108n5, **148**, 149n1, 170, 172,
  173–174, 174n1, 174n2, 174n3, 174n4,
  180, 181n1, 181n2, 181n4, **229–230**,
  230–231n2
Lorber, Dr. Harry 3, 101n1
Louise, Aunt (of Mabel Dodge) 69n3
  (dr. 2), **72**, 73n3, **75**, 107, 108n6, 127n4
Loy, Mina **198 (dr. 102)**, 199n1
Luhan, Antonio "Tony" (Dodge's fourth
  husband) *see* Dodge, Mabel: and
  Antonio Luhan
Luhan, Mabel *see* Dodge, Mabel

MacKaye children **109**, 110–111n9
MacKaye, Percy 109, 110–111n9,
  115–116, 170, **224 (dr. 127)**; *see also*
  Caliban
MacKaye, Robin **116**, 116n4
Mariana, Aunt (of Mabel Dodge) 69n3
  (dr. 3), 127n4
The Masses 55, 62, 206n4
Miller, Miss Frank (first name unknown)
  158–159, 159n2
Miss Graham's School 78n4
Montague ("Monty") (Sara Ganson's
  third husband) *see* Ganson, Sara:
  marriages
Morristown School 56, 142–143n1,
  165n2

Nervous and Mental Disease
  Monograph Series xv, xvii, 12
The New Republic 107, 107n1, 107n2
New Thought School 31, 55, 112, 113n2,
  113n3, 169n3

O'Brien, Joseph **205–206**, 206n5

Paget, Lady Violet **160**, 160n1 (dr. 64)
Palmer, May **141**, 143n6
Parmenter, Dr. John: affair with Dodge
  xx, 31, *see also* Dodge, Mabel: affair
  with Dr. Parmenter; affair with Sara
  Ganson xx, 122n4
Paterson Strike Pageant 61, 62
Pratt, Fred 122n4, 160n1 (dr. 63), 161n4
  (dr. 64)
Prince, Dr. Morton: Dodge's letter to
  xxvii, 35, 162–164, 175n9

Provincetown, Dodge in 32, 43, 65,
  166n3, 206n3
Provincetown Players50, 60, 113n4,
  199n1, 206n5, 222–223n1
Psychoanalytic Review xv, xvi, xvii,
  20–22, 117

Rauh, Ida 55, **112**, 113n4, **116**, 116n6
Reed, John 46, 61, 62, 74–75n5, **94**,
  94n2, 94–95n3, 100, 149, 153n11, **157**,
  157n1, 166n3, 170, 190n1 (dr. 92), **203**,
  206n5, **214**; and Dodge: first meets
  62, relationship with 31, 35, 50, 62,
  164, 214n2 (dr. 119), 215n3; *see also*
  Dodge, Mabel: and John Reed
Reeder, Admiral (Sara Ganson's second
  husband) *see* Ganson, Sara: marriages
Reicher, Emmanuel **103**, 103n1, 131,
  131n4, 131n5
Robinson, Edwin Arlington 46, **90**, 92n9,
  93n15, **172**, 172n1
Rudnick, Lois, *The Suppressed Memoirs
  of Mabel Dodge Luhan* xxviii
Rudnytsky, Peter 26n3; *Mutual Analysis*
  19, 26n2

Sachs, Dr. Bernard 31, **215**, 215n1
St. Margaret's School 78n4, 106n9,
  143n3
Saltonstall, Endicott Peabody 166n2,
  208 (dr. 114), 208n1
Sanger, Margaret 190n1 (dr. 92), 204n2,
  206n6
Scatchard, Dorothy 148, 149n2, 221,
  221n3
Scatchard, Emily 149n2, 221
Schroeder, Theodore **152**, 153n6
Scudder, Janet104–105n2, 111n10
Severn, Elizabeth: interview with Kurt
  Eissler 18–19; meets Freud 19; in
  psychoanalysis with Joseph Asch
  18; in psychoanalysis with Sandor
  Ferenczi xix, 18–19; in psychoanalysis
  with Jelliffe xix–xx, 18–20; in
  psychoanalysis with Otto Rank 18;
  writings by: *The Discovery of the
  Self* xix, 19–20; *The Psychology of
  Behavior* 19
Sohn, Mira 131–132n6, 203n1; *see also*
  Sterne, Maurice: and Mira Sohn
Steffens, Lincoln 60, 62, 74n3, 152,
  153n9; on Dodge's salons 62, 167n3

Stein, Gertrude 63, 65–66, 171n4, 199n1, 234n1 (dr. 133); first meets Dodge 63; plays by 52, 61; word portraits by: "Portrait of Constance Fletcher" 57, "A Portrait of F.B." 105n3, "Portrait of Mabel Dodge at the Villa Curonia" 57, 63, 66, 105n3

Stein, Leo 46, 63–64, **87**, 88n3, 95, **134**, 135n1, 135n4, 170–171, 171n4, 171n5, 188, 203n1, **216**; and Dodge 35: letters to xxvii, 64, 88n3, 133n6, 171n5, 171–172, 174n1; in psychoanalysis with Jelliffe 15, 16, 63–64; writings by: *Journey into the Self* 63, 88n3

Stekel, Wilhelm xviii, 12, 72n4

Sterne, Maurice (Dodge's third husband) 46, 64–65, 90n3, **102**, 102n2, **109**, 110n3, 111n12, 111n13, **112**, **121**, 121n1, **130**, 131n1, 131–132n6, 132, 133n3, **139**, **167**, **190 (dr. 92)**, **191 (dr. 94)**, **203**, **205 (dr. 110)**, 206n3, **211**, **214**, **226**, **237 (dr. 138)**, **241**; and Dodge: first meets 31–32, 64, letters to 121, 121–122n3, 122n6, 123, 138–139, marriage to 65, objection to Jelliffe's analysis with 102n3, 138–139, relationship with 39–42, 172, *see also* Dodge, Mabel: and Maurice Sterne; dreams of xxvii, 45, 138–139, 233; paintings by 90n3; photograph of (Figure 3.1) 32; resistance to psychoanalysis 15, 39, 121, 123, 167, 182–183n1; and Mira Sohn: planned visit to 203n1, 203n2, 214n1 (dr. 119), 232, 234n2, relationship with 131–132n6; syphilis of 47, 154n3; writings by: *Shadow and Light* 65, 121n1, 131n1

Stieglitz, Alfred 46, 48, 61, 65, **200**, 200n3 (dr. 104), 217n3; *see also* 291 Gallery; and Dodge, letters to xxvii, 95–96, 133n6

Streeper, Dr. Richard xxvi

Suppressed Desires, a play by Cook and Glaspell 222–223n1

Toklas, Alice B. 57, 63, 65–66, 82n1

291 Gallery 61, 65, 84n5, 200n3 (dr. 104)

Untermyer, Minnie **97**, 97n1

Untermyer, Samuel 97n1

Van Vechten, Carl 66, 86n5, 92–93n13, 177n3

Villa Curonia 50, 54, 56, 57, 63, 66, 91n5, 110n7, 137n4, 192n1 (dr. 95), 199n1, 215; haunted rooms at 109, 111n10; salons at 2, 54, 87n6

Villa, Pancho 152, 153n9, 153n11, 153n12

Vorse, Mary Heaton **205–206**, 206n4, 206n5

Waite, Dr. Arthur Warren 181, 182n1 (dr. 85)

White, William Alanson: and Freud, letter to xvii; and Jelliffe: friendship and collaboration with xv, xvii–xviii, 6, 11–12, 13, letter from xvii, letters to xxvii, 145–146; *see also* Jelliffe, Smith Ely and William Alanson White, writings by; and Jung, visit with 20

Wilcox, Nina *see* Nina Bull

Willard, Jess **179**, 180n2, 180n3

World War I 71n1 (dr. 6), 84n3, 94n1, 105n3, 126n8, 148n2

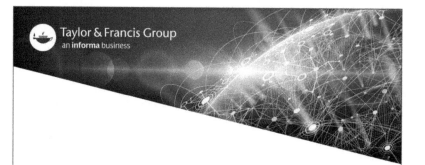